The Labor Progress Handbook

Early Interventions to Prevent and Treat Dystocia

Third Edition

The Labor Progress Handbook
Early Interventions to Prevent and Treat Dystocia

Third Edition

Penny Simkin, *BA, PT, CCE, CD(DONA)*
Senior Faculty, Simkin Center for Allied Birth
Vocations at Bastyr University
Independent Practice of Childbirth Education and
Labor Support

Ruth Ancheta, *BA, ICCE, CD(DONA),*
DONA-Approved Doula Trainer
Independent Practice of Childbirth Education
and Labor Support

with

contributions by

Lisa Hanson, *PhD, CNM, FACNM*
Suzy Myers, *LM, CPM, MPH*
Gail Tully, *BS, CPM, CD(DONA)*

Illustrated by **Shanna dela Cruz**

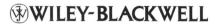
WILEY-BLACKWELL

A John Wiley & Sons, Inc., Publication

Wiley-Blackwell is an imprint of John Wiley & Sons, formed by the merger of Wiley's global Scientific, Technical and Medical business with Blackwell Publishing.

Registered office: John Wiley & Sons Ltd, The Atrium, Southern Gate, Chichester, West Sussex, PO19 8SQ, UK

Editorial offices: 2121 State Avenue, Ames, Iowa 50014-8300, USA
The Atrium, Southern Gate, Chichester, West Sussex, PO19 8SQ, UK
9600 Garsington Road, Oxford, OX4 2DQ, UK

For details of our global editorial offices, for customer services and for information about how to apply for permission to reuse the copyright material in this book please see our website at www.wiley.com/wiley-blackwell.

Library of Congress Cataloging-in-Publication Data

Simkin, Penny, 1938- author.
   The labor progress handbook : early interventions to prevent and treat dystocia / Penny Simkin, BA, PT, CCE, CD(DONA), Senior Faculty, Simkin Center for Allied Birth Vocations at Bastyr University, Independent Practice of Childbirth Education and Labor Support, Ruth Ancheta, BA, ICCE, CD(DONA), DONA-Approved Doula Trainer, Independent Practice of Childbirth Education and Labor Support; with contributions by Lisa Hanson, PhD, CNM, FACNM, Suzy Myers, LM, CPM, MPH, Gail Tully, BS, CPM, CD(DONA); illustrated by Shanna dela Cruz. – Third Edition.
      p. ; cm.
   Includes bibliographical references and index.
      ISBN 978-1-4443-3771-6 (pbk. : alk. paper)   1. Labor (Obstetrics)–Complications–Prevention–Handbooks, manuals, etc.   2. Birth injuries–Prevention–Handbooks, manuals, etc.   I. Ancheta, Ruth, author.   II. Title.
   [DNLM: 1.   Dystocia–prevention & control–Handbooks.   2. Birth Injuries–prevention & control–Handbooks.   3. Labor, Obstetric–Handbooks. WQ 39]
   RG701.S57 2011
   618.4–dc22
                     2010049407

A catalogue record for this book is available from the British Library.

This book is published in the following electronic formats: ePDF 9780470959367; ePub 9780470959374

Set in 9/11 pt Plantin by Toppan Best-set Premedia Limited

4   2013

Dedication

We dedicate this book to childbearing women and their caregivers in the hope that some of our suggestions will reduce the likelihood of cesarean delivery for dystocia; also to the wise, patient, and observant midwives, nurses, doulas, family doctors, and obstetricians whose actions and writings have inspired and taught us.

Contents

Foreword to the third edition   xv
Foreword to the second edition   xvii
Foreword to the first edition   xxi
Acknowledgments   xxiii

Chapter 1:   **Introduction**   **3**
        Penny Simkin, BA, PT, CCE, CD(DONA),
        and Ruth Ancheta, BA, ICCE, CD(DONA)

Some important differences in maternity
    care between the United States, the United Kingdom,
    and Canada   8
Notes on this book   12
Changes in this third edition   12
Material on epidurals   13
Conclusion   13
References   14

Chapter 2:   **Dysfunctional Labor: General
        Considerations**   **15**
        Penny Simkin, BA, PT, CCE, CD(DONA),
        and Ruth Ancheta, BA, ICCE, CD(DONA)

What is normal labor?   16
What is dysfunctional labor?   21
Why does labor progress slow down or stop?   23
    A role for the fetus in regulating labor?   23
The psychoemotional state of the woman: maternal
    well-being or maternal distress?   24
    Pain versus suffering   24

The "fight-or-flight" and "tend-and-befriend" responses to
distress and fear in labor   29
The environment for birth   31
Psychoemotional measures   31
Physical comfort measures   33
Physiologic measures   34
Why focus on maternal position?   35
Monitoring the mobile woman's fetus   37
Auscultation   37
When EFM is required: options to enhance
maternal mobility   37
Continuous EFM   38
Intermittent EFM   41
Telemetry   42
Techniques to elicit stronger contractions   45
Conclusion   46
References   46

Chapter 3:   Assessing Progress in Labor   51
                Suzy Myers, LM, CPM, MPH, with
                contributions by Gail Tully, BS, CPM,
                CD(DONA), and Lisa Hanson, PhD,
                CNM, FACNM

Before labor begins   52
Malposition   52
Leopold's maneuvers   57
Belly mapping   60
Other assessments prior to labor   64
Assessments during labor   66
Position, attitude, and station of the fetus   66
Vaginal examinations: indications and timing   66
Performing a vaginal examination during labor   67
Assessing the cervix   70
Unusual cervical findings   71
The presenting part   72
The vagina and bony pelvis   80
Quality of contractions   81
Assessing the mother's condition   84
Hydration and nourishment   84

Vital signs 85
Psychology 85
Assessing the fetus 86
Fetal heart rate 86
How to perform intermittent auscultation 87
When using continuous electronic fetal monitoring 89
The three-tiered fetal heart rate interpretation system 91
Putting it all together 94
Assessing progress in the first stage 94
Assessing progress in the second stage 96
Conclusion 96
References 96

Chapter 4: **Prolonged Prelabor and Latent**
First Stage **101**
Penny Simkin, BA, PT, CCE, CD(DONA),
and Ruth Ancheta, BA, ICCE, CD(DONA)

Is it dystocia? 101
When is a woman in labor? 102
Can prenatal measures prevent the fetal occiput position
during labor? 103
The woman who has hours of contractions
without dilation 106
The six ways to progress in labor 108
Support measures for women who are at home in
prelabor and the latent phase 109
Some reasons for excessive pain and duration of prelabor
or the latent phase 111
Iatrogenic factors 111
Cervical factors 111
Fetal factors 112
Emotional factors 112
Troubleshooting measures for painful prolonged prelabor
or latent phase 113
Measures to alleviate painful, nonprogressing, nondilating
contractions in prelabor or the latent phase 115
Synclitism and asynclitism 116
Conclusion 121
References 121

Chapter 7: Optimal Newborn Transition and Third and Fourth Stage Labor Management   **224**
Lisa Hanson, PhD, CNM, FACNM, and
Penny Simkin, BA, PT, CCE, CD(DONA)

Overview of the normal third and fourth stages of labor
for baby and unmedicated mother   225
Third stage management: care of the baby   227
   Oral and nasopharynx suctioning   227
   Delayed clamping and cutting of the umbilical cord   228
Third stage management: the placenta   229
   Expectant physiologic management of the third
     stage of labor   229
   Active management of the third stage of labor   230
The fourth stage of labor   234
   Keeping the mother and baby together   234
Baby-friendly (breastfeeding) practices   236
   Ten steps to successful breastfeeding   237
Routine newborn assessments   237
Conclusion   238
References   238

Chapter 8: Low-Technology Clinical Interventions to Promote Labor Progress   **242**
Lisa Hanson, PhD, CNM, FACNM

Intermediate-level interventions for management of
problem labors   243
When progress in prelabor or latent phase
remains inadequate   244
   Therapeutic rest   244
   Nipple stimulation   244
   Management of cervical stenosis or the "zipper" cervix   245
When progress in active phase remains inadequate   245
   Artificial rupture of the membranes (AROM)   246
   Digital or manual rotation of the fetal head   246
   Manual reduction of a persistent cervical lip   250
   Reducing swelling of the cervix or anterior lip   251
Fostering normality in birth   251
   Perineal management   251

When progress in second stage labor remains inadequate   257
   Duration of second stage labor   257
   Supportive directions for bearing down efforts   258
Hand maneuvers and anticipatory management
   of intrapartum problems   258
   Shoulder dystocia   258
   Somersault maneuver   265
Nonpharmacologic and minimally invasive techniques for
   intrapartum pain relief   267
   Acupuncture   267
   Sterile water injections   269
   Nitrous oxide   271
   Topical anesthetic applied to the perineum   271
Conclusion   271
References   272

Chapter 9:   **The Labor Progress Toolkit: Part 1.**
            Maternal Positions and Movements   277
            Penny Simkin, BA, PT, CCE, CD(DONA),
            and Ruth Ancheta, BA, ICCE, CD(DONA)

Maternal positions   278
   Side-lying positions   279
   Standing, leaning forward   289
   Kneeling positions   290
   Squatting positions   297
   Supine positions   306
Maternal movements in first and second stages   311
   Other rhythmic movements   323
References   324

Chapter 10: **The Labor Progress Toolkit: Part 2.**
            Comfort Measures   326
            Penny Simkin, BA, PT, CCE, CD(DONA),
            and Ruth Ancheta, BA, ICCE, CD(DONA)

General guidelines for comfort during a slow labor   327
Nonpharmacologic physical comfort measures   328
   Heat   328
   Cold   330

Hydrotherapy   332
Touch and massage   337
Acupressure   345
Acupuncture   347
Continuous labor support from a doula, nurse,
    or midwife   347
Psychosocial comfort measures   350
Assessing the woman's emotional state   351
Techniques and devices to reduce back pain   354
Counterpressure   354
The double hip squeeze   355
The knee press   357
Cook's counterpressure technique No. 1: ischial
    tuberosities (I-T)   359
Cook's counterpressure technique No. 2: perilabial (P-L)   361
Cold and heat   363
Hydrotherapy   365
Movement   366
Birth ball   367
Transcutaneous electrical nerve stimulation (TENS)   368
Sterile water injections for back pain   371
Breathing or moaning for relaxation and a sense of mastery   371
Bearing-down techniques for the second stage   374
Conclusion   376
References   376

Epidural Index   379
Index   381

Foreword to the third edition

Writing the foreword to the third edition of a successful book is a simple yet daunting task. Ellen Hodnett and Michael Klein so extolled the merits of the previous editions that there is little left to say. The core of the *Labor Progress Handbook* remains the same: a detailed description of labor as a physiologic process entwined with practical advice on how to help keep it that way. However, the third edition has been updated and newly referenced with some important additions: more practical guidance such as detailed descriptions of massage techniques and a complete analysis of directed versus spontaneous pushing. A beautifully written new chapter on the third and fourth stages of labor dispenses neatly with routine newborn suctioning and early cord clamping and gives a balanced discussion of active versus physiological third stage management. Another describes "intermediate interventions"—manual techniques and relatively low-level interventions to help avoid the need for medical or surgical management when labor is not progressing.

Labor is a dynamic neurohormonal dance and dramatic physical transition that transforms a woman's body, psyche, and soul. Labor is defined by dynamic and complex processes: psychological phenomena such as privacy and inhibition; the endocrine enigma of pulsatile oxytocin and endorphin surges; even the more tangible physiologic and anatomic changes of Ferguson's reflex and molding of the fetal skull. From a deductive scientific perspective, these remain poorly understood, even in 2011. Where science can no longer inform us, we must rely upon the experience, insight, and art of generations of skilled midwives and labor attendants, and this is where the *Labor Progress Handbook* is so helpful.

The authors demonstrate an excellent understanding of modern evidence-based practice; however, unlike in most medical texts, they are not constrained by the limits of science. Throughout the book, the highest level of evidence is sought and a multitude of current another "seven Ps," and I was pleased to find that many of them have been enumerated by the authors:

(4) The *Person*—the woman: her beliefs, preparation, knowledge, and "capacity" for doing the work of labor and birth.

(5) The *Partner*—how the woman is supported and the partner"s knowledge, beliefs, and preparation for the labor.

(6) The *People*—the "entourage"—others who may be involved in the pregnancy, labor, and birth process, and who are working with the woman. The entourage also have their beliefs, preparation, and knowledge of the process, and this interacts positively or negatively with those of the woman and her partner.

(7) The *Pain*—the influence and experience of pain and the sociocultural beliefs of the woman and her support system and her personal psychological environment. All this influences the woman's capacity for coping with labor and birth. Clearly pain interpretation and pain control impacts the progress of labor.

(8) The *Professionals*—the manner in which all members of the health care team support, inform and collaborate in care and information-sharing with the woman and her partner and support people, significantly influences the woman's response to the labor and birth process.

(9) The *Passion*—the journey of pregnancy, labor and birth, is one that is special and unique for all women. It is crucial for all involved in the care of women to recognize and honor this passion and allow this concept to guide us in our practice as we appreciate and guard the intimacy of this life-changing experience. And we need to control our anxiety and need for perfection so that the woman can fully experience the passion even when the birth is complex and requires considerable help from us.

(10) The *Politics*—You know it's true!

This book focuses on these concepts, while providing concrete information to help us facilitate the natural processes that are ready to be released, if we but give them time.

How refreshing to find a book that teaches how to stay out of trouble, how to prevent dysfunctional labors (and even to do so well before labor occurs) during prenatal care. It is liberating to have information on how to shift a fetus from an unfavorable to a favorable position, rather than waiting pessimistically to see an antenatal fetal malposition turn into an intrapartum OT or OP. New learners will benefit from the detailed descriptions of asynclitism and how to diagnose and treat it, as well as excellent descriptions of how to diagnose a flexed or extended head.

I have seen Penny teach these techniques in workshops for maternity caregivers, and seen the "Aha!" experience that results in the statement, "I can't wait to try these techniques in my next clinic or labor."

And now the information is available in accessible form to share with trainees and the women themselves. Thus, this book complements and augments the materials conventionally taught to medical students and specialist trainees. It will empower them with information that they can use in the labor suite. It will make them feel useful.

Epidural analgesia: the new reality. Who can argue with good pain relief? But at what price? And do women know, and have they been taught the full picture? The Cochrane Collaboration clearly demonstrates that it increases the length of the first and second stages of labor, increases the use of instrumentation and leads to excess perineal trauma. And while Cochrane reports no increase in cesarean section, most of us know that to be untrue. When used early and often (not the conditions of the major new trials in Cochrane)[1], epidural analgesia usually requires oxytocin augmentation (which is generally given in low dose regimes). Epidural analgesia clearly increases the frequency of cesarean section.

Therefore, I was particularly impressed with the way that the authors explained the influence of epidural analgesia on the course of labor. In fact, epidural analgesia is now so pervasive that we have forgotten how the entire shape of labor has been altered by its availability and omnipresence. Not to overstate the issue, there are places in North America and elsewhere where the staff either do not know or have forgotten how to look after women who do not have an epidural.

Unfortunately, it is this sad situation that makes it so necessary to describe how epidural analgesia alters labor and what techniques are needed to assist women who have an epidural. The authors have therefore elaborated on this new reality and provided the cautions and tools to assist caregivers do their best to let labor unfold in the presence of an epidural.

This little text, which will fit nicely in a back pocket or "lab coat," provides practical diagrams of normal and abnormal fetal positions that can be identified well before labor, and more importantly, corrected, so as to lessen the malpositions of labor that unleash the "cascade" of interventions that characterize the experience of so many women having their first babies. It will take much to turn society back from thinking of childbirth as an accident waiting to happen and to help women realize their power and competence, but the authors have given us a tool to help in that process, to help us keep normal birth normal. I am grateful that this book is available and entering its second edition.

Michael C. Klein, *MD, CCFP,*
FAAP(Neonatal-Perinatal), FCFP, ABFP
Emeritus Professor of Family Practice and Pediatrics
University of British Columbia

REFERENCE

1. Howell C. (2000). Epidural versus non-epidural analgesia for pain relief in labour. Cochrane Database Syst Rev (3), CD000331. doi:10.1002/14651858. CD000331.

Foreword to the first edition

At last, a book that offers practical advice for nurses and midwives who wish to help to prevent and treat dysfunctional labor! Penny Simkin and Ruth Ancheta have done a superb job of interweaving the clinical wisdom of observant, expert practitioners with the best available research evidence about what helps and does not help women during labor.

I wish this book had been available a long time ago. In the early 1970s when I was a novice labor and delivery nurse, I observed a common but puzzling problem. In those days we subjected women to an admission routine that included a variety of very unpleasant procedures. (Thankfully the worst of these procedures—perineal shaves, enemas, and rectal exams—have since been recognized as useless or harmful and have been eliminated from common practice.) Part of the admission routine involved assessment of the quality and strength of contractions. When I inquired about the contractions, I was often told, "My contractions were frequent and strong at home, but they seem to have gotten a lot weaker and further apart since I arrived."

I would reply, "Do not worry, this happens a lot. After we finish the admission procedures and you are settled in here, your labor will probably get going again."

Why did I say this? I believed it. I had observed it often and had overheard experienced colleagues reassure their patients in this way.

At some intuitive level I felt the decrease in labor intensity was caused by the woman's reaction to the stress of the hospital admission routine. But at the time almost nothing had been written about the role of stress hormones on uterine function, nor about the relationships between maternal anxiety, environmental influences, stress hormones, and labor complications. And the randomized controlled trials showing the substantial benefits of labor support had not even been conducted yet[1].

What about the instances in which labor did not return spontaneously to the strong, regular pattern that had been occurring prior to admission? Our repertoire of nursing interventions was limited primarily to advising the woman either to ambulate or to rest and wait. (Currently, in some settings the options may be even fewer, with ambulation restricted by the routine use of electronic fetal monitors.)

These women frequently ended up with a cascade of medical interventions—IV oxytocin, amniotomy, epidural analgesia, and forceps or cesarean delivery.

I now believe that there is much more I could have done to prevent or treat the problem of dysfunctional labor. Penny Simkin and Ruth Ancheta have described how "emotional dystocia" and stressful environmental influences may lead to complications, and they offer simple but potentially powerful nursing measures to ameliorate these problems. They have also persuaded me that many instances of dystocia or prolonged labor may be caused by subtle malpositions of the fetal head, potentially correctable with simple positioning techniques.

I can only imagine how much more effective I would have been if this book had been available when I was a labor and delivery nurse.

As a researcher, I am inspired to study these simple but potentially very powerful labor support techniques. Dystocia or dysfunctional labor is the most common reason for primary cesarean delivery. Given the high rates of cesarean delivery in North America and the United Kingdom, and the limitations and risks of medical treatments for dystocia, it seems long overdue that nurses and midwives take an active role in preventing and treating this common clinical problem. This book contains a wealth of information about and practical suggestions for preventing and correcting dysfunctional labor. It should be required reading for all who care for women in labor, and a reference text in every labor and birthing unit.

Ellen D. Hodnett, *RN, PhD*
Professor and Heather M. Reisman Chair
Perinatal Nursing Research
University of Toronto

REFERENCE

1. Hodnett E. (1998). Support from caregivers during childbirth (Cochrane Review). In: The Cochrane Library, Issue 3. Update Software, Oxford.

Acknowledgments

We have been helped in writing this book by many wonderful people, especially:

- Sally Avenson, Fredrik Broekhuizen, Roberta Gehrke, Joan Hintz, Lynn Diulio, Mary Mazul, Ann Neal, Jean Sutton, Karen Hillegas, Barbara Kalmen, Karen Kohls, Ann Krigbaum, and Karen Lupa for their helpful suggestions
- John Carroll, Alicia Huntley, Shauna Leinbach, Jenn McAllister, Sara Wickham, and Lisa Hanson for reviewing the text and giving us useful feedback
- Diony Young, for her assistance and support
- Anne Frye, midwife and author of Holistic Midwifery, for her stimulating conversation and generous sharing of ideas
- Shanna dela Cruz, our dedicated and meticulous illustrator
- The mother and child depicted in the cover photo
- The dozens of women and men who posed for our illustrations, including Robin Block, Asela Calhoun, Vic dela Cruz, Helen Vella Dentice, Carissa and Zsolt Farkas, Katie Rohs, Maureen Wahhab, Bob Meidl, and Lori Meidl Zahorodney, and class members in Penny Simkin's childbirth classes, staff members of Waukesha Memorial Hospital, Aurora Sinai Hospital, and St. Mary's Hospital of Milwaukee, Wisconsin, USA
- Celia Bannenberg, for permission to redraw the deBy birthing stool
- Jan Dowers, Lesley James, Tracy Sachtjen, and Heather Snookal, who provided support and assistance with manuscript preparation of previous editions, and Tanya Baer, Candace Halverson, and Molly Kirkpatrick, who provided extraordinary assistance in the preparation of this edition.
- Last but not least, we wish to acknowledge our families who have helped us in countless ways as we devoted ourselves to this larger than expected task.

The Labor Progress Handbook

**Early Interventions
to Prevent and Treat Dystocia**

Third Edition

Chapter 1

Introduction

Penny Simkin, BA, PT, CCE, CD(DONA),
and Ruth Ancheta, BA, ICCE, CD(DONA)

Some important differences in maternity care between the United
  States, the United Kingdom, and Canada, 8
Notes on this book, 12
Changes in this third edition, 12
Material on epidurals, 13
Conclusion, 13
References, 14

Labor dystocia, dysfunctional labor, failure to progress, arrest of labor, arrested descent—all these terms refer to slow or no progress in labor, which is one of the most vexing, complex, and unpredictable complications of labor. Labor dystocia is the most common medical indication for primary cesarean sections. Dystocia also contributes indirectly to the number of repeat cesareans, especially in countries where rates of vaginal births after previous cesareans (VBAC) are low. In fact, The American College of Obstetricians and Gynecologists (ACOG) estimates that 60% of all cesareans (primary and repeat) in the United States are attributable to the diagnosis of dystocia.[1] Thus, reducing the need for cesareans for dystocia is a strategic way to reduce the overall cesarean rate. Prevention of dystocia also reduces the need for many other costly and risky corrective obstetric

The Labor Progress Handbook: Early Interventions to Prevent and Treat Dystocia.
Edited by Penny Simkin, Ruth Ancheta
© 2011 by Penny Simkin and Ruth Ancheta; illustrations copyright Ruth Ancheta

measures and spares numerous women from the discouragement and disappointment that often accompany a prolonged or complicated birth.

The possible causes of labor dystocia are numerous. Some are intrinsic:

- The *powers* (the uterine contractions)
- The *passage* (size, shape, and joint mobility of the pelvis and the stretch and resilience of the vaginal canal)
- The *passenger* (size and shape of fetal head, fetal presentation and position)
- The *pain* (and the woman's ability to cope with it)
- The *psyche* (anxiety, emotional state of the woman).

Others are extrinsic:

- *Environment* (the feelings of physical and emotional safety generated by the setting and the people surrounding the woman)
- *Ethnocultural* factors (the degree of sensitivity and respect for the woman's culture-based needs and preferences)
- *Hospital or caregiver policies* (how flexible, family- or woman-centered, how evidence based)
- *Psychoemotional care* (the priority given to nonmedical aspects of the childbirth experience)

Please see Michael Klein's Foreword to the second edition (page xviii) for his discussion of factors influencing labor progress.

> *The Labor Progress Handbook* focuses on prevention, differential diagnosis, and early interventions to use with dysfunctional labor (dystocia). The emphasis is on relatively simple and sensible care measures or interventions designed to help maintain normal labor progress and to manage and correct minor complications before they become serious enough to require major interventions. We believe this approach is consistent with worldwide efforts, including those of the World Health Organization, to reserve the use of medical interventions for situations in which they are needed: "The aim of the care [in normal birth] is to achieve a healthy mother and baby with the least possible level of intervention that is compatible with safety."[2]

The suggestions in this book are based on the following premises:

- Progress may slow or stop for any of a number of reasons at any time in labor—prelabor, early labor, active labor, or during the second or third stage.
- The timing of the delay is an important consideration when establishing cause and selecting interventions.
- Sometimes several causal factors occur at one time.
- Caregivers and others are often able to enhance or maintain labor progress with simple nonsurgical, nonpharmacologic physical and psychological interventions. Such interventions have the following advantages:
  - compared to most obstetric interventions for dystocia, they carry less risk of harm or undesirable side effects to mother or baby.
  - they treat the woman as the key to the solution, not the key to the problem.
  - they build or strengthen the cooperation between the woman, her support people (loved ones, doula [trained labor support provider]), and her caregivers.
  - they reduce the need for riskier, costlier, more complex interventions.
  - they may increase the woman's emotional satisfaction with her experience of birth.

- The choice of solutions depends on the causal factors, if known, but trial and error is sometimes necessary when the cause is unclear. The greatest drawbacks are that the woman may not want to try these interventions; they sometimes take time; or they may not correct the problem.
- Time is usually an ally, not an enemy. With time, many problems in labor progress are resolved. In the absence of clear medical or psychological contraindications, patience, reassurance, and low or no risk interventions may constitute the most appropriate course of management.
- The caregiver may use the following to determine the cause of the problem(s):
  - *objective observations*: woman's vital signs; fetal heart rate patterns; fetal presentation, position, and size; cervical

performed and the results combined in meta-analyses, these common practices were found to be ineffective and to increase risks.[3]

Where possible, we will base our suggestions on scientific evidence and will cite appropriate references. However, numerous simple and apparently risk-free practices have never been scientifically studied. Some of these are based on an understanding of the emotional and physiologic processes taking place during childbirth. Others are applications of anatomy, kinesiology, and body mechanics to enhance the relationships between such separate but interdependent forces as pelvic shape, maternal posture, fetal position and station, uterine activity, and the force of gravity. Still others are based on a recognition of the importance of each laboring woman's personal and cultural values.

Some of the strategies suggested in this book will lend themselves to randomized controlled trials, while others may not. Perhaps readers will gather ideas for scientific study as they read this book and apply its suggestions.

SOME IMPORTANT DIFFERENCES IN MATERNITY CARE BETWEEN THE UNITED STATES, THE UNITED KINGDOM, AND CANADA

This book is being published simultaneously in North America and the United Kingdom, where the approaches to maternity care are quite different from one another. It may surprise the reader to learn about some of those differences, and it may also be interesting to learn that practices that are considered essential for safety in one country are considered ineffective or archaic in another. We hope that one indirect effect of our book will be to encourage a willingness to reconsider practices that are either entrenched or avoided in one's own workplace.

Table 1.1 compares some basic features of maternity care between the United States, Canada, and the United Kingdom. Because of such differences in maternity care as those listed in Table 1.1, the willingness to introduce new practices and the power to do so will vary among caregivers in different countries. We hope our readers will begin to use the simplest, most innocuous measures immediately and to educate themselves and change policies where necessary.

Table 1.1. Comparison of maternity care in the United States, Canada, and the United Kingdom

Feature	United States	Canada	United Kingdom
Primary maternity caregivers	Obstetricians for approximately 87% of women; midwives and family doctors for 13%. Maternity nurses provide most of the care during labor in the hospital, with the obstetrician managing any problems and the delivery. Two types of midwives—certified nurse midwives and certified professional midwives—provide care, the latter only for out-of-hospital birth.	Family doctors, with obstetricians and autonomous midwives now increasing in numbers. As in the United States, nurses provide most in-hospital care. One designation of midwife, the registered midwife, exists. They are not available in all provinces and still care for a small but growing minority of women.	Mostly midwives, some general practitioners, with obstetricians caring for women with complications. There are no maternity nurses. Midwives provide all intrapartum care and conduct most deliveries, with a small percentage providing home birth care.
Autonomy and independence of caregiver	Great variation in preferred routines among independent doctors. Nursing care varies according to the orders of each physician or hospital policies and protocol's. Insurance providers and health maintenance organizations now increasingly limit those doctors' practices that are not cost effective. Midwives are dependent on back-up services of doctors; in many areas, midwives' practices are severely limited because no doctors are willing to provide.	Government limits payment for some interventions, and regulates numbers of physicians and hospitals, giving doctors less autonomy than in the USA. Midwives are also closely regulated. They "follow the woman" and provide care in the birth place of the woman's choice.	Midwives have little autonomy, and practice according to the policies of their institutions. Those policies are established by authorities in maternity care and by the government.

(Continued)

Table 1.1. (*Continued*)

Feature	United States	Canada	United Kingdom
Participation by childbearing women in decision-making	'Informed consent' is the law, though most women (except assertive women with strong opinions) expect the obstetrician to make decisions and most obstetricians prefer that style of practice. Most midwives and family doctors share decision making with the woman.	Similar to the United States.	'Informed choice' and 'woman-centered care' are now standards of care, and extensive efforts are being made by government and childbirth activists to ensure that women are well informed for their role as partners in decision making.
Continuity of caregiver throughout the childbearing year	Not considered cost effective, feasible, or desirable by policy-makers in health care. Rarely available except for out of hospital births, though to many women it is a highly desirable option. Some assertive women try to obtain continuity of care through birth plans and doulas, and by verbalizing their concerns to each professional involved in their care.	Small group practices of family doctors or midwives are available in many parts of Canada. Continuity of caregiver during pregnancy and post partum is more likely than in the United States, although maternity nurses provide most care in labor.	Considered a very important feature of woman-centered care, programs ensuring continuity of caregiver are beginning to replace the old system of different midwives for pre- and postnatal and intrapartum care.

Influence of scientific evidence on maternity practices	Highly variable, but customs, peer practices, opinions, and prior experience of the practitioner and fear of litigation are more powerful influences. Failure to adhere to evidence-based practice may have contributed to increases in maternal and neonatal mortality and morbidity, cesareans, and labor inductions.	Leaders in obstetrics, family medicine, midwifery, and nursing are actively engaged in scientific evaluation of numerous unproved clinical practices. The national professional societies of midwives, family doctors, obstetricians, and nurses promote evidence-based practice.	Same as Canada, except that midwives are also actively involved in original research. There is widespread acceptance of a scientific approach to maternity care, where possible.
Influence of fear of malpractice litigation on maternity practices	The chances of physicians being sued for malpractice is a constant worry, and malpractice insurance premiums are extremely expensive, which has driven up costs of maternity care. In addition, insurers advise on how to reduce the likelihood of lawsuits. Such advice is not based on science, safety or effectiveness, but on risks of being sued.	Trends similar to the United States, although to a much lesser degree. Fear of litigation has less impact on care than scientific findings, costs, customs and other factors.	Similar to Canada.

1

NOTES ON THIS BOOK

This book is directed toward midwives, nurses, and doctors who want to support and enhance the physiologic process of labor with the objective of avoiding complex, costly, more risky interventions. It will also be helpful for students in obstetrics, midwifery, and maternity nursing; for childbirth educators who can teach many of these techniques to expectant parents; and for doulas, who are qualified and skilled in the use of many of the techniques. The chapters are arranged chronologically according to the phases and stages of labor.

Because a particular maternal position or movement is useful for the same problem during more than one phase of labor, we have included illustrations of these positions in more than one chapter. This will allow the reader to find position ideas at a glance when working with a laboring woman. Complete descriptions of all the positions, movements, and other measures can be found in the "Toolkit," Chapters 9 and 10.

The terms "caregiver" and "birth attendant" are used most commonly to refer to the maternity care professionals who provide care and support for the woman in labor.

CHANGES IN THIS THIRD EDITION

Besides updating the information, and adding new suggestions, 32 new illustrations, and references throughout this edition, we have asked Lisa Hanson, PhD, CNM, FACNM, associate professor at Marquette University College of Nursing, to author a chapter on intermediate interventions for use by midwives and doctors to enhance labor progress. This includes techniques for manually dilating a rigid cervix; digital or manual rotation of a malpositioned fetus in late labor or second stage; management of shoulder dystocia; the "somersault maneuver" for delivering a baby with a tight nuchal cord; and many others.

We also asked Lisa Hanson to co-author (with Penny Simkin) the new Chapter 7, "Optimal Newborn Transition and Third and Fourth Stage Labor Management," which includes a critical discussion of routine postpartum care practices in the context of holistic definitions of the third and fourth stages that are based on immediate and maximum skin-to-skin contact between mother and baby to foster family integration and facilitate breastfeeding and maternal behavior.

Suzy Myers, LM, CPM, MPH, chairperson of the Department of Midwifery at Bastyr University, near Seattle, Washington, has updated Chapter 3, "Assessing Progress in Labor." The innovative concept of "belly mapping," developed by Minnesota midwife and artist, Gail Tully, is also presented in this chapter. Gail Tully supplied the content and drawings for the "belly mapping" segment of the chapter, which is also coauthored by Lisa Hanson.

All of these midwives' contributions provide techniques and practical tips that are not taught in many schools of medicine, midwifery, and nursing.

MATERIAL ON EPIDURALS

In acknowledgment of the widespread use of epidural analgesia, we address the needs of readers who work extensively with women who have them and are unable to use many of the measures shown in this book. Labors with epidural analgesia are frequently accompanied by slow progress, maternal hypotension, maternal fever, the necessity for synthetic oxytocin, instrumental delivery, episiotomy, cesarean, prophylactic antibiotics for the newborn, and other undesired side effects. Usual care of women who have an epidural during a normally progressing labor (restriction to bed, limited movement, large amounts of intravenous fluids, supine position, and prolonged directed maximal bearing down during second stage) may actually add to the undesired effects of the epidural medication itself and increase the likelihood of labor dystocia. With that possibility in mind, we encourage our readers to treat a woman with an epidural as much as possible (within the realm of safety) like a woman who does not have an epidural. We have prepared a special "Epidural Index" (page 379) to help readers quickly identify measures that can safely be used for women with epidural analgesia to correct side effects and fetal malpositions and to aid progress.

CONCLUSION

The current emphasis in obstetrics is to find better ways to treat dystocia once it occurs. This book advocates prevention and a stepwise approach to interventions beginning with the least invasive approaches possible that will result in safe delivery. This approach is the focus of this book.

1

To our knowledge, this is the first book that compiles labor progress strategies that can be used by a variety of caregivers in a variety of locations. Most of the strategies described can be used for births occurring in hospitals, at home, and in freestanding birth centers.

We hope this book will make your work more effective and more rewarding. Your knowledge of appropriate early interventions may spare many women from long, discouraging, or exhausting labors; reduce the need for major interventions; and contribute to safer and more satisfying outcomes. The women may not even recognize what you have done for them, but they will appreciate and always remember your attentiveness, expertise, and support, which contribute so much to their satisfaction[4] and positive long-term memories of their childbirths.[5]

We wish you much success and fulfillment in your important work.

REFERENCES

1. American College of Obstetricians and Gynecologists (ACOG). (2003). Dystocia and augmentation of labor. ACOG Practice Bulletin No. 49. Obstet Gynecol 102, 1445–1454.

2. World Health Organization. (1996). Care in normal birth: A practical guide. In Safe Motherhood. Geneva, Author.

3. Hofmeyr GJ, Neilson JP, Alfirevic Z, et al. (2008). Pregnancy and Childbirth: A Cochrane Pocketbook. West Sussex, England, Wiley.

4. Hodnett E. (2002). Pain and women's satisfaction with the experience of childbirth: A systematic review. Am J Obstet Gynecol 186(5), s160–s172.

5. Simkin P. (1990) Just another day in a woman's life? Women's long term perceptions of their first birth experience. Part I. Birth 18(4), 203–210.

Chapter 2

Dysfunctional Labor: General Considerations

Penny Simkin, BA, PT, CCE, CD(DONA), and Ruth Ancheta, BA, ICCE, CD(DONA)

What is normal labor? 16
What is dysfunctional labor? 21
Why does labor progress slow down or stop? 23
A role for the fetus in regulating labor? 23
The psychoemotional state of the woman: maternal well-being or maternal distress? 24
Pain versus suffering, 24
The "fight-or-flight" and "tend-and-befriend" responses to distress and fear in labor, 29
The environment for birth, 31
Psychoemotional measures, 31
Physical comfort measures, 33
Physiologic measures, 34
Why focus on maternal position? 35
Monitoring the mobile woman's fetus, 37
Auscultation, 37
When EFM is required: options to enhance maternal mobility, 37
Continuous EFM, 38
Intermittent EFM, 41
Telemetry, 42
Techniques to elicit stronger contractions, 45
Conclusion, 46
References, 46

The Labor Progress Handbook: Early Interventions to Prevent and Treat Dystocia.
Edited by Penny Simkin, Ruth Ancheta
© 2011 by Penny Simkin and Ruth Ancheta; illustrations copyright Ruth Ancheta

WHAT IS NORMAL LABOR?

Normal labors may be long or short. They may very painful or hardly painful. They may occur after a high-risk or a low-risk pregnancy. They may result in the birth of a small or a large baby. They may take place within or outside the hospital.

Despite these variations, all such labors, if they meet the following criteria, would be considered normal by the World Health Organization (WHO),[1] which defines *normal labor* as having the following features:

- spontaneous onset of labor between 37 and 42 completed weeks of pregnancy
- low risk at the start, and remaining so throughout labor and delivery
- spontaneous birth of an infant in the vertex presentation
- mother and baby in good condition after birth

It is often stated that one can diagnose normal labor only in retrospect, leading many to conclude that it is preferable to treat all labors as high risk, even though WHO estimates that "between 70 and 80% of all pregnant women may be considered as low-risk at the start of labour."[1,chap1,p3] Because of the great expense, intensive training, and inherent risks of treating all labors as high risk, WHO states, "In normal birth there should be a valid reason to interfere with the normal process."[1,chap1,p3] However, assessment of risk must continue throughout pregnancy and labor: "At any moment early complications may become apparent and induce the decision to refer the woman to a higher level of care. ..."[1,chap1,p2] By emphasizing the need for ongoing surveillance of maternal and fetal well-being, WHO answers many of the concerns resulting from the impossibility of predicting which low-risk women will remain low risk throughout labor and birth.

Influential organizations and working groups in North America and Europe have taken up the challenge of defining *normal labor*.[2–7] Table 2.1 describes some of these efforts. Many others have taken on the task of developing tools to evaluate providers of maternity care (individuals and institutions) on how well or how poorly they promote normal birth.[8–12]

Table 2.1. Many ways to define "normal birth"

Defining Organization or Individual	Definition	Comments
World Health Organization (WHO), 1996[1]	"Spontaneous in onset, low-risk at the start of labor and remaining so throughout labor and delivery The infant is born spontaneously [without help] in the vertex position [head down] between 37 and 42 completed weeks of pregnancy. After birth mother and baby are in good condition."	This *retrospective definition* normal labor is based on healthy outcomes. Normal labor can only be diagnosed in retrospect
Society of Obstetricians and Gynecologists of Canada (SOGC), Association of Women's Health, Obstetric and Neonatal Nursing of Canada (AWHONN), Canadian Association of Midwives (CAM), College of Family Physicians of Canada (CFPC), and Society of Rural Physicians of Canada (SRPC)[2]	Same as WHO, above, plus: "**Normal birth includes** the opportunity for skin–skin holding and breastfeeding in the first hour after the birth. **A normal birth does not preclude possible complications** such as postpartum hemorrhage, perineal trauma and repair, and admission to the neonatal intensive care unit. **Normal birth may also include evidence-based intervention** in appropriate circumstances to facilitate labor progress and normal vaginal delivery; for example: ● Augmentation of labor and artificial rupture of the membranes (ARM) if it is not part of medical induction of labor ● Non-pharmacologic and pharmacologic pain relief (nitrous oxide, opioids and/or epidural) ● Managed third stage of labor ● Intermittent fetal auscultation **A normal birth does not include:** ● Elective induction of labor prior to 41+0 weeks ● Spinal analgesia, general anesthetic ● Instrumental delivery ● Cesarean delivery ● Routine episiotomy ● Continuous electronic fetal monitoring for low risk birth ● Fetal malpresentation"	This is a *prospective process-based definition of normal labor.* With this definition, one may have a normal labor, but a poor outcome. The group advocates ● Spontaneous of labor ● Freedom to move throughout ● Continuous labor support ● No routine intervention ● Spontaneous pushing in woman's preferred position ● Fetal surveillance by auscultation ● Good information for women ● Education on normal birth for childbirth educators and care providers

(Continued)

2

17

Table 2.1. (*Continued*)

Defining Organization or Individual	Definition	Comments
Coalition for the Improvement of Maternity Services (CIMS), 1996[6]	"Normalcy of the Birthing Process ● Birth is a normal, natural, and healthy process. ● Women and babies have the inherent wisdom necessary for birth. ● Babies are aware, sensitive human beings at the time of birth, and should be acknowledged and treated as such. ● Breastfeeding provides the optimum nourishment for newborns and infants. ● Birth can safely take place in hospitals, birth centers, and homes. ● The midwifery model of care, which supports and protects the normal birth process, is the most appropriate for the majority of women during pregnancy and birth."	CIMS published a ***Physiologic definition*** of normal birth. CIMS has published its TEN Steps to Mother-Friendly Childbirth, which are similar to the Lamaze Six Care Practices that Support Healthy Birth.
Debbie Gould, 2000 [7]	Who definition, plus: ● Labor and birth involves strenuous physical work by mother, ● Includes movement by mother (seeking comfort and progress), and ● Movement by fetus through the birth canal ● "Movement and the notion of hard work are crucial to a midwifery understanding of normal labor." PLUS: ● A healthy mother and baby who are ready to adjust together to their new roles; ● Empowerment of the woman ● Sense of achievement from her own productive efforts and her ACTIVE control (rather than passive role) in the birth.	This ***holistic definition*** includes references to the mother's and fetus's physical effort and emphasizes their shared roles in accomplishing the birth and postpartum adjustment together. With this definition, normal birth also includes psychological benefits for the mother.

2

A British midwife scholar, Debby Gould, has proposed a holistic definition of *normal labor*[7] that includes the WHO criteria but adds these other attributes:

- strenuous physical work by the mother
- movement by the mother (seeking comfort and progress)
- movement by the fetus (through the birth canal)

Gould believes "movement and the notion of hard physical work to be crucial to a midwifery understanding of normal labor."[7,p424] The consequences of a normal labor as defined by Gould include psychosocial outcomes:

- a healthy mother and baby who are ready to adjust together to their new roles in continuing the lifecycle of the woman and the family
- empowerment of the woman
- a sense of achievement that comes from the mother's productive efforts and her active central (rather than passive) role in her child's birth

Gould believes that acceptance of this definition of *normal birth* would lead to improved care of women and a reversal of the prevailing cultural trend of increasing passivity of women and medicalization of birth.[7] Gould's definition most closely embodies the approach to labor put forth in this book.

Although none of the organizations and individuals that have defined *normal birth* specifies rates of labor progress in their definitions, numerous authors consider adequate labor progress to be a defining characteristic of normality and a major focus of intrapartum care, along with monitoring and maintaining the well-being of mother and fetus. Given the wide range of normality, however, it is not surprising that there are many points of view on the meaning of abnormal progress and on how to prevent, identify, and correct this troublesome problem.

WHAT IS DYSFUNCTIONAL LABOR?

The term "dysfunctional labor" is a catch-all term that refers to protracted or arrested progress in cervical dilation during the active phase of labor, or protracted or arrested descent during the second stage. Other terms, such as "labor dystocia," "uterine inertia," "persistent malposition," "cephalo-pelvic disproportion," "failure to progress," "protracted labor," and, as some clinicians have said in frustration, "WCO" ("won't come out!"), have been used to refer to dysfunctional labor. In fact, Friedman compiled a list of 65 terms used to describe abnormal labor![13] Some caregivers are less patient than others and make the diagnosis of dysfunctional labor more quickly.

Diagnosis and management of dysfunctional labor vary, depending on the philosophy of the care provider.[14] For example, proponents of "active management of labor" begin high-dose oxytocin augmentation of nulliparas any time after labor is diagnosed, if the rate of dilation is less than 1 cm/hr for 2 hours.[15] Friedman's graphic analyses of labor progress, published between the mid-1950s and the 1970s, have profoundly influenced obstetrics in America and elsewhere for decades. He defined *dysfunctional labor* as a rate of dilation less than 1.2 cm/hr in nulliparas and less than 1.5 cm/hr in multiparas during the active phase of labor, which he defined as dilation from 3 to 10 cm.[13] This work still carries great influence, although more recent research shows that the mean rate of dilation is markedly slower.

Zhang and colleagues[16] replicated Friedman's graphic analyses of labor with 1200 contemporary women, who typically are larger and have larger babies than the women in Friedman's time. They also receive oxytocin augmentation and epidural analgesia more often. Zhang and colleagues concluded that new criteria are needed to allow a slower rate of dilation before resorting to cesarean delivery. They found that between 4 and 6 cm, the median rate of dilation was 1.2 cm/hr with contemporary women—a rate that Friedman would have diagnosed as "dysfunctional." Furthermore, the average duration of active labor (from 4 to 10 cm) was 5.5 hours, as opposed to Friedman's 2.5 hours.[13]

Albers and colleagues[17,18] conducted two studies of the length of labor in a total of 3984 midwife-attended healthy women at term who did not receive oxytocin or epidural analgesia. Their mean duration of active labor was 7.7 hours in nulliparas and 5.6 hours in multiparas. Active phase labors lasting as long as 19.4 hours in nulliparas and 13.8 hours in multiparas were associated with healthy outcomes. Along with Zhang et al., Albers and her colleagues call for revision of clinical expectations for the length of active labor.[16–18]

Other researchers report lower cesarean rates without additional risks to mother or baby when the diagnosis of dystocia is postponed until a delay in dilation exceeding at least 4 hours has occurred.[14,18,19] If the woman can be made comfortable and the fetus's status appears reassuring, these researchers feel less urgency to speed progress. Unfortunately, nonclinical factors often dictate the caregiver's decision on when, whether, and how to intervene. For example, these factors may include the adequacy of staffing now and later, their own availability, their personal threshold for patience, and the woman's needs or desires.

Many midwives and others embrace a "tolerance for wide variations in normal labor."[18] They try to preserve normality and avoid the need for augmentation with oxytocin by ensuring the privacy of the woman, remaining physically present but unobtrusive, nourishing the woman, supporting and reassuring her, using nonpharmacologic interventions (bath, movements, etc.), and exercising patience and watchful waiting while allowing the labor process to unfold at its own pace.

WHY DOES LABOR PROGRESS SLOW DOWN OR STOP?

Most cases of labor dystocia are caused by one or a combination of specific conditions, as listed in Table 2.2. Some of these etiologies disappear with changes in labor management. Others are corrected with skilled diagnosis and appropriate treatments based on the diagnosis. With time, patience, and trial and error, others may self-correct. And last, some will not respond and obstetric interventions will be indicated.

A role for the fetus in regulating labor?

Although scientific evidence is lacking, many maternity care professionals relate anecdotes of slow-progressing labors, which, when augmented with oxytocin, resulted in fetal intolerance of labor (also known as fetal distress and nonreassuring fetal heart rate tracings) and cesareans. One wonders whether practitioners who tolerate slower progress without augmentation are able to avoid cesareans for fetal distress that might be caused by augmentation with oxytocin. The intriguing question of whether the fetus, perhaps through

Table 2.2.   Etiologies and risk factors for dysfunctional labor (dystocia)

Etiology	Description	Comments
Cervical dystocia	Posterior unripe cervix at labor onset, scarred, fibrous cervix or "rigid os,""tense cervix" or thick lower uterine segment	Unripe cervix may prolong latent phase. Surgical scarring, damage from disease, or structural abnormality may increase cervical resistance
Emotional dystocia	Maternal distress or fear, exhaustion, severe pain	Increased catecholamine production may inhibit contractions
Fetal dystocia	Malposition, asynclitism, large or deflexed head, lack of engagement	Pendulous abdomen, size and shape of pelvis or fetal head may predispose fetus to malposition
Iatrogenic dystocia	Misdiagnosis of labor or second stage, elective induction (nulliparous), inappropriate oxytocin use, maternal immobility, drugs, dehydration, disturbance	Misdiagnosis or unneeded interventions or restrictions can slow or interfere with labor progress
Pelvic dystocia	Malformation, pelvic shape other than gynecoid, small dimensions	Maternal movement and upright positions increase pelvic dimensions
Uterine dystocia	Inadequate or inefficient contractions	May be secondary to fear, fasting, dehydration, supine position, cephalopelvic disproportion, lactic acidosis in myometrium, or structural abnormalities

catecholamine production or some other means, influences the labor pattern merits further scientific investigation.

THE PSYCHOEMOTIONAL STATE OF THE WOMAN: MATERNAL WELL-BEING OR MATERNAL DISTRESS?

Pain versus Suffering

Maternal well-being in labor is associated with numerous factors, but after safety for mother and baby, pain is probably the chief concern of women and their caregivers. What is it about pain that causes such concern? The distinction between pain and suffering is crucial to our understanding of women's emotional well-being in labor. For our purposes, the pain of labor might be defined as an unpleasant bodily sensation that one wishes to avoid or relieve. Suffering, however, is a distressing psychological state that includes feelings of helplessness, fear, panic, loss of control, and aloneness. Suffering may or may not be associated with pain, and pain may or may not be associated with suffering.

We postulate that it is *not pain, but an inability to cope with pain* that is at the root of the concern. In fact, in our discussions with pregnant women, it is not the pain of labor that worries them as much as how the pain will affect their behavior (losing control, crying out, writhing, showing weakness, or behaving shamefully) and whether they will find themselves in a state of helplessness (not knowing how long the pain will go on and being unable to do anything to reduce it). In other words, they are afraid of *suffering*. Suffering is similar in definition to *trauma* and can lead to emotional distress (even posttraumatic stress disorder) that sometimes continues long after the birth.

There are two main approaches to pain management: (1) use of medication to modify or eliminate the sensation of pain and (2) use of nonpharmacologic methods to keep the pain manageable, with the primary goal being the prevention of suffering.

In many hospitals, laboring women (and all other hospital patients) are asked periodically to assess their pain, using a visual analog scale of 0 ("no pain") to 10 ("worst pain imaginable"); it also includes images of faces indicating expressions ranging from smiling to somber to agony (Fig. 2.1). The woman indicates her pain level and is offered pain medications if it reaches a particular level.

More important than assessment of pain, however, is assessment of her ability to cope with it (Fig. 2.2). Here, the visual analog scale ranges from 10 ("no need to cope—very easy") to 0 ("totally unable to cope"). The mid-range denotes ability to cope, without or with help—usually demonstrated by maintaining some kind of rhythmic ritual during contractions and relaxing between (see page 160 for more on using relaxation, rhythm, and ritual—the "3Rs"—to cope with pain). The caregiver observes the woman's responses to her contractions. Another good way for the caregiver to assess coping is to occasionally ask the woman, after a contraction, "Could you tell me what was going through your mind during that contraction?" Her

Pain Intensity Scale

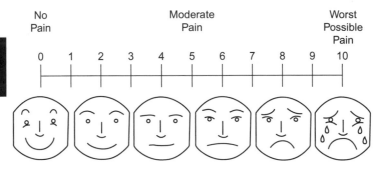

Fig. 2.1.   Pain intensity scale.

Pain Coping Scale

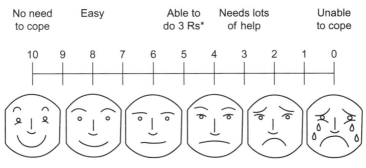

*Relaxation, Rhythm, and Ritual

Fig. 2.2.   Pain coping scale.

answer will indicate whether she is coping, is in distress, or some of both. If she is coping, all she needs is patience, encouragement, and approval. If her behavior indicates that she is in some degree of distress (crying out, whimpering, struggling, or giving up) or has lost her rhythm, or if her answers to your question indicate emotional distress ("This is much harder than I expected"; "I don't know how much longer I can go on"; "Please don't make me do this!"; "I don't know. I hate this;" or "That's it. I'm done!"), it may indicate or lead to suffering, and she will need intensive emotional and physical support and guidance in different comfort measures to recover a sense that she can cope. If she cannot respond to more intensive guidance, then she is probably a candidate for pain medications. The bottom line is that no woman should remain in a state of suffering. Chapters 9 and 10 ("Toolkits 1 and 2") offer numerous measures to enhance a woman's ability to cope with the pain and unpredictability of labor.

Labor progress and prevention of dystocia depend on harmonious interactions among a variety of psychoemotional, interpersonal, physical, and physiologic factors. As we shall see, progress is facilitated when a woman feels safe, respected, and cared for by her expert caregivers; when she can remain active, mobile, and upright; and when her pain is adequately and safely managed. Her sense of well-being is enhanced by a caring attentive partner or loved ones; competent, confident, compassionate caregivers and doulas; and a calm comfortable, and well-equipped birthplace. If these are not available to her, she may feel ashamed, embarrassed, inhibited, incompetent, alone, judged, unsafe, restricted, disrespected, ignored, or insignificant.[20] Such feelings may elicit a psychobiological reaction that interferes with efficient progress in labor.

The complex interplay of a variety of hormones influences—and is influenced by—the labor process as well as by the factors just named. These hormones—oxytocin, endorphins, catecholamines, and prolactin—have specific effects, which may either inhibit the effects of the others or facilitate them. It is the balance of hormones that determines the net effect on labor progress as well as maternal postpartum mental health, mother–infant interaction, and the initiation of breastfeeding. See Table 2.3.

Michel Odent, MD, an observer and student of normal birth since the early 1960s, suggests that when women give birth "in the method of the mammals" (that is, instinctively), their labors are more likely to proceed in a state of hormonal balance and without difficulty. He postulates that when the neocortex, the "newer," more uniquely human part of the brain—the thinking, reasoning part—is overstimulated, the birth process is inhibited. Because the birth process involves coordinated activity within the endocrine system and the "older," more primitive parts of the brain that humans share with other mammals, Odent advocates modifying present-day facilities and care practices to minimize stimulation of the neocortex. He notes that

Table 2.3. The hormones of labor and their functions in labor and early post partum

The following description of key hormones is synthesized from the published works of several prominent experts.[21–23]

- *Oxytocin.* Known as the hormone of "calm and connection" or the "love" hormone, oxytocin contributes to uterine contractions, the urge to push, and the "fetal ejection reflex,"[24] the "letdown" of breastmilk, maternal behavior, and feelings of well-being and love. It has opposite effects of catecholamines, as described later.
- *Endorphins.* These morphine-like hormones increase with pain, exertion, stress, and fear and tend to counteract associated unpleasant feelings. During labor, they are instrumental in creating the trance-like state (withdrawn, dreamy, and instinctual behavior) characteristic of women in active labor. They contribute to the "high" feelings that many unmedicated women have after birth. Once the stress or pain ends, the woman has the leftover euphoric effects of the endorphins.
- *Catecholamines.* These stress hormones (adrenalin or epinephrine, noradrenalin or norepinephrine, cortisol, and others) are secreted when a person is frightened or angry, is in danger, or feels she is in danger. These are the hormones of "fight-or-flight." Their physiologic effects enable the person's body to endure, defend against, or flee a dangerous situation. Catecholamines tend to counteract the effects of oxytocin and endorphins. First stage labor contractions may slow down or stop, the fetal heart rate may slow, and the woman becomes tense, alert, fearful, and protective of her unborn child. The term "fight-or-flight" accurately describes the physiologic response to danger of all mammals, as well as the behavioral response of males. Recent studies of female behavior when in fear or danger have shown that female behavior is often better described as "tend-and-befriend"—that is, protecting their offspring and reaching out for support.[25] In the second stage, a surge of catecholamines is physiologic and helps mobilize the strength, effort, and alertness needed to push out the baby. See pages 29–30 for further discussion of "tend-and-befriend."
- *Prolactin.* This "nesting hormone" prepares the breasts for breastfeeding during pregnancy and after birth, it promotes the synthesis of milk and has mood-elevating and calming effects on the mother. It seems to play a role in the altruistic behavior of a new mother—the ability to put the baby's needs before her own.

It is notable that the fetus and newborn also produce these hormones, which contribute to fetal well-being during labor, neonatal adaptation, initiation of breastfeeding, and other possible functions.

other mammals seek privacy in a comfortable, cozy, quiet space and dim light when they are about to give birth. Such an environment for humans would reduce activity in the neocortex and allow the mid-brain and brain stem to set in motion the processes, mediated by prostaglandins and hormones that allow labor to proceed undisturbed. Odent points out that in today's maternity facilities, the neocortex is constantly stimulated with bright lights, strangers, many questions, unfamiliar sights and sounds, and other disturbances, inhibiting primitive brain function and contributing to dystocia.[22,26]

The "fight-or-flight" and "tend-and-befriend" responses to distress and fear in labor

The well-known "fight-or-flight" response, a physiologic process that promotes survival of the endangered or frightened animal or human, is initiated by the outpouring of catecholamines or stress hormones. Triggered by physical danger, fear, anxiety, or other forms of distress, the fight-or-flight response has the potential of slowing labor progress (Fig. 2.3). During most of the first stage of labor, excessively high levels of circulating catecholamines cause maternal blood to be shunted away from the uterus, placenta, and other organs not essential for immediate survival to the heart, lungs, brain, and skeletal muscle, the organs essential to fight-or-flight. The decreased blood

Maternal Effects of Anxiety ('Tend and Befriend' Response) in Labor

Excessive maternal catecholamine levels in first stage of labor
Physiologic response in mother: decreased blood flow to uterus, suppression of oxytocin effects, decreased uterine contractions, increased duration of first stage of labor, decreased blood flow to placenta
Maternal psychological response: increased negative or pessimistic perception of events and the words of others, increased need for reassurance and support, protectiveness toward fetus
Physiologic response in fetus: increased fetal production of catecholamines, fetal conservation of oxygen, fetal heart rate decelerations

Excessive catecholamine levels in second stage labor
Maternal effects: Alertness, renewed energy and strength
Fetal effects: same as listed above, 'fetal ejection reflex' (rapid expulsion of fetus)

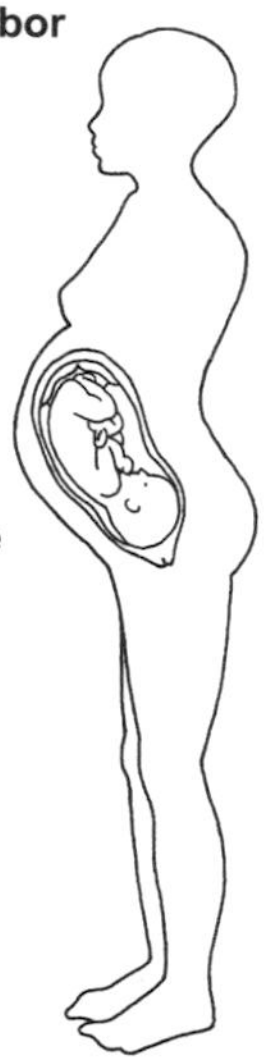

Fig. 2.3. Maternal effects of anxiety.

supply to the uterus and placenta slows uterine contractions[27] and decreases the availability of oxygen to the fetus.[28]

Fear or anxiety also causes the woman to interpret caregivers' words or labor events in a pessimistic or negative way. High levels of catecholamines prevent the woman from entering an instinctual mental state, sometimes called the "zone." Avoidance or reduction of maternal psychological distress or enhancement of the woman's sense of well-being appears to facilitate both the physiologic labor process and the sense of well-being that allows the woman to enter this instinctual trance-like state.

Interestingly, as the woman nears the second stage of labor, which requires alertness and great physical effort, an outpouring of catecholamines normally occurs and has the beneficial effect of speeding the birth by causing the "fetal ejection reflex."[29] In fact, many women briefly exhibit fear, anger, or even euphoria, typical catecholamine responses, just before the birth.[12,22]

Although the physiology of the fight-or-flight response is similar in men and women, behavioral differences exist between the sexes.[25] While fight-or-flight may characterize the primary physiologic responses to stress, behaviorally, males' responses follow the fight-or-flight pattern (fight to protect self, family, village, or country against dangerous attackers, or flee from danger if the odds are too great), but females' behavioral responses are often characterized by a pattern of "tend-and-befriend," which refers to protecting their young from harm and reaching out for help or affiliating with others to reduce the risks to themselves and their offspring. Observations of laboring women and some research support these tend-and-befriend behaviors. Women want and need supportive people around them during labor. In fact, the absence of this kind of support is one of the most frequently mentioned reasons for later dissatisfaction with childbirth[20] and is commonly associated with posttraumatic stress disorder after childbirth.[30-33] A woman's protectiveness toward her child is evident when she is told by a respected caregiver that her baby is in danger. She will quickly agree to whatever treatment is suggested, even if it does not fit with her prior preferences for her birth. On the other hand, if she does not trust the caregiver, she may try to protect her child by resisting suggested treatments.

Following are measures a caregiver may use or suggest to enhance the woman's feelings of security and trust and reduce the likelihood of emotional distress.

The environment for birth

Most hospital birth environments provide safety for mother and baby in the form of uniform care protocols and a large array of diagnostic and therapeutic equipment managed by skilled clinical professionals whose role is to quickly detect and treat problems if they arise. They also are designed for convenience and efficiency for the clinical staff. Last, and to a highly variable degree, some hospitals provide some amenities to enhance comfort and well-being of the woman and her support team. These amenities (baths, places to walk, comfort items, comfortable furniture for the woman and her family, and more) receive a low priority in the birth environment, partly because until recently, little was known about the importance of environment to the laboring woman. Yet, the "environment in which a woman labors can have a great effect on the amount of fear and anxiety she experiences. [The] hospital is an alienating environment for most women, in which institutionalized routines and lack of privacy can contribute to feelings of loss of control."[34,p2]

Scientific evidence of the positive or negative impact of environment on birth indicates that women report greater comfort and satisfaction where their needs are met, and they are more likely to labor out of bed and to avoid common obstetric interventions in environments designed to promote normal birth.[35,36]

Psychoemotional measures

Before labor, what the caregiver can do

Before birth, in childbirth classes, and in conversations with her midwife or doctor, encourage each woman to think about comforting things she and her partner might have during labor, for example, favorite music, scents, pictures, loved ones or a doula, her own clothing to wear during labor, visualizations, aromatherapy, massage, or relaxation techniques. Such things contribute to a woman's personal comfort in the birth environment. Of course, most of these are easily available in a home birth and may be do-able with some advanced planning and/or packing for a hospital birth.

Encourage parents to write a letter or "birth plan" to the staff, introducing themselves and describing their concerns, fears, preferences, and choices regarding their care.[37] Ask to review and discuss the birth plan with the woman during a prenatal appointment. This provides an opportunity to communicate as equals, identify and clear up misunderstandings, and establish trust. If, as in the United States and Canada (and some parts of the United Kingdom), the nurse and midwife or doctor are strangers to the woman, they should check her chart for her psychosocial history, her birth plan, and clinical notes.

During labor: tips for nurses and midwives, especially if meeting the woman for the first time in labor

- *Introduce yourself by name, and call her by name.* Greet her and her support team and orient them as appropriate to her needs and stage of labor. Introduce her to the unit (room, lighting, use of bed, bath or shower, call buttons, kitchen, nurses' station, lounge). Try to convey a sense of hospitality and friendliness, along with safety and competence.
- *Ask about her plans and preferences.* Try to be supportive of her wishes. Does she have a birth plan or preference list? If some of her wishes are unrealistic, discuss them kindly and respectfully, offering the choices you can provide.[37] Sometimes a detailed or negative birth plan reflects fear and mistrust of the staff. Try to reassure the woman and create rapport.
- *Encourage an atmosphere of privacy, comfort, and intimacy between her and her support people:*
  - knock before entering and keep the door closed
  - do not leave her body exposed
  - tell her what comfort devices you have available (ice pack, hot pack, warm blankets, birth ball, beanbag chair, bath, shower, squatting bar, birth stool, music tapes, juices, tea, others)
  - encourage cuddling, hugging, "slow dancing"
  - encourage and reassure the woman and try to remain with her as much as she wishes and as much as your other responsibilities allow

- Explain any clinical procedures or tests. Give her the results. If the woman's vital signs, her labor progress, and the fetal heart rate appear normal, it is reassuring to tell her so.
- Inform her of the signs of progress as you identify them. See pages 108–109 for information on the six ways to progress.

- Suggest comfort measures to help her cope with labor.

- Reassure her, not only with words, but also, as culturally appropriate, with praise, smiles, touch, hand-holding, or gestures of kindness and respect.

These measures create an atmosphere in which the woman feels well cared for and they have the added advantages of taking little time and costing next to nothing.

2

Physical comfort measures

Simple physical comfort measures may increase the woman's sense of mastery and reduce both her stress and the likelihood of a labor-slowing fight-or-flight response.

- Create an atmosphere (privacy, no sudden noises, dim light) that encourages the woman's spontaneous self-comforting behaviors and those learned in childbirth class:
  - relaxation techniques/rhythmic movements
  - calming vocalizations (moans, sighs)
  - rhythmic breathing (see Chapter 10, pages 371–373)
  - guided imagery/visualization

- Give her partner suggestions to use as long as they are acceptable to the woman:
  - massage and pressure techniques (see Chapter 10, pages 337–345)
  - timing contractions or counting her breaths through each one to help her know where she is in the contraction (middle or end)
  - encouraging rhythm in her movements, breathing, moaning, and even in mental activities
  - wiping her face and neck with a cool damp cloth
  - giving words of praise and encouragement
  - speaking rhythmically in a soothing low tone of voice

- Encourage the woman or couple to use available amenities (explained in Chapter 10), such as:
  - hot or cold packs
  - bath or shower
  - birth ball
  - cold or hot beverages, ice chips
  - lounge
  - music player, television

(a)

2

(b)

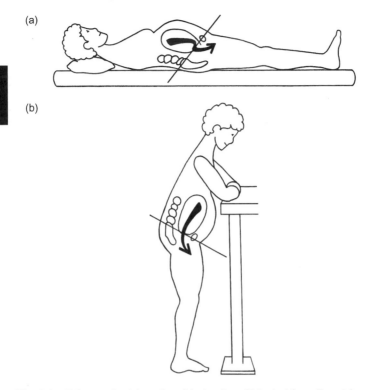

Fig. 2.4. Drive angle: (a) supine, (b) standing. (Adapted from Fenwick and Simkin.[49])

should allow freedom of movement, at least for those women who prefer to move around.

No single position is optimal for all situations or for hours at a time. Therefore, the woman should be encouraged to move, try various positions, and not to remain in one position when there is no apparent progress for long periods.

This book contains descriptions of various maternal positions and movements that may help in specific situations. See the Toolkit in Chapter 9 for a detailed description and discussion of each position and movement.

MONITORING THE MOBILE WOMAN'S F1

There sometimes appears to be a tradeoff between the a maternal mobility and the presumed advantages of cont ̲ ̲ ̲ ̲ tronic fetal monitoring (EFM), which usually requires the mother to remain lying in bed or semi-sitting. This tradeoff can be resolved in a variety of ways. One way is to discontinue the routine practice of continuous EFM, because it carries virtually no benefit for the low-risk woman or baby and does have some added risks.[51] For years, it was assumed that continuous EFM improved newborn outcomes, but numerous scientific trials have failed to confirm that assumption; in fact, these trials found that there were disadvantages associated with EFM, such as an increase in cesareans and instrumental deliveries, with no improvement in newborn outcomes for women at low risk (and who are not receiving oxytocin).[14,51]

Auscultation

The findings of these trials led the professional organizations of obstetricians in the United States (American College of Obstetricians and Gynecologists), Canada (Society of Obstetricians and Gynecologists [SOGC]), and the United Kingdom (Royal College of Obstetricians and Gynecologists), during the late 1980s and early 1990s, to support or promote intermittent auscultation as either equal to or preferred over EFM, for low-risk women with healthy pregnancies.[52-54] The organizations describe similar specific protocols for intermittent auscultation and offer strict guidelines on circumstances that require continuous EFM and/or fetal scalp blood sampling. The SOGC is firm in its recommendation that intermittent auscultation is preferable for normal labor.

When EFM is required: options to enhance maternal mobility

Despite these endorsements of intermittent auscultation, EFM has become well established in most hospitals in the United States, United Kingdom, and Canada. A high percentage still monitors continuously, even when the women are at low risk. Many doctors, nurses, and midwives who were trained in reading electronic monitor tracings remain uneasy with auscultation. In many cases, the nurse or midwife may work in an institution where policies or doctors' orders require continuous EFM, and the women, despite the doctrines of informed consent and informed choice, have little say on this issue. There also are high-risk situations in which continuous EFM is called for. In such situations, there is still much that can be done to encourage movement in women having continuous EFM.

Continuous EFM

The woman does not have to remain in any single position or in bed. She may lie on her side, sit up, kneel and lean forward, get out of bed and rock in a chair, stand and lean over the bed or a birth ball on the bed, sway or "slow dance" (Fig. 2.5) with her partner beside the monitor, kneel, lunge, or even sit in the bath. (The Toolkit in Chapter 9 describes many of these techniques.)

Even if the fetal heart rate is easier to detect in one particular position, the woman should not be required to remain in that position

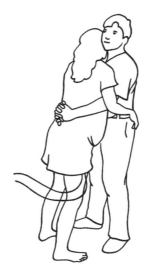

Fig. 2.5. Slow dancing with EFM.

for any longer than the time needed to document the heart rate. The woman's support person or a mesh garment may hold the transducer in place (Fig. 2.6) or a washcloth may be placed between the transducer and its belt (Fig. 2.7), so that it will not slip when the woman is in a standing, hands-and-knees, or other position. An internal scalp electrode usually has the advantage of not slipping out of place when the woman rolls over, kneels, or squats (Fig. 2.8), as the external monitor often does.

However, the scalp electrode is more invasive than the external ultrasound transducer, requires ruptured membranes, and is more likely to promote maternal–fetal transmission of the human immunodeficiency virus (HIV) in an HIV-positive mother. Because today's ultrasound devices can usually pick up the fetal heart rate very well, internal EFM is not often needed.

When an intrauterine pressure catheter (IUPC) is being used, a woman can also make use of upright positions, but it requires adjustment of the pressure gauge when the woman changes positions, in order to maintain accurate pressure readings. One should ask how important it is to record intrauterine pressure and avoid it if there are no compelling clinical reasons to do so.

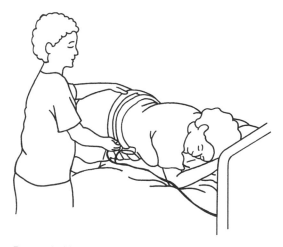

Fig. 2.6. Partner holding transducer in place.

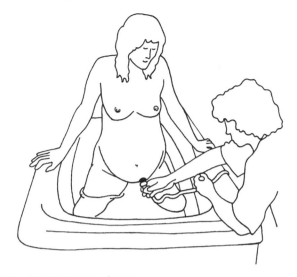

Fig. 2.10. Monitoring out of water.

Telemetry

If the woman must be monitored continuously and the birth setting has an EFM telemetry unit, the woman may walk in or outside her room or sit in the bath or shower (Figures 2.11a and b, 2.12, and 2.13). In the wireless telemetry units, both the ultrasound transducer and the contraction sensor have built-in radio transmitters, which are held on the woman's trunk with the elastic belts. All parts are watertight and safe to use in the bath or shower, as shown in Figures 2.12 and 2.13. The older radio telemetry system also consists of belts and transducers. These are connected to a portable radio transmitter that hangs around the mother's neck, clips to her robe, or hangs over the side of the bath. Again, check with the monitor manufacturer and your hospital engineering department to be sure that monitoring in the water is safe with your particular device.

Considering the documented benefits of walking[50] and hydrotherapy[55] in speeding slow progress and reducing pain, telemetry may be the optimal choice of monitoring methods when continuous monitoring is called for. (For more on the prevention of dystocia through

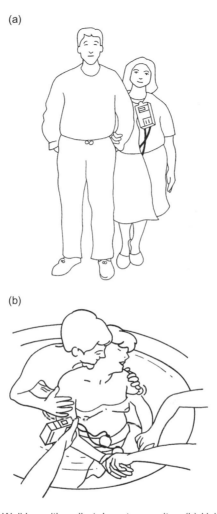

Fig. 2.11. (a) Walking with radio telemetry monitor. (b) Using radio telemetry in bath.

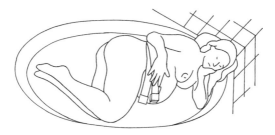

Fig. 2.12. Using wireless telemetry in bath.

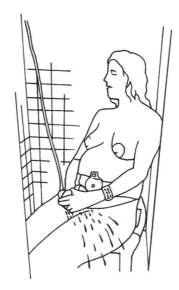

Fig. 2.13. Using wireless telemetry in shower.

movement and ambulation, see pages 33–36, 141–144, 196, 202, 210–211, 311–317, 323–324, 366; for more on hydrotherapy, see pages 332–337.)

By implementing these ideas, it may be possible to avoid some of the problems caused by immobility and the horizontal position that usually accompany EFM. These problems may include persistent occiput posterior position, less efficient contractions, supine hypotension (if the woman remains on her back), and excessive pain.[45]

TECHNIQUES TO ELICIT STRONGER CONTRACTIONS

The following techniques are associated with stronger or more frequent contractions.

- *Hydration.* Make sure that the woman is not dehydrated[22] or overhydrated.[38] See pages 34, 84–85, 146, 150–151 for a discussion of hydration.
- *Movement and positioning.* If progress is slow, ask the woman to walk for half an hour, change positions frequently (about every half hour), and avoid the supine position.
- *Comforting touch*, such as stroking, backrubs, hand-holding, etc., may increase endogenous oxytocin production (Fig. 2.14).
- *Immersion in warm water.* For a delay in active labor, ask the woman to enter a bath with water deep enough to cover her abdomen. She remains there for 30 to 90 minutes.[55]
- *Nipple stimulation* done by either the woman or her partner can be used to stimulate contractions because it increases oxytocin

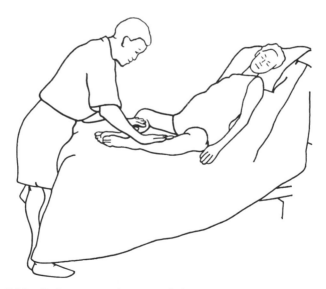

Fig. 2.14. Partner massaging woman's legs.

production.[56] The woman or her partner should start by stimulating one nipple, to see whether this will produce the desired effect. If not, both nipples may be stimulated. Contractions may become markedly longer and stronger so parents may need to be instructed to stop the nipple stimulation if contractions seem to become longer or stronger than is optimal for the fetus. See pages 45–46, 153, 244–245 for more discussion.

- *Acupressure* is sometimes suggested to augment contractions, although it requires trained professionals. See Chapter 10 for more information. Some midwives have received training in acupuncture for labor. See Chapter 8, page 269, for more on the use of acupuncture to speed labor.
- *Warm compresses* or a hot water bottle placed on the fundus may augment contractions. See Chapter 10, pages 328–330, for information on the use of heat.

CONCLUSION

This chapter describes practices that tend to prevent dystocia, with particular emphasis on minimizing maternal distress, promoting physiologic measures that maintain progress, and encouraging movement and position changes by the woman.

REFERENCES

1. World Health Organization. (1996). Care in Normal Birth: A Practical Guide. In Safe Motherhood. Geneva, Author, pp 1–7.
2. Society of Obstetricians & Gynecologists of Canada, Association of Women's Health, Obstetric and Neonatal Nursing of Canada, Canadian Association of Midwives, College of Family Physicians of Canada, Society of Rural Physicians of Canada. (2008). Joint policy statement on normal childbirth. J Obstet Gynaecol Can 30, 1163–1165.
3. UK Maternity Care Working Party including the Royal College of Midwives, Royal College of Obstetricians & Gynecologists, and National Childbirth Trust. (2007). Making normal birth a reality: Consensus statement from the Maternity Care Working Party. Accessed May 25, 2009, from http://www.rcmnormalbirth.org.uk
4. Amis D, Shilling T, Greene J, et al. (2009). Healthy Birth Practices. Washington, DC, Lamaze Institute for Normal Birth.

5. Declercq E, Sakala C, Corry MP, et al. (2006). Listening to Mothers, II: Report of the Second National U.S. Survey of Women's Childbearing Experiences. New York, Childbirth Connection.

6. Coalition for the Improvement of Maternity Services. (2007). Evidence basis for the ten steps of Mother-Friendly Care. J Perinatal Educ 165, 1–96.

7. Gould D. Normal labour: A concept analysis. (2000). J Adv Nurs 31, 418–427.

8. Chalmers B, Porter R. (2001). Assessing effective care in normal labor: The Bologna Score. Birth 28, 79–83.

9. Sandon-Bojo AK, Kvist LG. (2008). Care in labor: A Swedish survey using the Bologna Score. Birth 35, 321–328.

10. American College of Nurse Midwives, Division of Research, Optimality Index Work Group. (2009). The Optimality Index—US User Guidelines and Toolkit. http://www.acnm.org/dor_optimality_index.cfm

11. American College of Nurse Midwives, Division of Research, Optimality Index Work Group. (2009). Measuring outcomes of midwifery care: The Optimality Index—US. http://www.acnm.org/dor_optimality_index.cfm

12. Kennedy HP. (2006). A concept analysis of optimality in perinatal health. J Obstet Gynecol Neonat Nurs 35, 763–769.

13 Friedman E. (1978). Labor: Clinical Evaluation and Management, 2nd edition. New York, Appleton-Century-Crofts.

14. Enkin M, Keirse M, Neilson J, et al. (2000). Monitoring the progress of labour. In A Guide to Effective Care in Pregnancy and Childbirth, 3rd edition. Oxford, UK, Oxford University Press.

15. O'Driscoll K, Meagher D, Boylan D. (1993). Active Management of Labour, 3rd edition. London, Mosby.

16. Zhang J, Troendle J, Yancey M. (2002). Reassessing the labor curve in nulliparous women. Am J Obstet Gynecol 187, 824–828.

17. Albers L, Schiff M, Gorwoda J. (1996). The length of active labor in normal pregnancies. Obstet Gynecol 87, 355–59.

18. Albers L. (1999). The duration of labor in healthy women. J Perinatol 19, 114–119.

19. Cunningham F, Leveno K, Bloom S, et al. (editors). (2010). Williams Obstetrics, 23rd edition. New York, McGraw-Hill, p 468.

20. Hodnett E. (2002). Pain and women's satisfaction with the experience of childbirth: A systematic review. Am J Obstet Gynecol 186, s160–172.

21. Buckley S. (2008). Gentle Birth, Gentle Mothering: A Physician's Guide to Natural Childbirth and Gentle Early Parenting Choices. Berkeley, CA, Celestial Arts.

22. Odent M. (1999). The Scientification of Love. London, Free Association Books.

23. Uvnas-Moberg K. (2003). The Oxytocin Factor: Tapping the Hormone of Calm, Love and Healing. Cambridge, MA, Da Capo Press.

24. Odent M. (1987). The fetus ejection reflex. Birth 14, 104–105.

25. Taylor S. (2002). The Tending Instinct: Women, Men, and the Biology of Our Relationships. New York, Times Books.

26. Odent M. (1984). Birth Reborn: How Childbirth Can Be What Women Want It to Be—and How Mothers and Babies Both Benefit. New York, Pantheon Books.

27. Lederman RP, Lederman E, Work BA, et al. (1981). Relationship of psychological factors in pregnancy to progress in labor. Nursing Res 25, 94–98.

28. Lederman E, Lederman RP, Work BA, et al. (1981). Maternal psychological and physiologic correlates of fetal-newborn health status. Am J Obstetr Gynecol 139, 956–960.

29. Newton N. (1987). The fetus ejection reflex revisited. Birth 14(2), 106–108.

30. Creedy D, Shochet I, Horsfall J. (2000). Childbirth and the development of acute trauma symptoms: Incidence and contributing factors. Birth 27, 104–111.

31. Soet J, Brack G, Dilorio C. (2003). Prevalence and predictors of women's experience of psychological trauma during childbirth. Birth 30, 36–46.

32. Czarnocka J, Slade P. (2000). Prevalence and predictors of post-traumatic stress symptoms following childbirth. Br J Clin Psychol 39, 35–51.

33. Beck C. (2004). Post-traumatic stress disorder due to childbirth: The aftermath. Nurs Res 53, 216–224.

34. Royal College of Midwives (RCM). (2008). Birth environment. In Evidence-Based Guidelines for Midwifery-Led Care in Labour. London, Author, p 2.

35. Hodnett E, Stremler R, Weston J, et al. (2009). Re-conceptualizing the hospital labor room: The PLACE (Pregnant and Laboring in an Ambient Clinical Environment) Pilot Trial. Birth 36, 159–166.

36. Fahey K, Foureur M, Hastis C (editors). (2008). Birth Territory and Midwifery Guardianship: Theory for Practice, Education, and Research. London, Butterworth Heinemann (Elsevier), Books for Midwives, UK.

37. Simkin P, Whalley J, Keppler A, et al. (2010). Pregnancy, Childbirth, and the Newborn: The Complete Guide (5th edition). Minnetonka, MN, Meadowbrook Press.

38. Moen V, Brudin L, Rundgren M, et al. (2009). Hyponatremia complicating labour—Rare or unrecognised? A prospective observational study. BJOG 116, 552–561.

39. Singata M, Tranmer J, Gyte GML. (2010). Restricting oral fluid and food intake during labour. Cochrane Database Syst Rev (1)CD003930. doi:10.1002/14651858.CD003930.pub2.

40. Sharp DA. (1997). Restriction of oral intake for women in labour. Br J Midwif 5(7), 408–412.

41. The CNM Data Group. (1999). Clinical bulletin: Intrapartum nutrition. J Nurs-Midwif 44(3), 129–134.

42. Berry H. (1997). Feast or famine? Oral intake during labour: Current evidence and practice. Br J Midwif 5(7), 413–417.

43. Sleutel M, Golden S. (1999) Fasting in labor: relic or requirement. J Obstet Gynecol Neonatal Nursing 28, 507–512.

44. Roberts J. (1989). Maternal positions during the first stage of labour. In Chalmers I, Enkin M, Keirse M (editors). Effective Care in Pregnancy and Childbirth, vol. 2. Oxford, Oxford University Press.

45. Simkin P, O'Hara M (2002). Nonpharmacologic relief of pain during labor: Systematic reviews of five methods. Am J Obstet Gynecol 186, S131–S159.

46. Russell JGB (1969). Moulding of the pelvic outlet. J Obstet Gynaecol Br Commonw 76, 817–820.

47. Michel S, Rake A, Treiber K, et al. (2002). MR obstetric pelvimetry: Effect of birthing position on pelvic bony dimensions. AJR Am J Roentgenol 179, 1063–1067.

48. Simkin P. (2003). Maternal positions and pelves revisited. Birth 30, 130–132.

49. Fenwick L, Simkin P. (1987). Maternal positioning to treat dystocia. Clin Obstet Gynecol 30, 83–89.

50. Lawrence A, Lewis L, Hofmeyr GJ, et al. (2009). Maternal positions and mobility during first stage labour. Cochrane Database Syst Rev (2) CD003934. doi:10.1002/14651858.CD003934.pub2

51. Thacker S, Stroup D, Chang M. (2001). Continuous electronic heart rate monitoring for fetal assessment during labor (Cochrane Review). In: The Cochrane Library, Issue 3, 2004. Chichester, UK, John Wiley & Sons, Ltd.

52. American College of Obstetricians and Gynecologists. (2009). Intrapartum fetal heart rate monitoring: Nomenclature, interpretation, and general management principles. Practice Bulletin No. 106. Obstet Gynecol 144(1), 191–202.

53. Liston R, Sawchuck D, Young D, SOGC Fetal Health Surveillance Consensus Committee. (2007). Fetal health surveillance: Antepartum and intrapartum consensus guideline #197. JOGC 29(9, suppl 4), s29–s39.

54. Royal College of Obstetricians and Gynaecologists. (2001). The use of electronic fetal monitoring. The use and interpretation of cardiotocography in intrapartum fetal surveillance. Evidence-Based Clinical Guidelines No. 8. London, RCOG Press.

55. Cluett E, Burns E. (2009). Immersion in water in labour and birth. Cochrane Database Syst Rev (2):CD000111.

56. Kavanagh J, Kelly AJ, Thomas J. (2005). Breast stimulation for cervical ripening and induction of labour. Cochrane Database Syst Rev (3) CD003392. doi:10.1002/14651858.CD003392.pub2.

2

Chapter 3

Assessing Progress in Labor

Suzy Myers, LM, CPM, MPH, with contributions by
Gail Tully, BS, CPM, CD(DONA), and Lisa Hanson,
PhD, CNM, FACNM

Before labor begins, 52
Malposition, 52
Leopold's maneuvers, 57
Belly mapping, 60
Other assessments prior to labor, 64
Assessments during labor, 66
Position, attitude, and station of the fetus, 66
Vaginal examinations: indications and timing, 66
Performing a vaginal examination during labor, 67
Assessing the cervix, 70
Unusual cervical findings, 71
The presenting part, 72
The vagina and bony pelvis, 80
Quality of contractions, 81
Assessing the mother's condition, 84
Hydration and nourishment, 84
Vital signs, 85
Psychology, 85
Assessing the fetus, 86
Fetal heart rate, 86
How to perform intermittent auscultation, 87
When using continuous electronic fetal monitoring, 89
The three-tiered fetal heart rate interpretation system, 91
Putting it all together, 94
Assessing progress in the first stage, 94
Assessing progress in the second stage, 96
Conclusion, 96
References, 96

The Labor Progress Handbook: Early Interventions to Prevent and Treat Dystocia.
Edited by Penny Simkin, Ruth Ancheta
© 2011 by Penny Simkin and Ruth Ancheta; illustrations copyright Ruth Ancheta

Many important assessments help determine when labor is progressing normally and when it is not. These assessments inform and guide midwives, doctors, and nurses in promoting normal labor progress, preventing dysfunctional labors, and treating dystocia appropriately when it occurs. While training, mentorship, and practice are required to master these assessment skills, this chapter will provide descriptions, rationale, and practical tips.

Readers who do not have professional training in maternity nursing, midwifery, or medicine and who do not have clinical responsibility for the health of pregnant or laboring women (i.e., doulas and childbirth educators) do not use the hands-on assessment techniques because they are outside their scope of practice. Doulas and childbirth educators may, however, find this chapter helpful in understanding the reasons for and meanings of these assessments.

This chapter addresses labor progress assessment with a full-term singleton fetus in a longitudinal lie and a cephalic presentation (aligned vertically in the mother's torso, with the head lying over the pelvic inlet).

BEFORE LABOR BEGINS

Malposition

A primary cause of dysfunctional labor is fetal malposition,[1] and occiput posterior (OP) is the most common.[1]

Two questions should be considered: Can the fetal position be assessed accurately before labor begins? If so, does doing so provide an opportunity to correct some problems before labor begins?

- Can malposition accurately be determined antenatally?

Simkin[2] reviewed studies that examined whether certain prenatal assessments could identify the OP position in labor. These prenatal assessments offer clues to the location and orientation of the fetal back, which is presumed to correlate with the position of the fetal head in the maternal pelvis.

The assessments include:

1. observing the contour of the maternal abdomen
2. locating the point of maximum intensity (PMI) of the fetal heart tones via auscultation
3. performing abdominal palpation using Leopold's maneuvers

Table 3.1. Fetal positions—abdominal views. Fetal position i
by the location of the occiput (the back of the fetal head) in re
mother's left or right, and to the front (anterior) or back (poste
pelvis, as shown in Table 3.1

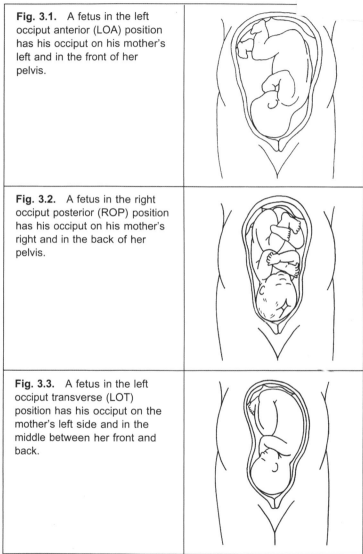

Fig. 3.1. A fetus in the left occiput anterior (LOA) position has his occiput on his mother's left and in the front of her pelvis.

Fig. 3.2. A fetus in the right occiput posterior (ROP) position has his occiput on his mother's right and in the back of her pelvis.

Fig. 3.3. A fetus in the left occiput transverse (LOT) position has his occiput on the mother's left side and in the middle between her front and back.

3

Although many experienced midwives believe in their utility as indicators of fetal position, the reliability of neither the maternal abdominal contour nor the PMI of the fetal heart tones has ever been assessed with well-designed studies.

1. Abdominal contour

When the fetus is lying with the back anterior (toward the woman's front), the maternal abdominal wall looks convex and the umbilicus may appear "popped out," as in Figure 3.4. The mother reports fetal movement predominantly in the upper quadrant opposite the fetal back.

When the fetal back is oriented more posteriorly (toward the mother's spine), the abdomen looks concave, especially depressed in the region of the umbilicus or below, as shown in Figure 3.5. The mother may report she feels fetal movement in the midline, or "everywhere." These are signs that the fetus is more likely to enter the maternal pelvis in the less favorable OP position, as shown in Table 3.1 and Figure 3.2. These observations may be difficult in obese women.

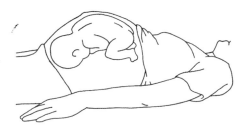

Fig. 3.4. Abdominal contour with fetal back anterior.

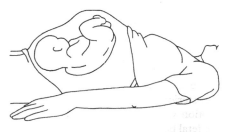

Fig. 3.5. Abdominal contour with fetal back posterior.

2. Location of the PMI of the fetal heart tones via auscultation

In most fetuses near term, the loudest sounds of the fetal heart are heard through the fetal back, at approximately the level of the scapula or shoulders. Locating this PMI of the fetal heart tones ...ps determine the orientation of the fetal back—either anterior ...sterior. The best tool for this purpose is a fetoscope (such ...De Lee-Hillis fetoscope or the Pinard Horn), which ... auscultation of the fetal heart (Fig. 3.6), rather ...(Dopplers use ultrasound to create an artificial ...affected by proximity to the heart valves.)

...t tones with a fetoscope.

...ear term is oriented with his curved ...ont, the heart tones are crisp and clear ...side of the maternal abdomen where ...the maternal umbilicus and several ...e (LOA or ROA [left or right occiput ...the fetus is oriented with his curved ...ine, the PMI is in the right or left ...l abdomen (LOP or ROP [left ...Fig. 3.7). Rarely, if the fetal back is ...e head completely extended (face ...nes may be heard through the fetal ...it, and difficult to hear.[3]

1. The first maneuver (Fig. 3.8) helps identify what part of the fetus is in the fundus (the top of the uterus). Facing the woman's head, the caregiver places both hands on the woman's upper abdomen and, using firm but gentle pressure, feels the fundus and the height, shape, size, and consistency of the fetal parts in that area. When the lie is longitudinal and the presentation is cephalic, the breech is palpated in the fundus. It may feel bony and relatively large but is differentiated from the head by feeling continuous with the spine and moving with it. In contrast, when the head is in the fundus (breech presentation), it usually feels ballotable— it "bounces" between the palpating hands because it can be moved independently from the fetal back. When the lie is transverse, neither a head nor a breech can be palpated in the fundus.

2. The second maneuver (Fig. 3.9) helps determine the location of the fetal back. Still facing the woman's head, the caregiver places her or his hands, palm down, on either side of the woman's abdomen. By keeping both hands in contact with the abdomen and alternating pressure from one hand to the other, the caregiver can palpate the shape and bulk of fetal parts on either side of the maternal torso and around toward the maternal spine. With this maneuver, the caregiver may differentiate the feel of smooth back from knobby limbs ("small parts") and amniotic fluid from fetal body parts. When the lie is transverse, the head or breech may be palpated on one or the other side of the maternal torso.

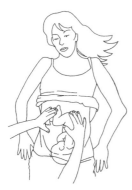

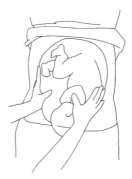

Fig. 3.8. Leopold's maneuver No. 1.

Fig. 3.9. Leopold's maneuver No. 2.

The final two Leopold's maneuvers are used to confirm the presentation and lie and to assess the presenting part and its descent into the pelvis.

3. For the third maneuver (Fig. 3.10), the caregiver uses the thumb and forefinger of the dominant hand to gently palpate the lower pole of the uterus, just above the symphysis. The nondominant hand may be used to grasp the fundus at the same time. If the lie is longitudinal and presenting part is cephalic, the examiner should feel the large bony skull, which is often mobile if not yet deeply engaged. If the presenting part is the breech, although it may feel bony, it is much smaller than the head and does not move independent of the body. When the lie is transverse, the lower pole, like the fundus, feels empty of fetal parts.

4. For the fourth maneuver (Fig. 3.11), the examiner turns to face the woman's feet and places one hand on each side of the woman's abdomen. With the fingers pointing toward the woman's feet, the caregiver presses the fingertips gently and firmly toward the maternal spine and around the presenting part.

A term head that is floating above the pelvic brim is easily palpated. It feels round, large, and mobile. As the head descends into the bowl of the pelvic inlet, it becomes more difficult to palpate. When the fetal head is deeply engaged prior to labor, it may be nearly impossible to feel with external palpation and sometimes requires internal assessment or ultrasound to confirm a cephalic presentation.

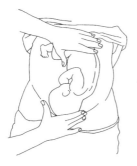 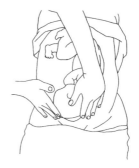

Fig. 3.10. Leopold's maneuver No. 3.

Fig. 3.11. Leopold's maneuver No. 4.

Not only do we need to know more about the utility of ultrasound as a tool to assess fetal position, we also need more information about "low-tech" methods. There is a significant gap in the research addressing whether observation, auscultation, and palpation by experienced caretakers can aid in determining the fetal position. Should these techniques show promise, they could be taught more effectively and used more appropriately (i.e., during labor).

- Even if accuracy could be improved, does the ability to determine fetal position antenatally make a difference in labor?

In Simkin's review,[2] only two published trials examined whether the OP position could be changed by prenatal maneuvers. These small and methodologically weak studies showed that although maternal positioning could change the fetus from OP to OA for short periods, there was no evidence that these changes were maintained during labor and birth.[7,8]

Belly Mapping

Belly mapping is a three-step process conceived by Gail Tully to identify fetal position, integrating mothers' observations, palpation, and auscultation of the fetal heart. It is an effective way to record the fetal position and explain it to mothers. Midwives, doctors, and nurses may find it helpful to combine belly mapping with Leopold's maneuvers to involve women in their care and enhance communications. We include here a description of this process, condensed from Tully's 2010 book,

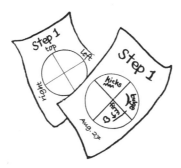

Fig. 3.B1. "Pie" map form.

The Belly Mapping Workbook: How Kicks and Wiggles Reveal Your Baby's Position.

Step 1: Make a pie

Belly mapping involves mentally dividing the maternal abdomen into quadrants ("pie pieces") and drawing it on paper as shown in Figure 3.B1. The woman can often contribute much of the information needed to identify the position of her fetus, including:

- Which side of her belly is firm (if either)
- Where she feels the "big bulge" of the fetal buttocks or head
- Where she feels stronger kicks (fetal feet or knees)
- Where she feels stretching from fetal leg movements
- Where she feels smaller movements (hands, elbows)

Figure 3.B2 shows a woman's experiences and how the belly map represents them.

The midwife, doctor, or nurse uses clinical skills (Leopold's maneuvers, auscultation, and possibly ultrasound) to confirm and/or add to the mother's subjective information on fetal position and marks all this in more detail on the belly map. (The "heart" represents where fetal heart tones are heard using a fetoscope or Pinard Horn. Because Doppler ultrasound fetoscopes can detect fetal heart tones farther from their point of origin, they are not as useful for this purpose.)

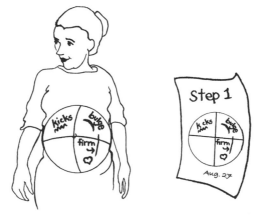

Fig. 3.B2. Example of a belly map.

Step 2: Visualize the baby

Putting all the information together, the care provider gets a good picture of the baby in the womb. When they are certain of the fetal position, some providers actually draw an outline of the fetus on the woman's abdomen with a nontoxic marker so that she can visualize how her baby is positioned. Or they may position a fetal doll over her abdomen to show the woman how her baby is positioned (Fig. 3.B3).

Step 3: Name the position

Both the woman and her care provider will gain a clear picture of the fetus' position and will be able to discuss it. Figures 3.B4 and 3.B5 show the correlation between belly maps, see-through views, and fetus-in-the-pelvis views for fetuses in LOA and ROP.

If the provider identifies an unfavorable position in late pregnancy, the mother may be able to use maternal positioning and exercises to reposition the fetus before labor. These may be more successful if they can be done in the last weeks of pregnancy before the fetal head is engaged. Sutton[9] and Scott[10] have devised an approach, "optimal fetal positioning" (OFP), that combines late pregnancy and intrapartum positions to facilitate and maintain favorable fetal positions. This approach should be studied scientifically for its effectiveness. Tully's *Spinning Babies* approach uses OFP concepts (see pages 103–106) plus other positions, movements, and devices that have been learned either from traditional midwives, physical therapists, chiropractors or from her

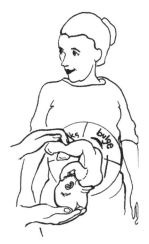

Fig. 3.B3.   Using a doll to explain the position.

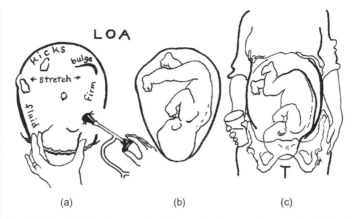

(a)   (b)   (c)

Fig. 3.B4. LOA belly map showing mother's experience and clinician's findings (**a**), LOA fetus (**b**), and LOA fetus in the pelvis (**c**).

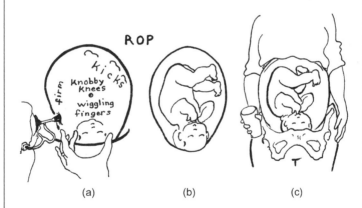

(a)   (b)   (c)

Fig. 3.B5. ROP belly map showing mother's experience and clinician's findings (**a**), ROP fetus (**b**), and ROP fetus in the pelvis (**c**).

own original discoveries while working with laboring women. See Chapter 4 for more information on repositioning the fetus.

Text and illustrations by Gail Tully, reprinted by permission. Condensed from Tully G. (2010). The belly mapping workbook: How kicks and wiggles reveal your baby's position. Bloomington, MN, Maternity House Publishing. See also www.SpinningBabies.com/baby-positions/belly-mapping

Other assessments prior to labor

Estimating fetal weight

Although most women with large babies deliver them without diffi-culty,[11] fetal macrosomia can complicate labor.[12,13] Additionally, when the fetus is large, problems associated with malposition may be compounded.

Methods of estimating fetal weight at term are imprecise. Fundal height measurement is a poor predictor of fetal weight, although it may be useful to screen for further investigation.[14] Ultrasound assess-ments and palpation have equivalent accuracy, with an estimated margin of error of ±10% to 20%. The accuracy of palpation is signifi-cantly increased when the examiner is experienced[15,16] but reduced when the fetus is macrosomic.[13] Furthermore, an inaccurate predic-tion of fetal macrosomia may influence a diagnosis of labor dysfunc-tion, leading to cesarean delivery.[17]

The best way to refine palpation skills for estimating fetal weight is to practice palpation on every available woman at term or in labor, commit oneself to an estimated fetal weight, and verify it when the baby is born.

The birth weight prediction equation

There may be promise in a "birth weight prediction equation" described by Nahum and Stanislaw.[18] Based on maternal and pregnancy-specific characteristics, it predicted the birth weights of term, healthy Caucasian infants within an average of ±8%, better than ultrasound. For predicting macrosomia, the equation was equivalent to ultrasound.

To summarize, the value of estimating fetal weight is questionable because of these problems: current methods of predicting birth weight are not reliable; the impact of macrosomia is variable, and it is not possible to reverse excessive fetal weight at or near term. Nonetheless, when labor progress is poor, caregivers may use an estimation of fetal weight as just that: an *estimation* and one of many variables factored into the complex problem-solving needed to help resolve dysfunctional labors.

Assessing the cervix prior to labor

During pregnancy, the cervix is composed of dense collagen fibers providing a firm, inelastic tubular structure that helps keep the uterine contents safely contained. In labor, the role of the cervix is reversed. It must become elastic enough for the muscular activity of the uterus to open it and expel the fetus. To accomplish this, hormonal changes cause alterations in the composition of the cervical tissue. Collagen fibers break down; elastin fibers in the internal os provide stretch; and the water content of the connective tissue increases, making the cervix soft and stretchy. These changes, called *cervical ripening,* begin weeks before labor's onset and are caused by hormonal influences distinct from the mechanisms of effacement and dilation.[19] Some labor problems, both preterm labors and prolonged labors at term, may be the result of *cervical* dysfunction, rather than *uterine* dysfunction, when the cervix undergoes these changes too soon or does not complete them.[20–22] Some reasons for *cervical dystocia* are scarring from procedures such as cautery, cryosurgery, or other surgery or congenital abnormalities.

In 1964, Bishop[23] published his 15-point scoring system for evaluating the "induce-ability" of labor based on five factors: cervical dilation, effacement, consistency, position in the vagina, and station of the head. A ripe, or favorable-for-induction, cervix has a Bishop's score of 6 to 8. The Bishop score has also been used more recently to assess the need for preinduction cervical ripening agents.

Some caregivers use Bishop's five variables to evaluate the cervical ripeness of women who are not necessarily candidates for induction, sometimes with weekly routine cervical examinations in the last month of pregnancy. How useful are these examinations? Assessing the prelabor cervix in women at term may help identify those more likely to experience short or prolonged latent phases.[24] Many people agree that, especially in nulliparas, women who begin labor with cervices that are long, firm, closed, and posterior are more likely to experience prolonged latent phases, while those whose cervices are thin, stretchy, and partially dilated are likely to progress more rapidly to the active phase. However, the value of prelabor cervical assessment in predicting the onset of labor or active phase disorders is not substantiated in any research literature.

It may be tempting to tell a woman whose cervix is soft, thin, anterior, and 2 cm dilated that she will surely be in labor in the next day or two or to tell a woman with a closed, uneffaced cervix that she will still be pregnant next week. However, the condition of the cervix late in pregnancy does not predict when labor will begin or how it will progress, and these statements are inaccurate often enough to cause patients unnecessary distress. The decision to examine the cervix before the onset of labor should be based on a balanced assessment of the value of the information provided and client preference, rather than routine.

The role of cervical ripening in the etiology of problem labor—both prolonged and preterm—deserves further study.

ASSESSMENTS DURING LABOR

3

It is important to assess labor progress holistically, taking into account the many complex factors and their interactions that influence labor progress. These include:

- position, attitude (whether the fetal chin is well flexed toward the chest), and station of the fetus
- cervical change over time
- quality of contractions
- condition of the mother
- condition of the fetus

Position, attitude, and station of the fetus

These are assessed during labor, primarily via internal vaginal examinations. Vaginal examinations also provide essential information about cervical change when repeated over time.

Vaginal examinations: indications and timing

Each woman in labor should be treated individually and her labor assessed as her needs dictate. This means that rather than being done in all labors at a predetermined time interval or according to a protocol, vaginal examinations are done as the need for information about the cervix and fetus arises, and with the woman's understanding and consent. Appreciating that this examination is a significant intrusion for most women, the caregiver should take time to establish rapport before performing a vaginal examination and, of course, to avoid doing it if she refuses. Reasons that justify assessing labor progress using vaginal examinations include:

- At the beginning of caring for a woman, to establish a baseline so that future progress or lack of progress can be better assessed.

- When a period of time in active labor has elapsed, usually more than 3 hours, and the labor pattern does not seem to be progressing (contractions are not becoming longer, more frequent, or more intense) or when there are no other outward signs of progress (mother's affect, spontaneous bearing down efforts, etc.), and a decision must be made about interventions to speed labor progress.
- After an intervention has been implemented for some time (i.e., a period of stair climbing to aid in rotation of the fetal head or time in the bath), to assess whether the desired effect has been achieved.
- When the woman in labor requests an assessment of her progress or expresses discouragement or a desire for pain medication.
- When there is a spontaneous urge to push without other signs of fetal descent over a reasonable time.
- When there are nonreassuring fetal heart rate (FHR) changes or any other concerning signs, such as excess vaginal bleeding.
- When an internal monitor (scalp lead or intrauterine pressure catheter) is needed.

Performing a vaginal examination during labor

Preparing to do the examination

Ideally, caregivers not only are making clinical assessments but also are mindful of the laboring woman's needs for emotional support and accurate information. The vaginal examination in labor should be approached with these principles in mind.

First, it is helpful to sit with the woman and observe her labor pattern and her responses to it.

- What are the frequency, duration, and quality of the contractions?
- How is the woman coping with them? (See Chapter 2, pages 24–30.)
- Is she moving with, or between, contractions?
- What positions does she spontaneously assume?

After making these basic observations, the caregiver should ask the woman if she thinks it would be helpful to assess her progress with a vaginal examination. Some women will welcome this information, while others are not yet ready. It is important to explain the benefits of having this information and not to act without her permission.

Ask the woman to empty her bladder before the exam. Next, she should lie down on a firm comfortable surface, preferably on her back with her head supported by not more than one pillow as shown in Figure 3.12a. The mother's legs should be well-supported, with her knees flexed and wide apart, and the soles of her feet either together or flat on the bed's surface. If lying on her back is too uncomfortable, she can rest in a supported semiprone position with a pillow wedged under one hip with her upper knee and hip flexed and supported (Fig. 3.12b). Some experienced practitioners perform vaginal exams with the mother in other positions (on hands and knees, standing, sitting, or squatting). This allows them to assess the station and cervical dilation. However, it is difficult to gain more detailed information, such as the often challenging position of the presenting part, with the mother in these positions. When detailed information is needed, it is better to ask the mother to lie down briefly than to have to repeat the exam.

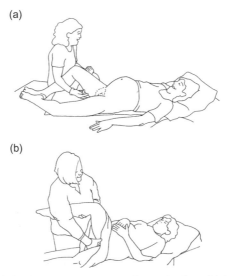

Fig. 3.12.   (**a**) Supine position for vaginal examination. (**b**) Side-lying position for vaginal examination.

After the woman gives permission, it is important to explain each step, offer to stop at any point if the woman requests it, and request her feedback about anything that hurts. The woman's ability to relax during this exam is important if the provider is to obtain the necessary information. But it is also a quality of care issue. Good care is defined as being both sensitive to the woman's needs and effective in obtaining the needed data. Some women experience fear during vaginal exams and may not be able to tolerate them, especially when performed by unfamiliar people or done without consideration of their discomfort. Often, these are women who have experienced previous trauma (i.e., sexual abuse or rough and inconsiderate vaginal exams). In order to be examined, they need patience, gentleness, and understanding from their providers and a sense of being in control over whether, when, by whom, and how the exam will be done.[25]

The vaginal examination, and other assessments, step by step

- The clinical caregiver washes and warms her or his hands and starts with firm, but gentle abdominal palpation, using the basic Leopold's maneuvers.
  - As in the prenatal examination (page 53), the caregiver determines the location and orientation of the fetal back (toward the woman's abdominal wall or toward her spine).
  - The caregiver estimates fetal weight, using palpation as well as historical information about the woman and her pregnancy. (Labor is the perfect opportunity to refine this skill—verifying the estimate will be possible very soon!)
  - The next step is to assess uterine tone, between and during contractions, by gently palpating at the fundus with the fingertips (see *Assessing Contraction Quality*).
  - This is also a good time to assess the FHR and maternal vital signs. Consolidating necessary assessments allows the woman to labor undisturbed for longer periods.

- Next, the caregiver asks the woman's permission to begin the vaginal exam. Of course, if permission is not granted, the caregiver does not do it.

- Between contractions, the caregiver inserts first one (the forefinger) and then two fingers (adding the middle finger) into the vagina, putting firm but gentle pressure on the posterior vaginal wall and avoiding pressure on the urethra. At the same time, the examiner asks the mother to relax her vaginal muscles. Without the mother's cooperation and active relaxation, this exam may be uncomfortable for her, and accurate assessment may be difficult.

- If the fingers were inserted with the pads down, when they have reached the bulbocavernosus muscle, or about 3 to 4 cm into the vagina, the examiner explains that she or he will rotate the fingers so that the wrist is face up. This position allows for better assessment of the cervix, the presenting part, the vagina, and the pelvis.

Assessing the cervix

- *Position:* Is the os anterior, posterior, or midline? When the cervical os is posterior, sometimes it is just barely possible to reach it, but not enough to assess dilation. In this case, the caregiver may be able, by applying gentle, steady pressure, to reach the os and manually pull it forward. Another aid is to ask the woman to place a fist under each buttock to help tilt the pelvis. This should bring the cervix into a more "reachable" position.

- *Consistency:* Are the cervical tissue and os stretchy and soft or firm? As labor progresses, the cervix should become softer and more yielding. A thick, rigid cervix is abnormal.

- *Effacement:* How long is the cervical canal? It is difficult, if not impossible, to assess effacement digitally without being able to insert at least one finger into the cervix. Since the length of the cervix prior to labor varies from 1 to 4 cm, effacement is best expressed in terms of the length of the cervical canal, in centimeters or fractions of centimeters (rather than using the older method of expressing effacement as a percentage).[26] A completely effaced cervix is "paper thin."

- *Dilation:* How open is the cervix, measured in centimeters, without manual stretching? The first 6 to 7 cm are assessed by evaluating how open the cervix is. It takes practice to know the approximate number of finger breadths, or the distance between fingers, and the corresponding dilation. Practice tools include plastic models made for this purpose, as well as household objects, such as jars with various sized mouths. The last 3 cm (from 7 cm to fully dilated) are easier to assess, because they are measured by evaluating how much of the cervix remains on *one* side, between the open edge of the os and where the cervix meets the lower uterine segment. Although "10 cm" has been used to express complete dilation, measurable full dilation could vary between 9 and 12 cm depending on the diameters of the head.

- *Membranes:* Are they intact or ruptured? A large bulging forebag is easy to feel and may make assessment of fetal position difficult. When there is no bulging bag of fluid presenting, the examiner should learn to discern the feel of the slippery membrane over the head compared to the way the scalp feels when membranes are ruptured.

Unusual cervical findings

- *The "zipper" cervix:* While the cervix is quite thin, the os is adherent and closed. Sometimes, after near complete effacement is achieved, this can be overcome by inserting one or two fingers and massaging the os open during a contraction. As the adhesion releases, the os opens like a zipper, sometimes dilating from 1 to 3 or 4 cm in one contraction! Expect bloody show as capillaries rupture with stretching. See Chapter 8, page 245, for more on this procedure.

- *The rigid os:* The cervix may be partially dilated but has thickness and lacks a feeling of elasticity. It does not yield easily with contractions. This may be a sign of primary cervical dysfunction[20] or a consequence of edema in the cervix caused by a poorly fitting head or uneven pressure on the cervix during contractions. In the former, the cervix never softens and effaces; in the latter, the cervix may be thinned and dilated during the latent phase or early active phase but becomes swollen in late active phase.

- *The os is not palpable at all!* The lower uterine segment is thinned, the head is well applied with a low station, and exam findings may mimic full dilation. Sometimes, with careful examination, it is possible to find a small depression where the os is, but this author has encountered one case in which several experienced examiners were unable to locate even this landmark.

- *Persistent anterior cervical "lip":* This occurs when most of the cervix has retracted behind the head (no rim of cervix is palpated around the lateral or pos*terior aspects of the head)* but the anterior portion of the cervix is caught between the head and the symphysis pubis. Position changes, time, and patience usually resolve the situation. If the tissue feels stretchy, it may be reduced manually as explained in Chapter 8, on pages 250–251.

The presenting part

- Is it a head? It is important to consider that the presenting part may *not be* a head; otherwise, one risks missing an undiagnosed breech presentation. Exam findings with a frank breech may mimic those with an extremely malpositioned head: no sutures or fontanelles are felt and the leading part feels soft and spongy, as with a caput. One way to clarify this situation, short of ultrasound, is to perform a sterile speculum examination. The presence of hair confirms a cephalic presentation.

- What is the fetal station? In relation to the imaginary transverse plane between the ischial spines, where is the leading edge of the bony skull (Fig. 3.13)?

- To assess station by vaginal examination:
  - Stations of descent are expressed in centimeters above or below the level of the ischial spines, which is designated as zero station. When the head has not yet entered the pelvis, the leading edge is said to be "floating."
  - The examiner first finds the approximate location of one ischial spine. It is easiest to do this by reaching with one's dominant hand diagonally across the mother's pelvis (so a right-handed provider will palpate the right maternal spine). In a woman with a normal midpelvis, the spine will be blunt

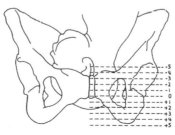

Fig. 3.13. Stations of descent.

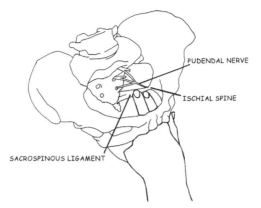

PUDENDAL NERVE

ISCHIAL SPINE

SACROSPINOUS LIGAMENT

3

Fig. 3.14. Finding the sacrospinous ligament.

and not easily palpated, so approximating its location takes practice. It helps to find the sacrospinous ligament and follow it with two fingers from the midline to the place of insertion on the sidewall as shown in Figure 3.14. Because this insertion point is also the location of the pudendal nerve, the mother may report an achy sensation when the examiner's fingers press there.

o   Second, the examiner compares the level of the leading edge of the head with the level of the ischial spines. It is imperative to use enough pressure to feel the *bone*, to avoid mistaking a large spongy caput for a head at a lower station.

●   To assess station by abdominal palpation:

According to the World Health Organization, "When there is a significant degree of caput or molding, assessment by abdominal palpation is more useful than assessment by vaginal exam."[27] Using abdominal palpation, an experienced clinician can:
   o   assess descent with a minimum of intrusion
   o   avoid the infection risks of a vaginal examination with ruptured membranes
   o   make more accurate assessments when considering the relative safety of cesarean surgery, operative vaginal delivery, or watchful waiting in a given situation

To assess descent by abdominal palpation, the examiner mentally divides the fetal head into five sections, each about the width of one of the examiner's fingers.

- When the entire fetal head is above the pubic symphysis, as in Figure 3.15a, it can be palpated with all five fingers and is said to be "five fifths" palpable (5/5). See Figure 3.15b. (At this height, the head is mobile.)
- When the head can only be felt with two fingers above the symphysis, it is said to be "two fifths" palpable (2/5) as shown in Figure 3.15c.
- When the head is entirely below the symphysis, it is said to be "zero fifths" palpable (0/5).

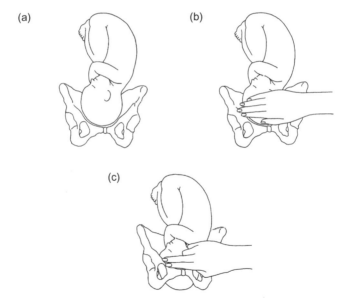

Fig. 3.15. Fetal head above pubic symphysis (**a**), palpating fetal head at 5/5 (**b**), and palpating fetal head at 2/5 (**c**). (Adapted from Publication Department of Reproductive Health and Research. [2003]. *Managing Complications in Pregnancy and Childbirth: A Guide for Midwives and Doctors*, p. 82, World Health Organization, Geneva.)

  ◦ A less precise measure, but one that is useful when learning to assess station, is how deeply the examiner's fingers may be inserted before reaching the head.[28] Assuming average-sized fingers:

    a. if the station is floating, the fingers will be inserted completely into the vagina and not reach the leading edge of the head (Fig. 3.16a).

    b. With station −4 to −2, the examiner's fingers will be inserted completely and will be able to palpate the head with the tips of the fingers.

    c. At zero station, the fingers are inserted about halfway before meeting the head (Fig. 3.16b), and at lower stations, the fingers reach the head easily (Fig. 3.16c).

Assessment of station, like many other internal examinations in labor, is not precise and varies from examiner to examiner. In a slow second stage, progress may be incremental, in millimeters, rather than in centimeters. When progress is in question, sequential evaluation by the same examiner is important.

(a) Floating, or well above spines

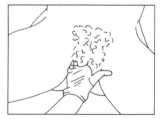

(b) At level of spines − O station

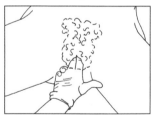

(c) Below the spines

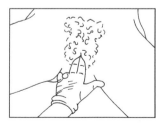

Fig. 3.16. Vaginal examinations to assess descent. (**a**) Floating, or well above spines. (**b**) At level of spines—O station. (**c**) Below the spines.

A high station in active phase, especially in a nullipara, may suggest malposition or true cephalopelvic disproportion (CPD).

- Evaluating fetal position: Identifying fetal position is perhaps the single most difficult assessment to make during intrapartum vaginal examinations. It is commonly determined by the caregiver palpating bony landmarks on the fetal head through a reasonably dilated cervix, to determine the location of the occiput in relation to the maternal pelvis. The accuracy of digital identification of bony landmarks of the fetal skull has been studied by numerous researchers, using comparisons with ultrasound findings as the standard. All these studies, in both first stage and second stage, found a low level of accuracy with digital exams (defined as within 45 degrees of the ultrasound determination of position).[2] Simkin[2] summarized these findings in a recent review article.

  The lack of demonstrable benefit may be difficult for experienced midwives, nurses, and doctors to accept. Simkin suggests that care providers compare some of their digital assessments with ultrasound results to confirm their accuracy or inaccuracy and also use ultrasound comparisons to refine and improve their skills. Misdiagnosis of fetal position may cause more harm than no diagnosis, due to the use of inappropriate action resulting from the misdiagnosis.

  With that caveat, and despite the negative findings regarding accuracy, we offer a description of the technique as taught to midwives in a leading midwifery school in the United States. We offer it here in hopes that those who are reluctant to accept the findings reported here will use this careful and methodical approach to digital assessment, with a healthy skepticism and an open mind to the very real possibility that their assessments will be wrong. They should maintain a willingness to question their findings and resort to trial and error if and when their corrective actions do not result in improved labor progress.

  Here is the step-by-step approach to digital assessment of position of the fetal skull:
  - The first step is to find the most easily palpated landmark—the sagittal suture. Some degree of asynclitism is normal as the head comes into the pelvic brim in early labor. But with a well-positioned head, throughout most of labor the sagittal suture is usually in the right or left oblique diameter and

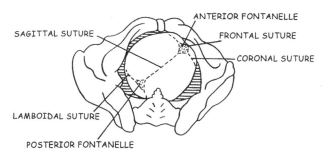

Fig. 3.17. Landmarks on the OP fetal head (sagittal suture in oblique diameter).

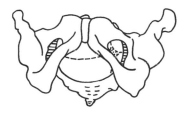

Fig. 3.18. Asynclitic fetus in occiput transverse.

roughly in the middle of the pelvis (Fig. 3.17). It may also be in a transverse diameter. During the second stage of labor when internal rotation normally occurs, it rotates 45 to 90 degrees to the anterior-posterior diameter of the pelvis.

If the sagittal suture in palpated just below the pubic arch, it indicates asynclitism (Fig. 3.18).

If the sagittal suture cannot be felt at all, there probably is significant asynclitism, usually posterior, with the posterior parietal bone (i.e., the parietal bone next to the woman's back) leading and the sagittal suture tucked under the symphysis pubis.

○ Next, the fontanelles are assessed by following the sagittal suture line in both directions from the midline. The posterior fontanelle is smaller and has three points. It does not actually feel like a triangular space as much as the joining of three

ture lines. The anterior fontanelle is much larger; it has four
ints and is shaped like a diamond. See Table 3.2, including
Figure 3.19, a–f.
o Even when it is not possible to accurately locate fontanelles,
   malposition can often be detected. It is important to notice
   whether the head fits more or less symmetrically. When the
   fetal head is malpositioned, it does not fill the pelvis. On

Table 3.2. Fetal positions viewed from below and from front of pelvis

Position	Vaginal view	Front view of fetus in pelvis
LOA	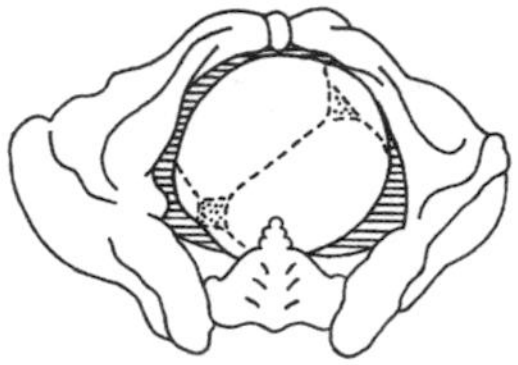 Fig. 3.19a	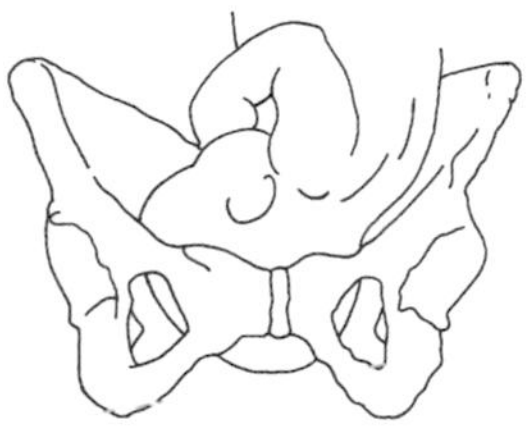 Fig. 3.19b
ROP	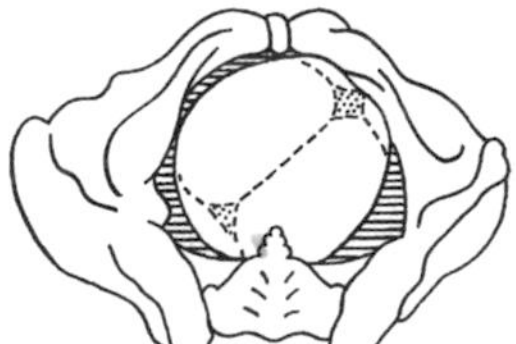 Fig. 3.19c	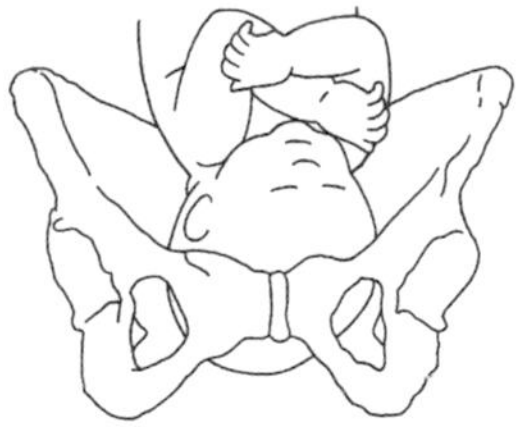 Fig. 3.19d
LOT	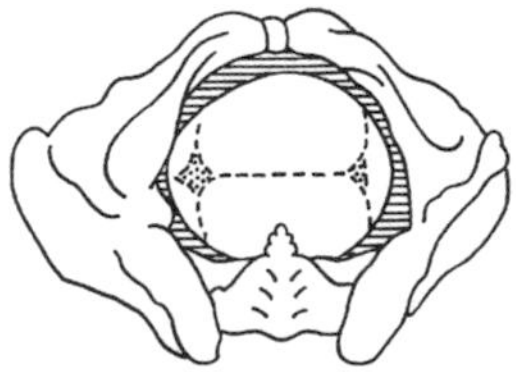 Fig. 3.19e	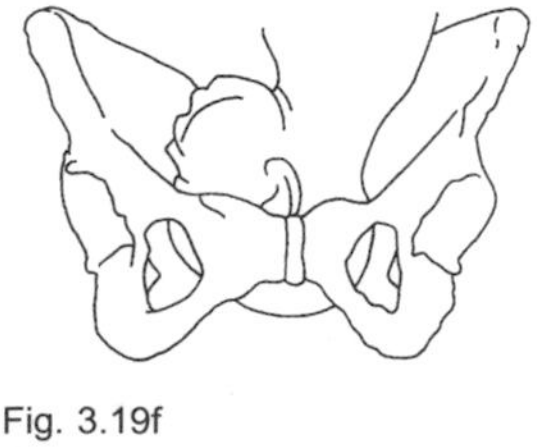 Fig. 3.19f

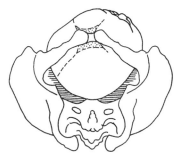

Fig. 3.20. Asynclitic fetus in ROP.

examination, the head feels tight in the front of the pelvis, as if it is sitting over the pubic symphysis, while there is room in the back of the pelvis (Fig. 3.20).

What is known about the accuracy of these digital examinations in labor? Simkin reviewed studies comparing digital assessments of fetal position with ultrasound assessments, concluding that digital assessment of position was often impossible, especially in the first stage.[29–31] In one study, digital assessment was accurate only 54% of the time when the occiput was posterior or lateral.[29] This research suggests that digital examination is useless for determining fetal position in labor and advocates for ultrasound as the "gold standard." However, Lieberman et al.[32] found that in about 10% of intrapartum ultrasound examinations, all performed by expert sonographers, the scans were "uninterpretable," raising the question of whether this technology, used by maternity care providers who are not ultrasound experts, would be as useful. Furthermore, are there care providers who *are* expert in digital assessment for fetal position? If so, can their skills be systematically evaluated and used to teach others to improve the accuracy of this lower-cost, less-invasive method? In the end, the 10% error rate found with the use of ultrasound is still far better than the error rates with digital assessment of fetal position, described above.

- Evaluating flexion of the fetal head: With a well-flexed head in the OA position, the small posterior fontanelle is palpable in the right or left oblique diameter of the pelvis while the anterior fontanelle is not. When a large fontanelle is easily palpated, the fetus is usually in a posterior, deflexed position.

Evaluating the presence of molding

Molding, the overlap of the bones of the head as a response to pressure during labor, permits the fetal head to better accommodate the tight fit through the maternal pelvis. Molding is often necessary for fetal descent. However, if excessive and occurring early in labor, molding may be a sign of difficulty.[33,34] Evaluating the degree of molding, together with the stage of labor, the station, estimated fetal size, and other variables, can aid in the assessment of dysfunctional labor. Molding obscures fontanelles and makes sutures feel more prominent.

Evaluating caput

Caput formation, the accumulation of fluid in the tissue of the scalp, is also a result of pressure on the fetal head. It normally occurs in second stage labor with active descent but may be present in the active phase of the first stage if the membranes have ruptured The finding of "caput formation" with a high station could actually represent an undiagnosed breech (soft and spongy) rather than caput! It might also signify OP position or disproportion. Extensive caput also makes assessment of position and station more difficult and is sometimes mistaken for descent. As the caput forms, the swelling expands lower in the pelvis, but the fetal head may not have descended at all.[33]

Evaluating the application of the head to the cervix

Is the head well applied to the cervix, or does the cervix feel like an "empty sleeve"? With a malpositioned head, it is common to find that the cervix is soft and stretchy but that, during contractions, the head does not press against it. This gives the impression of a poor fit, rather than a "rigid" cervix.

The vagina and bony pelvis

- Do the vaginal muscles feel soft and stretchy or tight and unyielding?

- Are there any obvious bony abnormalities (i.e., flat sacrum, short diagonal conjugate, prominent ischial spines, narrow pubic arch or rigid, prominent coccyx), or does the pelvis feel generally normal (i.e., exhibiting none of these abnormalities)?
- When all of these factors seem normal, it is reassuring to the care provider.

Quality of contractions

- Normal labor is characterized by uterine contractions that are involuntary and intermittent and that increase in frequency, duration, and intensity over time. A contraction can be visualized as a bell-shaped curve consisting of three phases: the *increment*, as the intensity builds; the *acme*, or peak; and the *decrement*, or relaxation as the intensity diminishes.

Normal coordination of the myometrium during labor causes the uterus to differentiate into a thick, muscular upper segment and a thinning, stretchy lower segment. *Retraction*, the continual shortening of the vertical muscle fibers, enables the uterus to decrease intrauterine space, thus opening the cervix and pushing the fetus down and out.

When labor is dysfunctional, it is important to evaluate uterine activity. Poor uterine activity can be a primary cause of dysfunctional labor, or it may be an effect of some other problem, such as a malpositioned fetus.[23] The expression "the uterus has a brain" aptly describes this interplay. When the fetus does not fit well through the pelvis, uterine contractions often diminish in response to this relative obstruction.[35]

The following features of contractions should be assessed:

- **Frequency** is measured from the start of one contraction to the start of the next. Some providers note this as the number of minutes from onset to onset, i.e., "q 5 minutes." Others record the number of contractions in a 10-minute period. Contractions of active labor are characterized by a frequency of two to five in 10 minutes. Concerns arise when contractions are more frequent than five contractions in 10 minutes (tachysystole). Because placental blood flow is markedly diminished during the most intense contractions of labor, a minimum rest of 30 seconds between

- **Mother's perception**. Because pain perception is highly variable from woman to woman, this alone is a poor indicator of contraction quality. However, the mother is able to report whether contractions are becoming more intense over time, a feature of normally progressing active phase labor. Dysfunctional labor may be characterized by contractions becoming less frequent, lasting less time, or feeling less intense.

ASSESSING THE MOTHER'S CONDITION

Trained clinicians assess many factors in a laboring woman's condition. This section addresses factors in the woman's condition that may influence labor progress. Progress may be positively or negatively affected by the degree to which the woman's physical and emotional well-being are attended to.

Hydration and nourishment

Chapter 2, page 34, provides a discussion of the adverse effects of dehydration during labor. Women in labor also require approximately 50 to 100 kcal/hr to maintain adequate muscle function.[38] Research literature firmly supports the free use of oral intake—both fluids and solids—during labor.[39] Given access, some women will naturally take in the necessary calories and nutrients to sustain them during labor, but some may need to be reminded. Prolonged labor may be both a cause and an effect of dehydration and insufficient caloric intake. Therefore, the caregiver should focus on prevention. Having non-acidic, easy-to-digest carbohydrate snacks and drinks available (broth, electrolyte-balanced sports drinks, fruit, honey, toast, etc.), offering beverages to the mother, and encouraging her to drink according to her thirst represent an effective strategy to prevent both hyponatremia (which may cause prolonged labor due to overhydration from forced oral fluids [see Chapter 5, page 150]) and maternal exhaustion caused by dehydration and poor caloric intake. Assessment of adequate hydration and nourishment includes:

- **Urine:** The laboring woman should void at least every 2 hours and produce urine that is light in color. Dark, concentrated, or scant urine suggests inadequate fluid intake.

- **Ketonuria:** Ketosis, the accumulation of ketones as a result of metabolizing stored fat in the absence of adequate carbohydrate availability, occurs normally in response to both exertion and fasting.[38] Controversy exists about whether the presence of ketone bodies in urine during labor is a sign of maternal compromise.[3,39]

- **Temperature:** A slight rise in temperature is normal during labor, but if elevated more than 0.5°C or 1°F and labor has been prolonged, it may signal dehydration. Significant increase in temperature (>38°C, 100.4°F), especially in the presence of ruptured membranes, may signal infection, a serious intrapartum complication.

- **Emesis:** Vomiting is common in labor. However, when it is prolonged or persistent, dehydration may result. Replacing fluids lost in this way requires additional intake, either oral or intravenous.

- **Fluid loss through perspiration:** Women laboring in warm conditions, especially those in warm water baths, need additional fluids. They should be reminded to drink to satisfy their thirst. Offering, but not pushing, liquids after each contraction or two is preferable to asking if she wants a drink.

- **Maternal distress:** Women who become seriously compromised due to inadequate intake may feel anxious, exhausted, and sick. Severe dehydration can exacerbate nausea and vomiting. Intravenous rehydration may be necessary.

Vital signs

During prolonged labor, maternal vital signs should be assessed at regular intervals between contractions. The presence of elevated blood pressure, pulse, or abnormal respiration rate must be noted and addressed. When maternal and fetal vital signs are normal, there is more leeway for patience.

Psychology

Much has been written about the *positive effects of confidence and wellbeing* and the *adverse effects of psychological distress* on the progress of labor.[40-46]

The mother's psychology works synergistically with the physical parameters of labor. Poor labor progress can be caused by psychological distress, and psychological distress can be a result of a long and difficult labor. When there are no apparent physical reasons for poor labor progress, a psychological source should be considered.

The caregiver's ability to communicate with the woman is essential. Establishing a trusting and supportive relationship provides the foundation for positive communication. This is easier when there has been a prenatal relationship, but many skilled intrapartum caregivers are able to establish good rapport quickly with women they have never met before.

The importance of minimizing psychological stress for laboring women, including information about creating a supportive labor environment, assessing a woman's emotional state, and building trust through good communication, is given in Chapter 2 and elsewhere in this text.

ASSESSING THE FETUS

Most of the time, the term fetus of the otherwise healthy woman tolerates prolonged or dysfunctional labor well. When the information about fetal well-being is reassuring, caregivers and parents can focus on the challenges of coping with and resolving the dysfunction. Injecting a bit of humorous reassurance ("Your baby is enjoying this labor more than you are!") reminds the mother who is working hard in her labor that she has a healthy fetus who is not becoming compromised.

Conversely, when signs of fetal compromise are present, attention to resolving the distress becomes paramount. Most parents are keenly aware of the potential for fetal compromise during labor and appreciate accurate information from caregivers when concern about the baby arises.

Elements of fetal assessment discussed here are the FHR, gestational age, and the presence or absence of meconium in the amniotic fluid.

Fetal heart rate

The primary source of information about fetal well-being during labor is the FHR and the fetus' response to contractions. For this reason, clinicians receive training and continuing education on interpreting FHR patterns according to the 2008 guidelines of the National Institute of Child Health and Human Development (NICHD).[47] The relative benefits and risks of continuous electronic fetal monitoring (CEFM) using external or internal instrumentation, versus intermittent auscultation (IA) using a fetoscope or hand-held Doppler, are summarized in Chapter 2.

This section provides an overview of both CEFM and IA. It is not meant to be a text on fetal surveillance, but rather, a learning tool for those who will use CEFM and/or want to restore the use of auscultation for healthy low-risk pregnant women.

IA is the method of fetal assessment used in home and free-standing birth center settings. In many hospitals, auscultation has been largely abandoned, although it is a reliable method of monitoring fetal well-being.[14] However, as mentioned in Chapter 2, telemetry can be employed, or the electronic fetal monitor can be used intermittently in order to promote mobility for hospitalized laboring women. The technique for IA is described here in detail.

Appropriate candidates for intermittent auscultation

- Healthy full term pregnancy[48] with the absence of medical or obstetric risk factors
- Absence of medical interventions such as oxytocin and/or epidural anesthesia[48]
- Presence of care provider(s) skilled in the use of IA

How to perform intermittent auscultation

A handheld Doppler device or a fetal stethoscope may be used. Ultrasound detects motion of the heart valves and converts this into a manufactured sound that replicates the fetal heartbeat. The fetal stethoscope is specially designed to use the bone conduction of the examiner's skull to transmit the subtle sounds of fetal cardiac activity through the ear pieces. It generally requires more practice than the Doppler to use correctly.

The Doppler offers these advantages:

- allows easier auscultation in a variety of maternal positions
- allows auscultation during contractions

- enables parents and others to hear the FHR
- does not require pressure on the woman's abdomen, so it is more comfortable
- can be adapted for use in water (requires special waterproof probe)
- compared to fetoscope, some studies showed improved neonatal outcome[48]

The fetal stethoscope (fetoscope) offers these advantages:

3

- detects true sounds of fetal heart, including dysrhythmias, avoiding risks of artifact or detecting maternal pulse in error
- provides no additional ultrasound exposure
- requires no battery or mechanical parts than can malfunction
- can also be used to help verify fetal position, as discussed earlier in this chapter

The following guideline is derived from published IA guidelines of the American College of Nurse-Midwives,[49] Association of Women's Health, Obstetric and Neonatal Nurses,[50] and Society of Obstetricians and Gynecologists of Canada.[48] These organizations publish updated guidelines periodically.[51]

General principles of IA

- **Frequency of auscultation:** There is limited evidence concerning recommendation for the frequency of IA during the latent phase of labor. However, it is prudent to monitor the fetus at the time of assessments, approximately every hour during latent labor.[48] During active first stage labor, IA should be accomplished every 15 to 30 minutes[49,51] and every 5 minutes with active bearing down during the second stage.[49,51] If an abnormality is detected, more frequent auscultation should be performed.

- **Timing of auscultation:** Contractions should be palpated, and auscultation should be done between contractions, counting the FHR for 60 seconds.[48]

- **Method of counting:** Counting the FHR for a full 60 seconds provides the most accurate rate.[46] While auscultating for 30 seconds may be easier during active labor, it is not considered Au reliable.[48] The maternal pulse should be evaluated periodically to ensure that the rate that is being counted is fetal and not maternal. This distinction should be documented in the woman's medical record.

Intermittent auscultation technique[49]

- Use Leopold's maneuvers to locate the fetal back, the point of maximal ability to auscultate the FHR.
- Palpate for contractions.
- Palpate the maternal pulse.
- Place the fetal stethoscope or Doppler over the fetal back.
- Determine the FHR baseline by listening for 60 seconds between contractions.
- Record findings including any accelerations or decelerations.

Reassuring signs of fetal well-being that can be assessed without CEFM

- normal baseline FHR
- absence of decelerations
- absence of FHR arrhythmia
- accelerations of the FHR with or without fetal scalp or vibro-acoustical stimulation[50]
- fetal movement reported by the woman or palpated by the examiner
- clear amniotic fluid

When using continuous electronic fetal monitoring

When using CEFM, it is critical to establish and maintain vigilance that it is the FHR, not the mother's that is being recorded on the tracing.[52] In 2008, the NICHD published revised guidelines that provide "specific recommendation for FHR pattern classification and intrapartum management actions."[47,p661] A major change is the new "three-tiered fetal heart rate interpretation system"[47,p664] that will allow more standardized interpretation of fetal status during labor as well as recommendations for interventions. The following are the NICHD definitions of these components of FHR interpretation.

While the NICHD guidelines are specific to CEFM, the definitions also apply to IA,

Baseline FHR definitions:

- Normal FHR baseline rate is 110 to 160 beats per minute (bpm).
- Tachycardia is a baseline rate that exceeds 160 bpm.
- Bradycardia is a baseline rate that is less than 110 bpm.

3

Variability defined:

- Defined as "fluctuations in the baseline FHR that are irregular in amplitude and frequency."[47,p663] This can only be assessed with CEFM, not through the use of IA.[48]
- Classifications of variability[47]
  - ○ Absent: No variability detectible
  - ○ Minimal: less than 5 bpm
  - ○ Moderate: 6 to 25 bpm
  - ○ Marked: greater than 25 bpm

Accelerations defined:

- According to the NICHD guidelines, an acceleration is a visually apparent abrupt increase in FHR of 15 or more beats for 15 seconds or longer.[47] In the preterm fetus (<32 weeks' gestation), accelerations are defined as 10 or more beats for 10 seconds or longer.[47]
- Accelerations are considered a sign of fetal well-being.
- To determine the presence of accelerations, the FHR can be counted for segments of 5 to 15-second duration. The rates between the segments can be compared for the presence of an increase that would indicate an acceleration.[49] Accelerations can and should be listened for and documented during IA.

Decelerations defined:

- Decelerations are periodic changes in the FHR that fall below the baseline and are defined by their onset, timing, and shape on the

CEFM tracing. The types of decelerations are not well-distinguished by the use of IA.

- *Early decelerations* are considered a normal finding during labor. They are symmetrical, gradual declines in FHR with the lowest point of the deceleration occurring >30 seconds from onset of the contraction.[47] The onset and recovery to baseline are both early compared to the start and end of the contraction. Early decelerations mirror the shape of the contraction. Early decelerations are associated with compression of the fetal head that leads to vagal nerve stimulation. Therefore, early decelerations are most common in late active and second stage labor.

- *Variable decelerations* are irregularly shaped and irregularly timed abrupt decelerations with the lowest point of the deceleration occurring less than 30 seconds from the onset of the contraction. Variable decelerations indicate mechanical compression of the umbilical cord that may lead to fetal compromise. Changing the mother's position often reduces pressure on the umbilical cord and is the first step in appropriate care. The significance of variable decelerations depends of the entire context of the CEFM tracing according to the three-tiered categorization system.[47]

- *Late decelerations* are gradual uniform declines in the FHR with the lowest point of the deceleration occurring more than 30 seconds from the onset of the contraction.[47] A defining characteristic is their timing, because they occur *late* in the contraction and return to baseline *following* the end of the contraction. They are considered an indication of potential uteroplacental insufficiency (diminished blood and oxygen flow to the baby). The significance of late decelerations depends of the entire context of the CEFM tracing according to the three-tiered categorization system.[47]

The three-tiered fetal heart rate interpretation system

- The three-tiered FHR interpretation system is described in Table 3.3.
- It is incumbent on care providers to have skill in using this system for assessment and documentation of fetal status.

Table 3.3. Three-tiered fetal heart rate (FHR) interpretation system

Features	Implications
Category I	
Baseline: 110–160 bpm Baseline FHR variability (BLV): moderate Accelerations: present or absent Decelerations • Early decelerations: present or absent • Late or variable decelerations: absent	• Normal • Strongly predictive of normal fetal acid-base status at the time of observation • No specific action is required.
Category II *[These include all FHR tracings that are not Category I or III. Examples below]*	
Baseline variability • Minimal variability • Absent variability not accompanied by recurrent decelerations • Marked variability Accelerations • Absence of induced accelerations after fetal stimulation: Periodic or episodic decelerations • Recurrent variable decelerations with minimal or moderate BLV • Prolonged deceleration (≥2 minutes but <10 minutes) • Recurrent late decelerations with moderate BLV • Variable decelerations with other characteristics, such as slow return to baseline, "overshoots," or "shoulders"	• Indeterminate • Not predictive of abnormal fetal acid-base status • Requires evaluation, continued surveillance, and reevaluation • Take into account the entire associated clinical circumstance

Table 3.3.   (continued)

Features	Implications
Category III	

Baseline variability: Absent BLV AND Any of the following:
• Decelerations
 	
   o Recurrent late decelerations
   o Recurrent variable decelerations
 	
• Bradycardia
• Sinusoidal pattern
 	
   o Smooth, sine wave–like, undulating pattern of the FHR baseline
   o of regular frequency of 3–5 cycles per minute
   o that persists for ≥20 minutes
	• Predicts abnormal fetal acid-base status
	• Requires prompt evaluation
	• Warrants efforts to expeditiously resolve the abnormal FHR pattern including but not limited to intrauterine resuscitation:
	
	   o Provide maternal oxygen
	   o Change maternal position
	   o Discontinue labor stimulation
	   o Treat hypotension

Based on Macones GA, Hankins GDV, Spong CY, et al. (2008). The 2008 National Institute of Child Health and Human Development Workshop Report on Electronic Fetal Monitoring: Update on Definitions, Interpretation, and Research Guidelines. J Obstet Gynecol Neonat Nurs 37(5), 510–515. Reprinted with permission.

Here is a brief overview of gestational age, meconium, and indications for consultation.

• **Gestational age:** Both preterm (<37 completed weeks) and post-term (>42 completed weeks) fetuses are more vulnerable to the stress of labor.

With premature fetuses:

   o Decelerations of the FHR are more ominous.
   o Additional risk to the fetus may be related to the etiology of the preterm labor (i.e., infection or placental abruption).

With post-term fetuses:

- o   There are increased risks of oligohydramnios, meconium passage, meconium aspiration syndrome, and cord compression.[19] There is an increased likelihood of macrosomia, with its attendant labor risks (cephalopelvic disproportion and malposition).[13]
- o   Some studies have also found a positive association between postdates and shoulder dystocia. Other studies have not confirmed this association, except when there is macrosomia.[53]
- o   There is increased risk for placental insufficiency, resulting in growth restriction and higher rates of stillbirth.

- **Meconium:** The fetus may pass meconium in utero when there is a brief episode of hypoxia that causes relaxation of the anal sphincter. Meconium in the amniotic fluid during labor may indicate a compromise in fetal oxygenation. However, it is more often a normal maturational event, occurring more frequently as gestational age reaches and exceeds 40 weeks, and in 35% to 50% of all post-term pregnancies.[19]

  Meconium should be considered a sign of fetal compromise if it is:

  - o   associated with a nonreassuring FHR pattern
  - o   associated with maternal fever or other signs of infection
  - o   thick, dark colored, or particulate (containing discrete pieces or chunks)

- **Consultation:** Midwives who attend births in out-of-hospital settings (home and birth centers) consider the following fetal conditions to be indications for intrapartum consultation and/or transfer to a hospital[54–58]:
  - o   nonreassuring FHR assessment
  - o   gestational age less than 37 weeks
  - o   gestational age greater than 42 weeks
  - o   significant (dark, thick, or particulate) meconium in the amniotic fluid

PUTTING IT ALL TOGETHER

Assessing progress in the first stage

As discussed in Chapter 2, clinicians and researchers use a variety of definitions of normal labor progress. In Chapter 4, we discuss some distinctions between prelabor and latent phase contraction. *prelabor* characterized by contractions that do not change in qu. or change the cervix over time. The *latent phase* is characterized by persistent contractions that do effect change, albeit slow and sometimes subtle. *Active phase* is defined as the time when contractions are more intense and frequent and the rate of change becomes more accelerated. With this is mind, different criteria should be used to assess labor progress for latent phase than for active phase.

- **Features of normal latent phase**

  - The cervix softens and effaces slowly but progressively.
  - Fetal station may or may not change.
  - Dilation is slow, up to 4 to 5 cm.[59]
  - Contractions may be regular or irregular, with varying frequency and duration, but are usually mild to moderate in intensity.
  - Normal duration is up to 20 to 24 hours. This is the longest phase of labor for most nulliparas.[60] The woman may be distractible during contractions and carry on "normal" activities between contractions.
  - Mother does not become exhausted.

- **Features of normal active phase**

  - Cervical effacement becomes complete, later in multiparas than in nulliparas.
  - The rate of cervical change increases over time, although progress may not be uniform from hour to hour.
  - Dilation progresses over time to full dilation, but the rate of dilation varies tremendously between women.
  - The fetal head engages, particularly in the nullipara.
  - The fetal head descends to lower stations, especially toward the completion of first stage.
  - The woman's behavior becomes serious and focused, both during and between contractions. Her coping behaviors may become more dramatic.
  - If there is back pain, the place that hurts moves downward over time.
  - Normal symptoms during rapid dilation may include an increase in bloody show, nausea, vomiting, shaking, irritability, anger, or feelings of desperation.

3

○ This phase lasts longer for nulliparas than for multiparas.

○ The upper limits of normal duration vary from author to author (see Chapter 5).

○ Mother and fetus fare well with the work of labor.

Assessing progress in the second stage

There is often a latent phase after full dilation and before the fetus descends enough to trigger a pushing urge (see Chapter 6). If the active phase of second stage is defined to include full dilation *and spontaneous active pushing efforts,* active second stage progress is assessed by linear descent of the head and concludes with the birth of the baby.

• **Features of normal second stage**

○ The mother has spontaneous pushing urges (unless she has regional anesthesia).

○ Contractions increase or remain strong and intense, though they may be shorter or less frequent than those in late first stage.

○ The fetal head may rotate, mold, and form a caput.

○ All of the mechanisms of labor are accomplished: descent, flexion, internal rotation, birth of the head, restitution, external rotation, and birth of the shoulders and body of the fetus.

○ Upper limits of normal duration vary but are longer for nulliparas than for multiparas.

○ The mother and the fetus fare well with pushing.

CONCLUSION

This chapter has covered methods of assessment of mother and fetus that are relevant to diagnosis and management of dystocia. These techniques enable the clinical care provider not only to identify dystocia but also its specific etiology.

REFERENCES

1. Blasi I, D'Amico R, Fenu V, et al. (2010). Sonographic assessment of fetal spine and head position during the first and second stages of labor for

the diagnosis of persistent occiput posterior position: A pilot study. Ultrasound Obstet Gynecol 35(2), 210–215.

2. Simkin P. (2010). The fetal occiput posterior position: State of the science and a new perspective. Birth 37(1), 61–71.

3. Varney H. (2003). Varney's Midwifery, 4th edition. Boston, MA, Jones & Bartlett.

4. Peregrine E, O'Brien P, Jauniaux E. (2007). Impact on delivery outcome of ultrasonographic fetal head position prior to induction of labor. Obstet Gynecol 109(3):618–624.

5. McFarlin B, Engstrom J. (1985). Concurrent validity of Leopold's maneuvers in determining fetal presentation and position. J Nurs-Midwif 30(5), 280–284.

6. Sharma J. (2009). Evaluation of Sharma's modified Leopold's maneuvers: A new method for fetal palpation in late pregnancy. Arch Gynecol Obstet 279:481–487.

7. Andrews C, Andrews E. (1983). Nursing, maternal postures, and fetal position. Nurs Res 32(6), 336–341.

8. Karaminia A, Chamberlain ME, Keogh J, Shea A. (2004). Randomised controlled trial of effect of hands and knees posturing on incidence of occiput posterior position at birth. BMJ 328, 490–493.

9. Sutton J. (2001) Let Birth Be Born Again: Rediscovering and Reclaiming Our Midwifery Heritage. London, UK, Birth Concepts.

10. Scott P. (2003) Sit Up and Take Notice: Positioning Yourself for a Better Birth. Tauranga, New Zealand, Great Scott Publications.

11. Gregory K, Henry O, Ramacone E, et al. (1998). Maternal and infant complications in high and normal weight infants by method of delivery. Obstet Gynecol 92(4 pt 1), 503–513.

12. American College of Obstetricians and Gynecologists. (2003). Dystocia and the augmentation of labor. In ACOG Practice Bulletin No. 45. Washington, DC, Author.

13. American College of Obstetricians and Gynecologists. (2000). Fetal macrosomia. In ACOG Practice Bulletin No. 22. Washington, DC, Author.

14. Enkin M, Neilson MK, Crowther J, et al. (2000). A Guide to Effective Care in Pregnancy and Childbirth, 3rd edition. Oxford, Oxford University Press.

15. Baum J, Gussman D, Wirth J. (2002). Clinical and patient estimation of fetal weight vs. ultrasound estimation. J Reprod Med 47(3), 194–198.

16. Nahum G. (2002). Predicting fetal weight: Are Leopold's maneuvers still worth teaching medical students and house staff? J Reprod Med 47(4), 752–760.

17. Levine A, Lockwood C, Brown B, et al. (1992). Sonographic diagnosis of the large for gestational age fetus at term: Does it make a difference? Obstet Gynecol 79(1), 55–58.

18. Nahum G, Stanislaw H. (2002). Validation of a birth weight prediction equation based on maternal characteristics. J Reprod Med 47(9), 752–760.

19. Gabbe S, Niebyl J, Simpson J. (2002). Obstetrics: Normal and Abnormal Pregnancies. Edinburgh, Churchill Livingstone.

20. Olah K, Gee H. (1992). The prevention of preterm delivery: Can we afford to continue to ignore the cervix? Br J Obstet Gynecol 99(4), 278–280.

21. Olah K, Gee H, Brown J. (1993). Cervical contractions: The response of the cervix to oxytocic stimulation in the latent phase of labour. Br J Obstet Gynaecol 100(7), 635–640.

22. Granstrom L, Ekman G, Malmstrom A. (1991). Insufficient remodelling of the uterine connective tissue in women with protracted labour. Br J Obstet Gynecol 98(12), 1212–1216.

23. Bishop E. (1964). Pelvic scoring for elective induction. Obstet Gynecol 24(2), 266–268.

24. Peisner D, Rossen M. (1985). Latent phase of labor in normal patients: A reassessment. Obstet Gynecol 66(5), 644–648.

25. Neumann Y. (2004). Doing a pelvic exam with a woman who has experienced sexual abuse, Chapter 12. In Simkin P, Klaus P, editors. When Survivors Give Birth. Seattle, Classic Day Publishing.

26. Holcomb W, Smeltzer J. (1991). Cervical effacement: Variation in belief among clinicians. Obstet Gynecol 78(1), 43–45.

27. Publication Department of Reproductive Health and Research. (2003). Managing Complications in Pregnancy and Childbirth: A Guide for Midwives and Doctors. Geneva, World Health Organization, p 82.

28. Flint C. (1986). Sensitive Midwifery. Oxford, Heinemann Nursing.

29. Akmal S, Kametas N, Tsoi E, et al. (2003). Comparison of transvaginal digital examination with intrapartum sonography to determine fetal head position before instrumental delivery. Ultrasound Obstet Gynecol 21(5), 437–440.

30. Sherer D, Miodovnik M, Bradley K, Langer O. (2002). Intrapartum fetal head position, II: Comparison between transvaginal digital examination and transabdominal ultrasound assessment during the second stage of labor. Ultrasound Obstet Gynecol 19, 264–268.

31. Nizard J, Haberman S, Paltieli Y, et al. (2009). Determination of fetal head station and position during labor: A new technique that combines

ultrasound and position-tracking system. Am J Obstet Gynecol 200, 404.e1–404.e5.

32. Lieberman E, Davidson K, Lee-Parritz A, Shearer E. (2005). Changes in fetal position during labor and their association with epidural analgesia. Obstet Gynecol 105(5 pt 1), 974–982.

33. Oxorn H. (1986). Human Labor and Birth, 5th edition. New York, McGraw-Hill.

34. Bennett V, Brown L, editors. (1999). Myles Textbook for Midwives, 13th edition. London, Churchill Livingstone.

35. Neilson J, Lavender T, Quenby S, Wray S. (2003). Obstructed labour. Br Med Bull 67, 191–204.

36. Crane J, Young D, Butt K, et al. (2001). Excessive uterine activity accompanying induced labor. Obstet Gynecol 97(6), 926–931.

37. Whitely N. (1975). Uterine contractile physiology: Applications in nursing care and patient teaching. J Obstet Gynecol Neonat Nurs 4(5), 54–58.

38. Sinclair C. (2004). A Midwives' Handbook. St. Louis, Saunders.

39. Ludka L, Roberts C. (1993). Eating and drinking in labor: A literature review. J Nurs-Midwif 38(4), 199–207.

40. Odent M. (1992). The Nature of Birth and Breastfeeding. Westport, CT, Bergin & Garvey.

41. Odent M. (1999). Birth reborn, Chapter 6. In The Scientification of Love. London, Free Association Books.

42. Lederman R, Lederman E, Work B, McCann D. (1979). Relationship of psychological factors in pregnancy to progress in labor. Nurs Res 28(2), 94–97.

43. Lederman E, Lederman R, Work B, McCann D. (1981). Maternal psychological and physiologic correlates of fetal-newborn health status. Am J Obstet Gynecol 139(8), 956–960.

44. Wuitchik M, Bakal D, Lipshitz J. (1989). The clinical significance of pain and cognitive activity in latent labor. Obstet Gynecol 73(1), 35–42.

45. Simkin P. (2002). Supportive care during labor: A guide for busy nurses. JOGNN, 31(6), 721–732.

46. Simkin P, Klaus P. (2004). When Survivors Give Birth: Understanding and Healing the Effects of Early Sexual Abuse on Childbearing Women. Seattle, Classic Day Publishing.

47. Macones GA, Hankins GDV, Spong CY, et al. (2008) The 2008 National Institute of Child Health and Human Development Workshop Report on Electronic Fetal Monitoring: Update on definitions, interpretation, and research guidelines. J Obstet Gynecol Neonat Nurs 37(5), 510–515.

48. Liston R, Sawchuck D, Young D, SOGC Fetal Health Surveillance Working Group. (2007). Fetal health surveillance: Antepartum and intrapartum consensus guideline. J Obstet Gynaecol Can 29(9), S2–S56.

49. American College of Nurse-Midwives. (2007). Intermittent auscultation for intrapartum fetal heart rate surveillance. J Midwif Womens Health 52(3), 314–319. ACNM Clinical Bulletin No. 9.

50. Paine L, Johnson T, Turner M, Payton R. (1986). Auscultated fetal heart rate accelerations, Part II. An alternative to the non-stress test. J Nurs Midwif 31(2), 73–77.

51. Association of Women's Health, Obstetric and Neonatal Nurses. (2009). Fetal Heart Monitoring Principles and Practices, 4th edition. Dubuque, IA, Kendall/Hunt.

52. Hanson L. (2010). Risk Management in intrapartum fetal monitoring: Accidental recording of the maternal heart rate. J Perinat Neonat Nurs 24, 7–9.

53. Lewis D, Edwards M, Asrat T, et al. (1998). Can shoulder dystocia be predicted? J Reprod Med 43(8), 654–658.

54. College of Midwives of British Columbia. (1997). Standards of Practice and Indications for Discussion, Consultation and Transfer of Care. Vancouver, BC, College of Midwives of British Columbia.

55. National Health Insurance Board of the Netherlands. (2000). Final Report of the Obstetric Working Group of the National Health Insurance Board of the Netherlands. In Obstetric Manual: National Health Insurance Board of the Netherlands. Diemen, the Netherlands.

56. Midwives Association of Washington State. (2002). Indications for Consultations in an Out-of-Hospital Midwifery Practice. Seattle, Author.

57. Tennessee Midwives' Association. (2001). Practice Guidelines. Memphis, TN, Author.

58. Massachusetts Midwives Alliance. (1998). Transfer Criteria. Stoneham, MA, Author.

59. Zhang J, Troendle J, Yancey M. (2002). Reassessing the labor curve in nulliparous women. Am J Obstet Gynecol 187(4), 824–828.

60. Friedman E. (1978). Normal labor. In Labor: Clinical Evaluation and Management, 2nd edition. New York, Appleton-Century-Crofts.

Chapter 4

Prolonged Prelabor and Latent First Stage

Penny Simkin, BA, PT, CCE, CD(DONA), and
Ruth Ancheta, BA, ICCE, CD(DONA)

Is it dystocia? 101
When is a woman in labor? 102
Can prenatal measures prevent the fetal occiput position during labor? 103
The woman who has hours of contractions without dilation, 106
The six ways to progress in labor, 108
Support measures for women who are at home in prelabor and the latent phase, 109
Some reasons for excessive pain and duration of prelabor or the latent phase, 111
Iatrogenic factors, 111
Cervical factors, 111
Fetal factors, 112
Emotional factors, 112
Troubleshooting measures for painful prolonged prelabor or latent phase, 113
Measures to alleviate painful, nonprogressing, nondilating contractions in prelabor or the latent phase, 115
Synclitism and asynclitism, 116
Conclusion, 121
References, 121

4

IS IT DYSTOCIA?

A diagnosis of dystocia is usually based on the rate of labor progress, which, as one might expect, would depend on the time of the onset of labor. Ironically, diagnosing the onset of labor, as fundamental as it may seem, is not easy, and wide disagreement exists among experts on how to decide when labor begins.

The Labor Progress Handbook: Early Interventions to Prevent and Treat Dystocia.
Edited by Penny Simkin, Ruth Ancheta
© 2011 by Penny Simkin and Ruth Ancheta; illustrations copyright Ruth Ancheta

When is a woman in labor?

Two obstetricians whose teachings have dominated Western obstetrics for half a century represent the extremes of opinion regarding the definition of *labor*. Emmanuel Friedman defined *labor* as follows:

> The onset of labor is defined simply as that time at which the patient first perceived regular uterine contractions. There is no way to distinguish true labor from false except by hindsight (when the contractions cease or when active dilation begins).[1]

This definition is still used today.[2,3] At the other end of the spectrum, Kieran O'Driscoll, master obstetrician at the National Maternity Hospital in Ireland in the 1960s and 1970s, introduced, and his successors to this day have continued to use, a very precise definition of *labor*: painful contractions occurring at least every 10 minutes or closer, accompanied by at least one of the following: bloody mucous vaginal discharge; spontaneous rupture of the membranes; or complete cervical effacement.[4] A woman may have regular painful uterine contractions for many hours or even days before meeting O'Driscoll's criteria for labor. These widely varying definitions of *labor* result in different management styles. According to Friedman, the latent phase in nulliparas averages 9 hours and is considered "prolonged" at 20 hours. O'Driscoll and colleagues would deny that a woman in Friedman's "latent phase" is even in labor unless she exhibits one of the other signs or symptoms mentioned earlier. Friedman suggested drug-induced rest for women with a prolonged latent phase, whereas O'Driscoll and colleagues do not admit her to the labor ward or acknowledge any clinical significance to these contractions, regardless of what the women feel and think.

In this book, our definition of *labor* is based on distinguishing between progressing and nonprogressing contractions. Progressing contractions increase over time in one or more of the following measures: intensity, duration, and frequency. Nonprogressing contractions remain the same over time. We define *prelabor* as a period of regular, nonprogressing contractions, without an increase in cervical dilation, which may or may not continue without interruption into the latent phase. We define the *latent phase* of labor as the period beginning with continuous progressing contractions accompanied by cervical effacement and dilation and ending at 4 to 5 cm.[5] When the onset of labor is spontaneous, the woman or her partner is the informant regarding the time of onset. They should be taught to time her contractions with watch, pencil, and paper or by using one of the online contraction recording systems and to differentiate between progressing and nonprogressing contractions.

Use of a definition of *labor* based on more specific characteristics than Friedman's "regular contractions" recognizes that "false," or prelabor, contractions can be differentiated from true labor as they occur, not only in retrospect. This may aid the caregiver as he or she considers management options. It is important to recognize that from the woman's point of view, continuing contractions must be dealt with, whether or not they are becoming more frequent, intense, or longer, or are accompanied by bloody show or ruptured membranes. Prelabor must not be discounted; nor, however, should it be treated as labor.

4

Can prenatal measures prevent the fetal occiput posterior position during labor?

Chapter 3 describes methods used to assess fetal position before labor. If an occiput posterior (OP) position is diagnosed before labor, what, if anything, can be done to facilitate rotation to an occiput transverse (OT) or occiput anterior (OA) position? What can be done to maintain the OA position once it is achieved? First, spontaneous rotation, without intervention, occurs in most labors, although this rotation may often be accompanied by greater discomfort and prolonged labor. One study found that 87% of fetuses who were OP at the onset of labor rotated to OA by delivery; but 68% of fetuses who were OP at delivery had been OA at the onset of labor and rotated to OP during labor.[6] In other words, of 100 fetuses, 20 are OP at the onset of labor, but only 2 of those would still be OP at delivery. The other 3 fetuses who are OP at delivery would have begun labor in the OA position.

Factors that cause rotation from OA to OP during labor may include the shape and size of both the fetal head and maternal pelvis but also maternal position during labor.[7–9] Other factors, such as the use of epidural analgesia and the woman's bearing-down efforts, are discussed in Chapters 5 and 6.

The concept of "optimal fetal positioning" (OFP), originally described by Sutton and Scott,[7–9] refers to maternal positions that can be used during the final weeks of pregnancy to improve the likelihood of the fetus being in the left OA or transverse (LOA or LOT) position at the onset of labor, which are considered optimal for comfort and progress during labor. (OFP also includes intrapartum techniques to encourage or maintain an LOA position during labor. These will be discussed in Chapter 5.)

Sutton and Scott advocate that the woman spend very little time during late pregnancy in supine or semireclining positions, as these encourage an OP fetal position. They recommend that she spend most of her time in forward-leaning, vertical, and lateral positions, such as those seen in Figure 4.1. Sutton and Scott state that such postures use gravity to increase the space at the pelvic brim, within the pelvis, and at the outlet.

They advocate exercise, such as walking, swimming in a prone position, and yoga, while discouraging prenatal squatting and long car trips sitting in a bucket seat. These low-risk but rather extensive lifestyle changes are widely practiced in hopes of averting one of the most troublesome deterrents to normal progress and vaginal birth.

Although Sutton and Scott's prenatal recommendations are widely practiced, they have not been adequately studied for their effectiveness in achieving an OA fetal position before labor. Only two studies have examined the effectiveness of the prenatal use of the hands-and-knees position.[10,11]

In one study including 100 women with OP or OT fetal positions, the use of one or two 10-minute periods in a hands-and-knees position with or without pelvic rocking, abdominal stroking, or both was more likely to result in an OA fetal position immediately after the intervention compared to a sitting position. There was no follow-up on whether the fetuses remained in the OA position after the study period.[10] The other study, a randomized controlled trial, included 2547 women with unknown fetal positions. It compared the incidence of OP position at birth in two groups of women: the experimental group, who, beginning at 37 weeks' gestation, spent two 10-minute periods per day in a hands-and-knees position combined with pelvic rocking, and the control group, who took a daily walk. They found no differences between groups in the incidence of OP at birth.[11]

Lieberman and others[12] discovered that the fetus changes position frequently during labor. Using ultrasound, they assessed fetal position three times while the woman was in labor and visually assessed the position at birth. Fetal position changes were common: 80% of

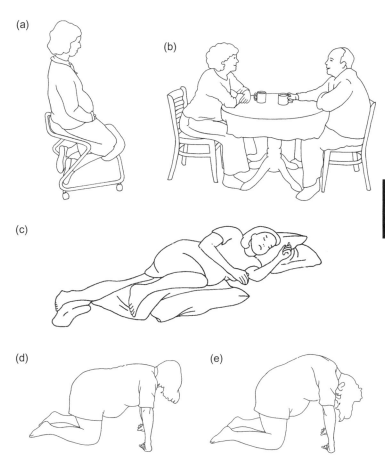

Fig. 4.1 Helpful positions for later pregnancy: (**a**) sitting straight; (**b**) sitting leaning forward; (**c**) semiprone on left side; (**d, e**) doing the pelvic rocking exercise ("cat-cow" in yoga).

the fetuses who were OP at 8-cm dilation rotated to OA or OT at delivery, and of those who were OA at 8 cm, 5.4% rotated to OP by delivery.

The authors did not mention the use of any low-technology interventions to rotate the OP fetuses.

Lieberman et al.'s study,[12] along with those mentioned earlier,[6,13–15] demonstrate that fetal position at the onset of labor does not predict fetal position at birth. It seems unlikely, therefore, that prenatal attempts to ensure an OA or OT position at the onset of labor, even if successful, will improve the likelihood of an OA position at birth.[16]

In Chapter 5, we examine studies of intrapartum measures to attain or maintain an OA position during labor.

The woman who has hours of contractions without dilation

Sometimes it takes many hours, even days, of contractions before a woman's cervix dilates to 4 or 5 cm. To a great extent, the duration of prelabor (sometimes referred to as "false labor") or of latent first stage depends on the state of her cervix at the onset of contractions. The more unripe, uneffaced, and posterior a woman's cervix is, the greater the likelihood that her prelabor or latent phase will last longer than it would with a more favorable cervix.

Although there is disagreement on definitions of the *onset* of labor, most authors of obstetric and midwifery textbooks and practice guidelines agree that very little should be done to try to speed either prelabor or the latent phase in the absence of medical problems requiring imminent delivery.[1,4,17–21] Because most slow-starting labors eventually resolve into normal labor patterns, a diagnosis of dystocia or dysfunctional labor cannot accurately be made before the active phase[20] (i.e., in a nullipara before 4 to 5 cm dilated and nearly 100% effaced; in a multipara, before 4 to 5 cm dilated and 70% to 80% effaced). Special supportive measures, in addition to those listed in Chapter 1, may be needed to help the woman through the time it takes for her cervix to change. Chart 4.1 illustrates a step-by-step approach to the problem of a prolonged prelabor or latent phase. Some of these same supportive measures apply when a woman is undergoing cervical ripening and induction of labor, which may take place over several days.

In this section we suggest ways to assess and meet the woman's support needs during a prolonged prelabor or latent phase, especially when she describes or appears to have more pain than women usually report at this degree of cervical dilation.

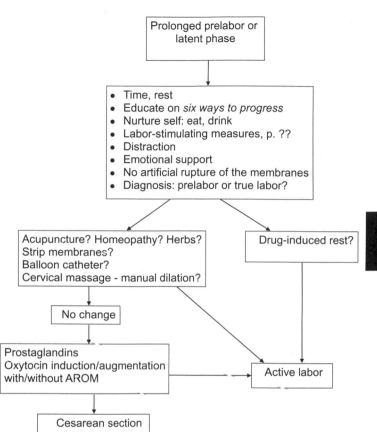

Chart 4.1 Prolonged prelabor or latent phase.

WAYS TO PROGRESS IN LABOR

Contractions without dilation are discouraging to the woman, who believes she is not making progress. She needs to understand that significant dilation can occur only when the cervix has already undergone preparatory changes. The caregiver should explain the reasons for predilation (prelabor) contractions in the context of the *Six Ways to Progress*. Although health care providers know these six ways, they often ignore the fact that when the cervix has not undergone the first three steps (ripening, effacement, and anterior movement), significant dilation (beyond 4 cm in the nullipara, more in the multipara) rarely occurs. There is a tendency among caregivers to minimize the importance of these three cervical changes when, in fact, progress in those areas is a very good sign and a necessary precursor to dilation. If such progress is ignored, an incorrect diagnosis of dysfunctional labor may be made before the woman is even in labor!

The following six steps must be accomplished for a baby to be born vaginally. For most women, the first three steps take place gradually, simultaneously, and almost unnoticed over a period of weeks before labor begins. For a minority of women, however, hours or days of nonprogressing prelabor contractions are necessary to prepare the cervix for dilation. Sometimes these contractions are intense enough to prevent sleep, and the woman becomes discouraged and exhausted.

Here are the six ways to progress:

1. The cervix moves from a posterior to an anterior position.
2. The cervix ripens or softens.
3. The cervix effaces.
4. The cervix dilates.
5. The fetal head rotates, flexes, and molds.
6. The fetus descends, rotates further, and is born.

If the woman's cervix is not yet dilating, even though she is having contractions, she will need reassurance and education from her caregiver that these prelabor contractions are accomplishing the important job of preparing her cervix to dilate. She is making necessary progress. Before dilation begins, support measures should focus on educating the woman about the six ways to progress, encouraging her to engage in distracting activities, helping her to accept the slow progress of early labor as a normal variation, preventing exhaustion, meeting her nutritional needs, and keeping her comfortable.

Rotation, flexion, molding, and descent of the fetal head take place in active labor and second stage. These will be discussed in Chapters 5 and 6.

SUPPORT MEASURES FOR WOMEN WHO ARE AT HOME IN PRELABOR AND THE LATENT PHASE

While most women remain at home during this phase, some will come to the hospital and some will call for telephone advice. It helps if they have been taught in advance or given a list of ways to cope with early labor. In the absence of medical contraindications, these suggestions will help the woman maintain normal progress and confidence:

- She should continue normal activities—restful activities (even if she cannot sleep) at night, pleasant distracting activities during the day—for as long as possible, while avoiding overexertion.
- She should have her partner, a friend, a relative, or a doula remain with her.
- If it is nighttime and the woman can rest, she should lie down or relax in the bathtub. (*Please note:* Immersion in water in early labor may temporarily stop contractions and give the woman some rest.[22-26] This is an advantage if she needs rest but may be a disadvantage if conditions exist that make it important that her labor progresses, e.g., prolonged pregnancy or prolonged rupture of membranes.)
- If she is unable to rest, or it is daytime, she should try distraction measures, such as:
  - going for a walk or having someone take her for a drive
  - visiting with friends or family
  - going to a movie or other entertainment, shopping
  - reading aloud to a companion, and being read to
  - preparing meals for after the birth or baking bread
  - preparing the baby's clothing, bedding
  - watching videotapes, television
  - doing a "project"—sorting photographs, writing in a journal, cleaning a closet, drawing or painting
  - playing games, and others

- She should eat when hungry, unless she knows she is having a cesarean section (e.g., because of a herpes lesion, a complicated presentation, or other preexisting condition). Best food choices are easily digested complex carbohydrates (starchy foods, fruits and vegetables). She should avoid greasy or highly spiced foods, which are more difficult to digest.

- She should drink to thirst. Water, broth, fruit juice, caffeine-free teas, or electrolyte-balanced beverages are good choices. Do not encourage her to drink more than she willingly accepts. Offer a beverage periodically, but if she refuses, do not urge her to drink more. A recent study[27] compared the volume of fluids drunk during labor with blood sodium levels of 287 women. Of those who drank more than 2.5 liters of fluid, one in four developed hyponatremia (too little sodium in the blood). The authors report that, contrary to usual advice, women normally have a lower tolerance for a water load during labor and should not drink excessively. Prolonged second stage, instrumental delivery, and cesarean delivery are some of the risks of hyponatremia.

- She should begin using labor coping techniques during her contractions when distraction is no longer possible and she cannot walk through or talk through her contractions without pausing at the peaks. Relaxation and self-calming techniques, slow breathing (sighing), and attention-focusing are appropriate at this time.

- She should periodically time four or five consecutive contractions in a row for duration, frequency, and interval to determine if her contractions are progressing. Online computer recording applications allow both parents to focus more on other things than the mathematical calculations required to detect a contraction pattern.

- She should know her providers' guidelines on when to come to the hospital (including guidelines on ruptured membranes).

Some women, having no idea of what to expect from early labor, "overreact"—that is, they are preoccupied with every contraction, and they may rush to use learned coping techniques that are more appropriate for active labor. They often expect to be 5 or 6 cm dilated when they are first checked and are crushed when they are examined and found to be only 1 to 2 cm! They do not see how they are going to cope with the more intense contractions to come. A woman in this situation needs a chance to express her disappointment. The caregiver can help by acknowledging her disappointment, giving her some suggestions to reduce the intensity of the contractions, and proceed to calm and relax her. She will need help to get her head "back where her cervix is."[28]

If a woman arrives at the hospital earlier than necessary, she is often encouraged to return home. The way this is handled can make her feel either more confident, knowledgeable, and willing to go home or ashamed, angry, or afraid to leave the hospital. If the mentioned support measures are followed, the former is more likely. Before sending her home, however, be sure she has coping techniques and a clear idea of the circumstances that will indicate that she should return. Chapter 4 contains many appropriate coping techniques for early labor.

4

SOME REASONS FOR EXCESSIVE PAIN AND DURATION OF PRELABOR OR THE LATENT PHASE

For some women, prelabor or latent phase is extremely painful and prolonged for a variety of reasons:

Iatrogenic factors

Oxytocin-induced contractions are sometimes painful and debilitating, especially when the cervix is unripe, or when the woman's contractions come every 2 or 3 minutes and her cervix is only 1 or 2 cm dilated.

There may be policies or practices that restrict the woman to bed. Reasons given for such a policy include ruptured membranes (see page 114), continuous electronic fetal monitoring (see pages 37–44), pregnancy-induced hypertension (see page 114), or hospital custom. In many cases, restriction to bed is not required, but the woman is not encouraged to get out of bed.

Cervical factors

An unripe cervix at term may indicate insufficient remodeling of the connective tissue, which causes cervical resistance[29-31] to increasing intrauterine pressures, or the presence of muscle fibers in the cervix,[32] which cause cervical contractions during uterine contractions.

Scar tissue in the cervix, possibly from previous surgery (e.g., cauterization, cryosurgery, cone biopsy, loop electrosurgical excision procedure [LEEP], or other procedures), sometimes increases the resistance of the cervix to effacement and the first few centimeters of dilation.[17,33] Contractions of great intensity for many hours or days, cervical massage, or manual dilation (see Chapter 10) may be required to overcome this resistance, after which dilation often proceeds normally.

Fetal factors

These include OP position of the fetus or brow, face presentation, or large unengaged fetal head.

Emotional factors

Extreme fear, anxiety, loneliness, stress, or anger before or during labor may lead to a buildup of catecholamines and a resulting slowdown in progress[34] (see Chapter 2 pages 29–30). Women who are not supported emotionally or who have experienced previous difficult childbirths; traumatic experiences such as emotional, physical, or sexual abuse; substance abuse; multiple hospitalizations; or other experiences may find early labor unexpectedly painful or traumatic.[35-37]

Exhaustion, discouragement, and feelings of hopelessness may result from a long prelabor or latent phase. The woman's optimism and coping ability diminish and her pain worsens as time goes on without apparent progress.

It is sometimes helpful to ask the woman about her emotional state during latent labor. Her answer may assist the caregiver in diagnosing emotional distress. Between contractions, questions such as "What was going through your mind during that contraction?" or "How are you feeling right now?" or "Why do you think this labor is going slowly right now?" may reveal that the mother is distressed or worried over specific concerns. Knowing these concerns will help the caregiver support the woman emotionally. See Chapters 5 and 10, pages 162–167, and 351–354, for more on how to help an emotionally distressed woman.

Women having painful nonprogressing prelabor or early labor often appear to be much further along in labor than they truly are. The contractions may be so intense that the women must rely on coping strategies that others might not use until late in the first stage. Of course, they also become discouraged and hopeless. It is important that caregivers not label these women as being frail or unable to cope or discount or minimize their pain at this early stage of labor. It does not help them cope and only results in their feeling inadequate or unsupported.

The next section offers suggestions to improve labor progress or reduce discomfort in early labor. Of course, if fetal distress, macrosomia, malpresentation, inadequate contractions, or other complications are diagnosed, the supportive measures will have to be tailored to the situation.

TROUBLESHOOTING MEASURES FOR PAINFUL PROLONGED PRELABOR OR LATENT PHASE

- Follow the general measures for early labor as described in Chapter 2.
- For the pain and discouragement that may accompany some labor inductions or an unripe or scarred cervix, reassure the woman that under these circumstances early labor is more challenging, but it does not necessarily mean that active labor will be abnormal.[29]

Such women also need validation, intense emotional support, and physical comfort. Try not to contribute to her self-doubt or worries by suggesting that something is wrong.

- If she is discouraged over slow dilation or nonprogressing contractions, remind the woman that before her cervix can dilate, it must move forward, ripen, and efface—each of which is a positive sign of progress. Be sure to disclose any progress in these areas to her whenever you check her cervix. See *six ways to progress* on pages 108–109.
- Avoid the term "false labor" because it implies that her contractions are somehow "not real" and that because her cervix is not dilating, the contractions are not accomplishing anything significant. Such implications are most discouraging to the woman who is experiencing them. In fact, if her cervix is changing at all, these prelabor contractions are preparing the cervix for dilation.

- Encourage her to seek and use positions or movements that she finds more comfortable. See *Monitoring the mobile woman's fetus*, pages 37–44, for suggestions on monitoring during induced labor.
- Offer a bath, shower, or massage as a temporary relaxer and pain reliever.
- Transcutaneous electrical nerve stimulation (TENS) may be especially useful to relieve back pain during early labor. TENS is more useful for back pain than for other labor pain and is more beneficial when introduced early in labor (see Chapter 10). If at all possible, do not restrict the woman to bed. Before restricting a woman with ruptured membranes to bed [which is a requirement in many hospitals even if the fetal head is engaged], the caregiver might auscultate the fetal heart and assess fetal movement with the woman in an upright position. Sometimes the upright position actually protects against a prolapsed cord, as gravity may keep the head applied to the cervix, thus preventing the cord from slipping through.)
- Many caregivers, especially in North America, restrict the woman with pregnancy-induced hypertension to bed in late pregnancy and in labor, because blood pressure is usually lowered while a woman lies on her left side. Whether such treatment has resulted in improved outcomes or less progression of preeclampsia is not known.[38] The topic has received too little study to draw conclusions. However, if you are caring for a woman who is in bed with pregnancy-induced hypertension, you can explain why left-sided bedrest is being asked of her (while acknowledging the lack of study in this area). Help her focus on comfort measures that she can use while in bed. Relaxation, rhythmic breathing, vocalization, guided imagery, visualizations, other attention-focusing measures, and massage of her back or feet may help. In addition, if limited walking is acceptable, she may walk to and from the bathroom, to use the shower or bath (both of which frequently lower high blood pressure). Having some choices regarding her position boosts her morale.
- Assess the woman's emotional state during early labor; if she is distressed, try appropriate measures to help improve her emotional state. See the Toolkit in Chapter 10, pages 351–354.
- For exhaustion, discouragement, and hopelessness, you can raise her spirits by suggesting a change: have her wash her face, comb her hair, brush her teeth, take a walk, play some upbeat music.

These measures are especially effective as the sun comes up after a long night with little progress. The new day can renew spirits.

- Have a good talk with her and her partner, encouraging them to express their feelings. Acknowledge and validate their feelings of frustration, discouragement, fatigue, or even anger at the staff for not "doing something" to correct the problem. She may benefit from a good cry, followed by a pep talk and perhaps a visit from a friend or family member who is rested and optimistic.
- If the above measures are unsuccessful, a drug-induced rest with alcohol, a sleep medication, or pain reliever may be an appropriate choice. This is discussed in Chapter 8.

MEASURES TO ALLEVIATE PAINFUL, NONPROGRESSING, NONDILATING CONTRACTIONS IN PRELABOR OR THE LATENT PHASE

If early contractions are painful and irregular with little or no progress in dilation, it makes sense to consider persistent asynclitism or another unfavorable fetal position, such as OP (Fig. 4.2).

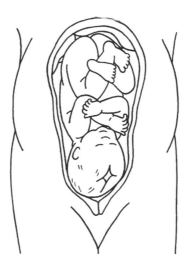

Fig. 4.2 Right occiput posterior, abdominal view.

Synclitism and asynclitism

Labor normally begins with the fetal head in asynclitism (i.e., the head is angled so that one of the parietal bones, rather than the vertex, presents at the pelvic inlet, as shown in Fig. 4.3). This facilitates passage of the fetal head through the pelvic inlet, and then the head usually shifts into synclitism (Fig. 4.4) so that the vertex presents as the head descends further. However, sometimes the asynclitism persists and, if so, it can keep the fetus from rotating and descending.[33] Without descent, the head may not be well applied to the cervix and contractions often become irregular and ineffective. At this stage of labor, it is difficult or impossible (and not considered very clinically important) to assess the angle and position of the fetal head. However, if contractions are irregular and ineffective for a long time, position changes and movements may correct the problem and improve the contraction pattern.

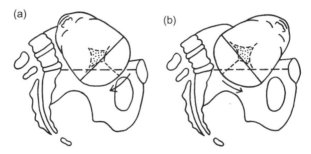

Fig. 4.3 (a) Posterior asynclitism. (b) Anterior asynclitism.

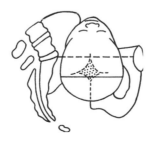

Fig. 4.4 Synclitism.

If the woman is having her first baby or has good abdominal muscle tone, having her lean forward often moves the fetus's center of gravity forward, encouraging his head to pivot into a more favorable position (Figs. 4.5 through 4.7). This may evenly disperse or increase the head-to-cervix force, leading to more regular, more effective contractions.

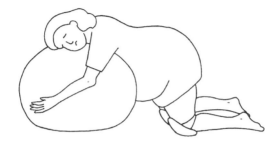

Fig. 4.5 Kneeling with a ball and knee pads to correct possible posterior asynclitism.

4

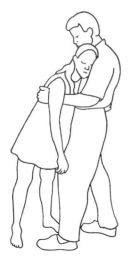

Fig. 4.6 Standing, leaning forward on partner.

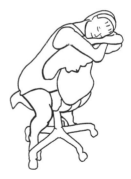

Fig. 4.7 Straddling a chair.

If the woman's abdominal muscle tone is poor and her abdomen is pendulous, the fetus' center of gravity may fall so far forward that the fetus is not well-aligned with the pelvic inlet. She might benefit from a semireclining position (Fig. 4.8). Having her "lean back" in this way may move the fetus's center of gravity toward her back, thus aligning the fetus with her pelvis and allowing the head to put more pressure on the cervix during the contractions, and this may lead to more regular, more effective contractions.

(a)   (b)

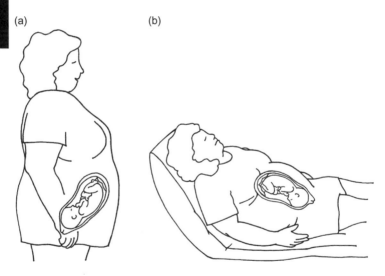

Fig. 4.8   (a) Woman with poor abdominal muscle tone and pendulous abdomen, standing. Fetal center of gravity falls away from pelvic inlet. (b) Woman with poor abdominal muscle tone and pendulous abdomen, semireclining. Fetal center of gravity aligns with pelvic inlet.

(a)   (b)

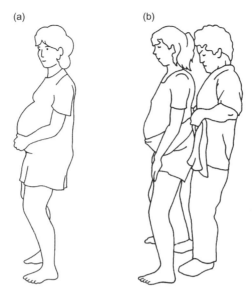

Fig. 4.9. (**a**) Abdominal lifting. (**b**) Abdominal lifting with a shawl.

King suggests abdominal lifting (Fig. 4.9) with a pelvic tilt during contractions at any time in labor if the woman has back pain in association with pendulous abdominal muscles, a short waist, a previous back injury, or a malpositioned baby.[39] Abdominal lifting, when it works well, realigns the baby's torso in relation to the angle of the pelvic inlet. The contractions then become more efficient in pressing the baby's head onto the cervix. See the Toolkit in Chapter 9, pages 318–320, for specific instructions. We suggest that fetal heart tones be checked periodically by the nurse or midwife during a contraction with abdominal lifting. In the remote possibility that the heart rate decelerates, it might be due to anterior placement of the umbilical cord. The fetus might become markedly more active if this is the case, or the heart rate may slow. If so, the pressure on the low abdomen could compress the cord, and abdominal lifting should not be used.

The open knee–chest position is another way to reposition the fetus in prelabor or early labor. The position takes advantage of gravity to allow the fetus to "back out" of the woman's pelvis, rotate, and descend again in a more favorable position.

El Halta,[40] an American midwife, teaches the open knee–chest position for specific symptoms in prelabor or the latent phase, when there is a long period of frequent, irregular, and brief uterine contractions, usually accompanied by severe persistent backache but resulting in little or no dilation. El Halta's experience is that this contraction pattern is associated with an OP position. She instructs the woman to spend 30 to 45 minutes in an open knee–chest position: that is, her hips are flexed to an angle greater than 90 degrees (Fig. 4.10). Because the position is difficult to maintain for 30 or more minutes, the woman will tolerate the position better if she can rest her shoulders against her partner's shins (padded with small towels), so that he can support much of the weight of her upper body (Fig. 4.10b).

The open knee–chest position tilts the pelvis forward with the inlet lower than the outlet. This allows gravity to encourage the unengaged OP fetal head out of the pelvis and may allow the head to reposition more favorably toward OA before reentering the pelvis. By contrast, a "closed knee–chest position" (Fig. 4.11) causes the woman's hips and knees to be flexed so that her thighs are beneath her abdomen and the pelvic inlet is higher than the outlet. This does not encourage the fetus to move out of the pelvis and removes the gravity effect.

(a) (b)

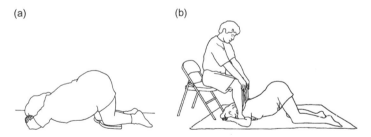

Fig. 4.10 (a) Open knee–chest position. (b) Open knee–chest position, shoulders resting on partner's shins.

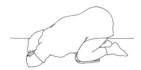

Fig. 4.11 Closed knee–chest position with knee pads. Pressure of the thighs on the abdomen may interfere with fetal rotation.

CONCLUSION

Prolonged prelabor and the latent phase of labor by themselves rarely indicate a complication, although they are discouraging and exhausting for the woman. Suggestions are given for coping with the discouragement, and early measures are described to correct possible fetal malposition. Most of the measures suggested here are well tolerated or favored by women, but if a woman finds them distressing or uncomfortable, she should be encouraged to do what she finds most helpful.

REFERENCES

1. Friedman EA. (1993). Dysfunctional labor. In Cohen WR, Friedman EA, editors. Management of Labor. Baltimore, University Park Press, p. 17.
2. Greulich B, Tarrant B. (2007). The latent phase of labor: Diagnosis and management. J Midwif Womens 52, 190–198.
3. MacKenzie S. (2004). Obstetrics: Labor. In University of Iowa Family Practice Handbook, 4th edition, Chapter 14. Iowa City, University of Iowa.
4. O'Driscoll K, Meagher D, Boylan P. (1993). Active Management of Labour, 3rd edition. London, Bailliere Tindall.
5. Zhang J, Troendle J, Yancey M. (2002). Reassessing the labor curve in nulliparous women. Am J Obstet Gynecol 187, 824–828.
6. Gardberg M, Laakkonen E, Salevaara M. (1998). Intrapartum sonography and persistent occiput posterior position: A study of 408 deliveries. Obstet Gynecol 91(5 pt 1), 746–749.
7. Sutton J, Scott P. (1996). Understanding and Teaching Optimal Foetal Positioning. Tauranga, New Zealand, Birth Concepts.
8. Sutton J. (2001). Let Birth Be Born Again: Rediscovering and Reclaiming Our Midwifery Heritage. Bedfont, UK, Birth Concepts UK.
9. Scott P. (2003). Sit Up and Take Notice! Positioning Yourself for a Better Birth. Tauranga, New Zealand, Great Scott Publications.
10. Andrews C, Andrews E. (1983). Nursing, maternal postures, and fetal position. Nurs Res 32, 336–341.
11. Kariminia A, Chamberlain M, Keogh J, Shea A. (2004). Randomised controlled trial of effect of hands and knees posturing on incidence of occiput posterior position at birth. BMJ. doi:10.1136/bmj.37942.594456.44, 1–5.
12. Lieberman E, Davidson K, Lee-Parritz A, Shearer E. (2005). Changes in fetal position during labor and their association with epidural analgesia. Obstet Gynecol 105(5 pt 1), 974–982.

13. Sizer A, Nirmal D. (2000). Occiput posterior position: Associated factors and obstetric outcomes in nulliparas. Obstet Gynecol 96(5 pt 1), 749–752.

14. Sherer D, Miodovnik M, Bradley K, Langer O. (2002). Intrapartum fetal head position, I: Comparison between transvaginal digital examination and transabdominal ultrasound assessment during the active stage of labor. Ultrasound Obstet Gynecol 19(3), 258–263.

15. Cheng Y, Shaffer B, Caughey A. (2006). The association between persistent occiput posterior position and neonatal outcomes. Obstet Gynecol 107(4), 837–844.

16. Simkin P. (2010). The fetal occiput posterior position: The state of the science and call for a new perspective. Birth 37(1), 61–71.

17. Davis E. (2004). Heart and Hands: A Midwife's Guide to Pregnancy and Birth, 4th edition. Berkeley, CA, Celestial Arts.

18. Varney H, Kriebs J, Gegor C. (2004). Varney's Midwifery, 4th edition. Boston, Jones and Bartlett.

19. Cunningham F, Leveno K, Bloom S, Hauth J, Rouse D, Spong C, editors. (2010). Williams Obstetrics, 23rd edition. New York, McGraw-Hill.

20. Oppenheimer L, Holmes P, Yang Q, Yang T, Walker M, Wen S. (2007). Adherence to guidelines on the management of dystocia and cesarean section rates. Am J Perinatol 24, 271–275.

21. Fraser W, Krauss I, Boulvain M, Oppenheimer L, Milne K, Liston R, et al. (1995). Dystocia. Society of Obstetricians and Gynecologists of Canada (SOGC) Clinical Guidelines, 40, 1–16.

22. Eriksson M, Mattsson LA, Ladfors L. (1997). Early or late bath during the first stage of labor: A randomized study of 200 women. Midwifery 13(3), 146–148.

23. Odent M. (1997). Can water immersion stop labor? J Nurs Midwif 42, 414–416.

24. Simkin P, O'Hara M. (2002). Nonpharmacologic relief of pain during labor: Systematic reviews of five methods. Am J Obstet Gynecol 186, S139–159.

25. Simkin P, Klein M. (2009). Nonpharmacological approaches to management of labor pain, parts 1 and 2. UpToDate 17(3), 1–11.

26. Cluett E, Burns E. (2009). Immersion in water in labour and birth. Cochrane Database Syst Rev (2)CD000111. doi:000110.001002/14651858.CD14000111.pub14651853.

27. Moen V, Brudin L, Rundgren M, Irestedt L. (2009). Hyponatremia complicating labour—Rare or unrecognised? A prospective observational study. Br J Obstet Gynecol 116, 552–561.

4

28. Wilf R. (1980). Personal communication.
29. Olah K. (1991). Measurement of the cervical response to uterine activity in labour and observations on the mechanism of cervical effacement. J Perinat Med 19(suppl 2), 245.
30. Olah K, Gee H, Brown J. (1993). Cervical contractions: The response of the cervix to oxytocic stimulation in the latent phase of labour. Br J Obstet Gynaecol 100, 635–640.
31. Ulmsten U. (1994). The forces of labor, resistance of the cervix and the contractions of the myometrium. Eur J Obstet Gynecol Reprod Biol 55(1), 7.
32. Olah K, Neilson J. (1994). Failure to progress in the management of labour. Br J Obstet Gynaecol 101, 1–3.
33. Oxorn H. (1986) Oxorn-Foote Human Labor and Birth, 5th edition. New York, McGraw-Hill.
34. Alehagen S, Wijma B, Lundberg U, Wijma K. (2005). Fear, pain, and stress hormones during childbirth. J Psychosomat Obstet Gynaecol 26, 153–165.
35. Waldenstrom U, Hildinsson I, Ryding E. (2006). Antenatal fear of childbirth and its association with subsequent caesarean section and experience of childbirth. Br J Obstet Gynaecol 113, 638–646.
36. Alehagen S, Wijma B, Wijma K, Rhydhstrom H. (2006). Fear of childbirth before, during and after childbirth. Acta Obstet Gynecol Scand 85(1), 56–62.
37. Nieminen K, Stephansson O, Ryding E. (2009). Women's fear of childbirth and preference for caesarean section—A cross-sectional study at various stages of pregnancy in Sweden. Acta Obstet Gynecol Scand 88, 807–813.
38. Enkin M, Keirse M, Neilson J, Crowther C, Duley L, Hodnett E, et al. (2000). Hypertension in pregnancy. In A Guide to Effective Care in Pregnancy and Childbirth, 3rd edition, Chapter 15. Oxford, Oxford University Press.
39. King J. (1993). Back Labor No More!! What Every Woman Should Know before Labor. Dallas, TX, Plenary Systems.
40. El Halta V. (1995). Posterior labor: A pain in the back. Midwif Today 36, 19–21.

Chapter 5

Prolonged Active Phase of Labor

Penny Simkin, BA, PT, CCE, CD(DONA),
and Ruth Ancheta, BA, ICCE, CD(DONA)

When is active labor prolonged? 125
Characteristics of prolonged active labor, 126
Possible causes of prolonged active labor, 127
Fetal and fetopelvic factors, 129
How fetal malpositions delay labor progress, 132
Problems in diagnosis of fetal position during labor, 133
Artificial rupture of the membranes with a malpositioned fetus, 134
Specific measures to address and correct problems associated with a "poor fit"—malposition, cephalopelvic disproportion, and macrosomia, 135
Maternal positions and movements for suspected fetal malposition, cephalopelvic disproportion, or macrosomia, 136
Forward-leaning positions, 136
Side-lying positions, 138
Asymmetric positions and movements, 141
Abdominal lifting, 144
An uncontrollable premature urge to push, 144
If contractions are inadequate, 146
Immobility, 147
Medication, 149
Dehydration, 150
Exhaustion, 151
Uterine lactic acidosis as a cause of inadequate contractions, 151
When the cause of inadequate contractions is unknown, 153
If there is a persistent anterior cervical lip or a swollen cervix, 156
Positions to reduce an anterior cervical lip or a swollen cervix, 156
Other methods, 158
Manual reduction of a persistent cervical lip, 158

The Labor Progress Handbook: Early Interventions to Prevent and Treat Dystocia.
Edited by Penny Simkin, Ruth Ancheta
© 2011 by Penny Simkin and Ruth Ancheta; illustrations copyright Ruth Ancheta

If emotional dystocia is suspected, 158
Assessing the woman's coping, 158
Indicators of emotional dystocia during active labor, 160
Predisposing factors for emotional dystocia, 161
Helping the woman state her fears, 161
How to help a laboring woman in distress, 162
Special needs of childhood abuse survivors, 164
Incompatibility or poor relationship with staff, 166
If the source of the woman's anxiety cannot be identified, 166
Conclusion, 167
References, 167

WHEN IS ACTIVE LABOR PROLONGED?

The active phase of labor (or active labor) usually refers to cervical dilation greater than 3 to 5 cm, accompanied by progressing contractions—that is, contractions that are becoming longer, stronger, and more frequent. See pages 22–23) for a discussion of various expert opinions on when normal active labor begins.

It is sometimes unclear whether a woman is in active labor. For example, multiparas sometimes reach 3, 4 or even 5 cm of dilation with only sporadic or nonprogressing contractions. If a caregiver is unaware that a woman has been at 4 or 5 cm dilation for several days and does not review her contraction pattern, he or she may assume incorrectly that the woman is in labor. Then, once the woman is admitted to the hospital, if she makes no further progress and her contractions seem inadequate, the caregiver may diagnose her with "failure to progress," when, in fact, she was never in labor. This illustrates why both dilation and the contraction pattern are crucial to a correct diagnosis of active labor.

The term "prolonged active labor" refers to an insufficient rate of dilation after active labor has been diagnosed. However, the diagnosis of "insufficient rate of progress" varies among authors: less than 1 cm/hr for at least 2 hours after labor progress has been well established[1]; less than 1.2 cm/hr in a primigravida and less than 1.5 cm/hr in a multipara[2,3]; and longer than 12 hours from 4 cm to complete dilation (which translates into 0.5 cm/hr).[4,5] An "arrest disorder" has been defined as no dilation for more than 2 hours at or beyond 4 cm dilation despite adequate contractions. *Adequate contractions* are defined as contractions exerting a pressure greater than or equal to 200 Montevideo units),[6] the amount considered necessary for adequate labor during active labor. Montevideo units are calculated by multiplying the number of contractions by the increase in uterine pressure above baseline tone (as measured with an intrauterine pressure catheter) in a 10-minute period.

Studies by Zhang and colleagues[5] and Albers and colleagues[7] have found that the criteria used today for the diagnosis of prolonged labor and arrest disorders in nulliparous women (largely derived from Friedman's work 30 to 50 years ago[1]) are too stringent and that women who give birth safely via the vagina may progress at a rate of less than 0.5 cm/hr between 3 and 7 cm and at less than 1 cm/hr at 7 to 10 cm dilation.[5,7]

CHARACTERISTICS OF PROLONGED ACTIVE LABOR

- The contractions stop progressing or slow down, becoming less intense, shorter in duration, and/or less frequent.
- Alternatively, they may take on a quality of sameness, neither progressing nor slowing down.
- The woman continues coping in the same way for hours, or finds labor easier to manage than it was previously.
- On a vaginal exam, the cervix is unchanged.

Clinical management of prolonged active labor varies, depending on the caregiver's philosophy and the woman's wishes—for example:

- One very common approach, once the diagnosis has been made, is to rupture the membranes (if that has not already been done) and start incremental doses of intravenous oxytocin. If these measures are unsuccessful in stimulating progress, a cesarean delivery is performed.[8]
- In the Active Management of Labor protocol,[1,9] as practiced at the National Maternity Hospital in Dublin and elsewhere, the membranes are ruptured as soon as labor is diagnosed. If dilation is less than 1 cm/hr for 2 hours at any time after labor is diagnosed (regardless of cervical dilation), high doses of oxytocin are administered incrementally until a rate of at least 1 cm/hr is achieved.
- With a low intervention model of maternity care, the caregiver assesses the rate of dilation but perceives a slow rate of dilation

in the active phase as an indication for evaluation rather than medical intervention. The midwife or other low-intervention caregiver is likely to make broader allowances for individual variations in progress of dilation, taking into account fetal and maternal tolerance of the delay and assessing signs of progress other than dilation, such as rotation of the fetal head, which is often a necessary precursor to further progress. (See Chapter 4, pages 108–109, for six ways to progress in labor.) Such an approach relies on preventive measures and time, patience, support, and primary and intermediate interventions such as those offered in this book. The goals are to support the woman through the delay and encourage labor progress.[3,10] Oxytocin and artificial rupture of the membranes (AROM) are reserved for later use if necessary.

POSSIBLE CAUSES OF PROLONGED ACTIVE LABOR

Slowing or arrest of dilation in the active phase may sometimes be prevented or corrected by first using simple, low-cost interventions that carry little or no known risk. If they are not successful, then the intermediate interventions (see Chapter 8) are used, and, if necessary, the more powerful and complex obstetric interventions that are also more expensive and associated with more potential risks. Chart 5.1 illustrates a step-by-step approach to the problem of a prolonged active phase of labor.

The choice of intervention depends on the apparent cause of the problem. Causes of prolonged active labor include the following:

Fetal and fetopelvic factors: Cephalopelvic disproportion (CPD—a poor fit between the fetal head and maternal pelvis). CPD may involve a large head or a malpositioned head, in which the malposition (i.e., occiput posterior, occiput transverse, or asynclitism) causes the presentation of a larger diameter (e.g., a deflexed head) than when the vertex presents in an occiput anterior position). CPD may also occur with a discrepancy between the shape of the fetal head and the dimensions and shape of the maternal pelvis.[11] A persistently high station in the presence of adequate contractions may indicate a poor fit of the head, but not necessarily too large a head, within the pelvis.

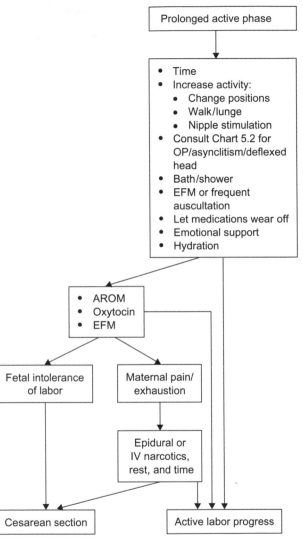

Chart 5.1. Prolonged active phase of labor.

Uterine factors: Inadequate intensity of contractions, uterine inertia

Cervical factors: Persistent cervical lip, rigid os

Emotional factors: Fear, anxiety, tension, or anger (see Chapter 2)

Iatrogenic factors: Dehydration; restriction of movement; pain medications, epidural analgesia, inappropriate or excessive use of oxytocin

Maternal factors: Exhaustion; short waist; lumbar lordosis, combined with lack of lumbar mobility; pendulous abdomen[12]

Combination of etiologies or unknown etiology: Sometimes the delay in progress results from a combination of the above, for example, a persistent malposition associated with a large baby, maternal fear or exhaustion, and inadequate contractions. Sometimes the cause is unclear. In such cases, the contractions appear adequate, fetal position appears favorable, fetal size seems average, and the woman appears to be coping well, but progress in dilation is slow. Patience and trial and error, using a number of the measures discussed in this chapter, may result in greater progress without anyone figuring out exactly what the problem was. For example, a subtle undetectable variation in position or another problem may be corrected with the passage of time and a variety of movements and comfort measures.

Fetal and fetopelvic factors

Malposition, macrosomia, and cephalopelvic disproportion

The usual ways to identify fetal position—observations of abdominal shape, abdominal palpation, location of fetal heart tones, the woman's symptoms, the contraction pattern, internal examination of the suture lines of the fetal skull—are notoriously undependable, according to a number of studies reviewed recently.[13] In fact, even ultrasound examinations are sometimes uninterpretable,[14] although ultrasound is the most useful diagnostic technique in use today. Because of the difficulty in determining fetal malposition, any time there is a delay in active labor, the caregiver should not rule out fetal malposition as an etiology, even if he or she cannot confirm it or differentiate it from other etiologies such as macrosomia, CPD, compound presentation, or others. Even with an uncertain diagnosis, the primary interventions for all of these conditions are very similar, so a trial-and-error approach is usually acceptable. These interventions are grouped in this section. See pages 133–135 for further discussion of the difficulties in diagnosis and the potential ramifications of a misdiagnosis.

Persistent asynclitism

At the onset of labor, most fetuses are in an asynclitic occiput transverse (OT) or occiput anterior (OA) position. This means the fetal head is angled so that one parietal bone enters the pelvis first, and the fetal biparietal diameter is not parallel to the plane of the inlet of the pelvis (Figs. 5.1 and 5.2).

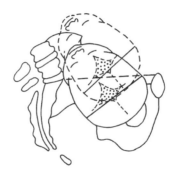

Fig. 5.1. Posterior asynclitism and persistent posterior asynclitism.

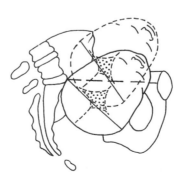

Fig. 5.2. Anterior asynclitism and persistent anterior asynclitism.

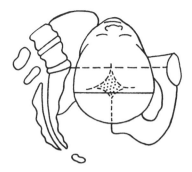

Fig. 5.3. Synclitism.

With contractions, the head usually pivots into synclitism, so that the fetal biparietal diameter is parallel to the plane of the inlet as it descends (Fig. 5.3). Only if asynclitism is persistent, that is, it *remains when the fetus is at a low station*, does it slow labor progress.

Occiput posterior

Estimates of the incidence of occiput posterior (OP) position at the onset of labor range between 10% and 20% of all labors. OP is more common in primigravidas.[15] (See Chapter 3, pages 52–63, for discussion of techniques used to identify an OP fetus before the onset of labor.) Many fetuses who are occiput anterior (OA) at the onset of labor rotate to OP during labor, and most fetuses who are OP at the onset rotate to OA spontaneously by late first stage or by delivery and are born without difficulty. The latter is a common scenario for women with anthropoid pelves.[15] In the end, approximately 5% of fetuses remain OP at delivery (persistent OP).[14–17] Contractions, gravity, resilience of the muscles in the pelvis, shape of the pelvis, the woman's position and movement, fetal efforts, and other forces combine to cause rotation of the fetal head.

If OP (Fig. 5.4) and occiput transverse (OT) (Fig. 5.5) positions and asynclitism persist, they usually become problematic, with increased chances of operative delivery. If the woman's pelvis is roomy enough, however, time, support, and specific measures by the woman and staff will usually allow a vaginal birth. As long as the fetus and

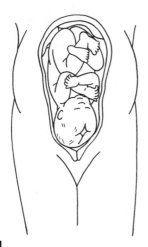

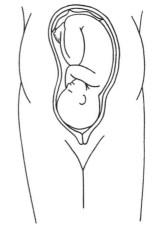

Fig. 5.4. Right occiput posterior, abdominal view.

Fig. 5.5. Left occiput transverse, abdominal view.

5

woman can tolerate them, these measures are often all that is necessary to solve the problem. But, if the problem persists despite these measures, that helps confirm the diagnosis of prolonged or arrested active labor. At this time, intermediate and tertiary (obstetric) interventions are instituted.

How fetal malpositions delay labor progress

When rotation or improved alignment is needed, it makes sense that labor will take more time than when the fetus is ideally positioned. Dilation may begin later or take longer because the pressure of the fetal head or forewaters on the cervix, which normally enhances dilation, may be uneven or generally reduced. Descent may also be delayed until the fetal head rotates, flexes, or aligns with the plane of the pelvis.

One should always suspect a malposition, asynclitism, CPD, or macrosomia if one or more of the following occurs:

- There is premature rupture of membranes at term.[18]
- Contractions are irregular (varying in intensity and duration in an unpredictable way).

- Contractions "couple" or "group" (two or three close together, followed by a relatively long interval).
- Contractions "space out" or slow down in active labor.
- The woman complains of back pain that may or may not go away between contractions.
- The rate of dilation plateaus in active labor.
- The woman has an uncontrollable urge to push long before dilation is complete.

Problems in diagnosis of fetal position during labor

The methods and challenges of diagnosing fetal position during pregnancy were discussed in Chapter 3. When making this diagnosis during labor, several symptoms are considered to be clues to fetal position, such as a delay in active labor dilation, presence of back pain, and coupling of contractions. Those, along with a digital pelvic exam to determine location of the fontanels and alignment of the sagittal suture, provide the information to make the diagnosis. However, one study found that back pain was as common among women with OA or OT fetuses as in women with OP fetuses.[14]

The most accurate method of assessment, the ultrasound examination, is not widely used during labor for this purpose. A review of the scientific literature[13] evaluating these methods has identified ultrasound as the only reliable method for detecting fetal position (and even ultrasound requires operator experience before it becomes a reliable technique).

In addition, the average percentage of agreement (within 45 degrees) between digital and ultrasound assessments in four comparison studies of fetal position in the first stage of labor was 42% (range, 31% to 49%).[19–22] The average percentage of agreement in 6 similar studies during the second stage was 60% (range, 27% to 80%).[21,23–27] More mistakes were made when the fetus was in the OP position than in other positions.[13]

How important is it to be able to diagnose fetal position correctly when there is a delay in active labor? If treatment is to be tailored to the etiology of the delay, a correct diagnosis is desirable. If the treatment is the same without regard for etiology (e.g., rupture of membranes and oxytocin), then knowing the position is less important. In the former, if a misdiagnosis of an OP position occurs, it is likely that the opportunity is lost to intervene with noninvasive corrective measures, which are presented on pages 135–144.

A common scenario: the consequences of misdiagnosis

Labor progress stalls.

The woman has no back pain.

A digital exam reveals the fetus to be direct OA.

Therefore, no effort is made to use positions or movements, which might rotate an OP fetus or correct a fetus in another malposition.

Artificial rupture of the membranes and oxytocin are tried but result in no change.

The baby is delivered with instruments or via cesarean, in an OP position or asynclitism, much to the surprise of all.

5

The presented scenario illustrates how a misdiagnosis of fetal position can be more problematic than no diagnosis at all, because with an uncertain etiology, trial and error with a variety of corrective measures is more likely to be used and may improve progress.

Many advocates believe that portable ultrasound, with its ability to make the fetus visible, should be used with any delay in labor. The knowledge gained allows the selection and use of corrective measures, and also makes it possible to measure success.

Furthermore, ultrasound may be a useful teaching technique to improve accuracy in clinical examination skills. Immediately after the digital exam (or Leopold's fetal heart tone location or another diagnostic method), a brief ultrasound examination could confirm or deny its accuracy. Of course, the woman's informed consent should be obtained beforehand.

Artificial rupture of the membranes with a malpositioned fetus

When there is a delay in active labor, caregivers often rupture the membranes and give oxytocin to speed it up. There is some concern over the wisdom of such a practice when the fetus is malpositioned. A Cochrane review of 12 randomized controlled trials that included 7792 women investigated the effects of routine early amniotomy plus oxytocin to prevent prolonged labor (10 trials) or to treat labors that are already prolonged (2 trials). There were no differences in maternal satisfaction with childbirth or maternal or neonatal condition. In the prevention group, labors were shortened by an average of 1.1 hours, and the cesarean rate was lowered by 1.5%.[28]

The meager results obtained from using routine artificial rupture of the membranes (AROM) and oxytocin, with their inherent risks and the increased need for intensive staff involvement, might persuade readers to rely first on low-technology practices (such as continuous labor support, movements, positions, and baths), which have been shown to speed labor and/or lower the likelihood of a cesarean, with fewer risks than amniotomy and oxytocin. There is little evidence of efficacy from using AROM plus oxytocin when a fetal malposition is impeding labor progress. The Cochrane review cited[28] found only two randomized controlled trials that investigated the efficacy of reserving AROM plus oxytocin only to treat labors that had already slowed down. There were no improvements in labor duration or in cesarean rates when AROM and oxytocin were used. Schwarcz, Caldeyro-Barcia, and colleagues raised these concerns years ago.[29] Others have also suggested that rotation to OA is more difficult after membranes rupture.[11,30] The explanatory hypothesis is as follows: When the fetus is poorly positioned, intact forewaters may provide some protection and maneuverability for the fetal head. When the forewaters are removed, the malpositioned fetus may be subjected to uneven head compression, excessive molding, more pronounced caput succedaneum, and a greater likelihood of operative delivery than would otherwise occur. Further large trials of amniotomy in labors with known OP positions or asynclitism are warranted to establish whether the malposition is more or less likely to self-correct with or without intact membranes. Without clear evidence of benefit, the potential risks (as well as other known risks of amniotomy—prolapsed cord and infection) remain a concern. It is surprising that the almost standard practice of performing amniotomy to augment slow labors associated with fetal malposition has not been adequately studied.[30–32]

Specific measures to address and correct problems associated with a "poor fit"—malposition, cephalopelvic disproportion, and macrosomia

In addition to the measures described here, see Chapter 1 for general measures to aid labor progress. Besides having the woman try the positions illustrated in this section, help her to deal with back pain, which occurs in about 30% of labors with fetal malposition or other types of "poor fit." Baths and showers, back pressure and massage, the knee press, kneeling and swaying on the birth ball, transcutaneous electrical nerve stimulation, cold or warm compresses (described in Chapter 10), and intracutaneous or subcutaneous sterile water injections (described in Chapter 8) are effective in relieving back pain.

Chart 5.2 (page 140) illustrates a step-by-step approach to be used when an OP position or asynclitism is suspected.

MATERNAL POSITIONS AND MOVEMENTS FOR SUSPECTED MALPOSITION, CEPHALOPELVIC DISPROPORTION, OR MACROSOMIA

Maternal positions and movements alter the forces of gravity, pelvic dimensions,[33,34] and the various pressures within the uterus and on pelvic joints. The position of the fetus is influenced by these changing forces. (See Chapter 9 for more information on each position and movement.)

Forward-leaning positions

Forward-leaning positions (Fig. 5.6) may help reposition the fetus during labor.[35] These positions are vigorously promoted by Sutton,[11] Scott,[36] Tully,[37] and others, for their contributions to optimal fetal positioning. See Chapter 9 for an explanation of how these positions may correct some problems of a "poor fit" between fetus and maternal pelvis.

Fig. 5.6. Forward–leaning positions. (**a**) Open knee–chest position, resting shoulders on partner's padded shins. (**b**) Kneeling with a ball and knee pads. (**c**) Hands and knees. (**d**) Kneeling over bed back. (**e**) Kneeling, with partner support. (**f**) Kneeling on bed with partner support and knee pads. (**g**) Standing, leaning on bed. (**h**) Standing, leaning forward on partner. (**i**) Straddling a toilet, facing backward. (**j**) Straddling a chair.

(a)

(b)

(c)

(d)

(e)

(f)

(g)

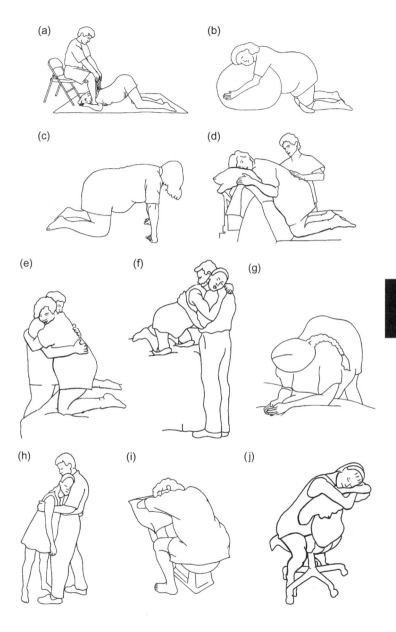

(h)

(i)

(j)

5

137

Side-lying positions

The effects of gravity on the fetus are quite different when a woman is in a pure side-lying versus a semiprone (Sims') position. When the fetus is thought (or known with ultrasound confirmation) to be OP:

- the woman using "pure side-lying" should lie on the side toward which the occiput is already directed, with the baby's back "toward the bed" (Figs. 5.7 and 5.8). This encourages the OP baby to OT.

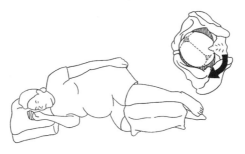

Fig. 5.7. Woman with a suspected or known OP fetus in pure side–lying on the "correct" side, with fetal back "toward the bed." If fetus is ROP, woman lies on her right side. Gravity pulls fetal occiput and trunk towards ROT.

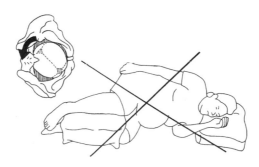

Fig. 5.8. Woman with a suspected or known OP fetus in pure side–lying on the "wrong" (left) side for an ROP fetus. Fetal back is toward the ceiling. Gravity pulls fetal occiput and trunk toward direct OP.

- if the woman is semiprone, she should lie on the side opposite the direction of the occiput, with the fetal back "toward the ceiling"[38] (Fig. 5.9).

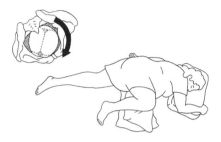

Fig. 5.9. Woman with a suspected or known OP fetus in semiprone on the "correct" side, with fetal back "toward the ceiling." IF fetus is ROP, the semiprone woman lies on her left side. Gravity pulls fetal occiput and trunk toward ROT, then ROA.

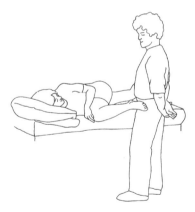

Fig. 5.10. Side–lying lunge.

With the "side-lying lunge" (Fig. 5.10), the woman lies semiprone and gentle pressure is applied to the sole of her upper foot, in the direction of her head, in order to increase hip flexion and abduction. This widens the pelvis, improving the chances of fetal rotation.

The side-lying lunge with support is useful for the woman with an epidural, who cannot hold her leg in place by herself. The support against her foot should be gentle, since she will not feel if the stretching of her hip joint is excessive.

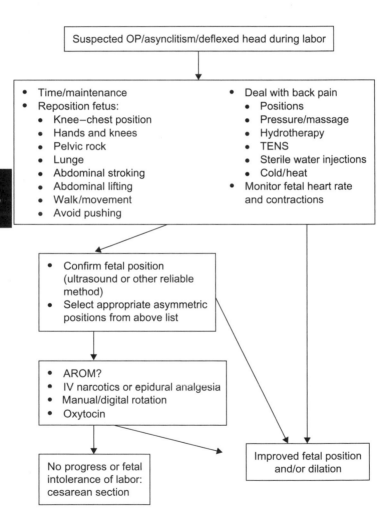

Chart 5.2.   Suspected fetal malposition in active labor.

Asymmetric positions and movements

Asymmetric positions, such as those pictured here (Fig. 5.11), enlarge the pelvis on the side where the leg is raised and slightly alter the internal shape of the pelvis. This may allow more space where it is needed for rotation. With these positions, it helps to know if the fetus is OA or OP and the direction of the occiput, so that the woman can enlarge the side of her pelvis where the fetus needs more space. If fetal position is uncertain, use trial and error—that is, alternate

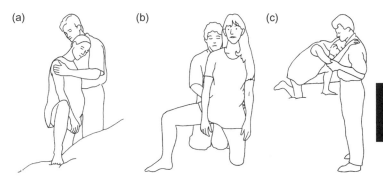

(a)   (b)   (c)

Fig. 5.11. (a) Standing with one leg elevated. (b) Asymmetrical kneeling. (c) Asymmetrical kneeling with partner support.

raising one leg for two contractions and the other for two contractions. If elevating one leg clearly feels more comfortable than elevating the other leg, she should continue with the more comfortable position for several more contractions. The rationale is that it should feel better to the woman when she is giving the fetus more room. If there is no difference in her comfort with either position, the woman should continue alternating after every 2 contractions for 30 minutes to 1 hour. The lunge (Fig. 5.12) uses weight-bearing and mild stretching of the hip abductors to create leverage to widen one side of the pelvis. To master the technique of the lunge, please see the instructions in Chapter 9, pages 283 and 313–314, before teaching it to the woman in labor. The same rationale applies: If fetal position is known, the woman should lunge in the direction of the occiput; if it is not known, she uses trial and error as described earlier.

(a) 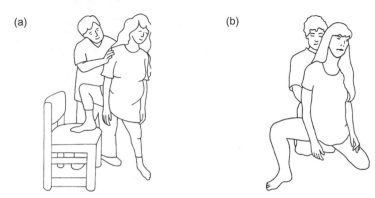 (b)

Fig. 5.12. (a) Standing lunge. (b) Kneeling lunge.

5

> *Supine and semisitting positions for occiput posterior*
>
> When a woman is fully supine or semisitting, gravity encourages the trunk of the OP fetus to lie next to the woman's spine, increasing the chances of compression of her inferior vena cava and causing supine hypotension but also minimizing the likelihood of rotation to OA. These positions also increase the pressure of the fetal occiput against the woman's sacrum and may worsen her back pain (Fig. 5.13a). There is a much greater likelihood of rotation and less back pain when the woman sits upright or leans forward (Fig. 5.13b).[11] When the woman is upright, the uterus tilts forward, thus encouraging flexion of the fetal head into the pelvic basin (Fig. 5.13c). When the woman is upright, the uterus, tilting forward, directs the fetal head into the pelvic basin (Fig. 5.13d).

Note: A woman with a pendulous abdomen may need to lean back in order to align the fetal head with her pelvic inlet; see page 118.

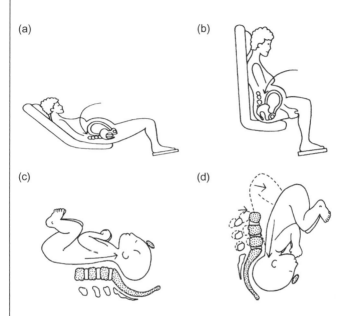

(a)

(b)

(c)

(d)

Fig. 5.13. (**a**) Woman reclining. Weight of uterus rests on her spine. (**b**) Woman upright. Fundus tilts forward. (**c**) Woman reclining. Head of OP fetus directed toward pubic bone. (**d**) Woman upright. Head directed into pelvic basin. [Adapted from Fenwick L, Simkin P. (1987) Maternal positioning to prevent or alleviate dystocia. *Clin Obstet Gynecol* **30**(1), 83–89.]

Abdominal lifting

To improve the alignment of the fetal trunk and head with the axis of the birth canal, during contractions, the woman bends her knees to tilt her pelvis, places her hands beneath her abdomen, and lifts her abdomen[12] (Fig. 5.14). The use of a shawl (woven cloth measuring approximately 45 cm wide [folded to about 15 cm wide] by 150 to 180 cm long) aids abdominal lifting. *Caution:* On rare occasions, the umbilical cord is located low and in front, and there is a small possibility that the cord would be compressed with abdominal lifting. It is wise for the midwife or nurse to check the fetal heart rate occasionally during contractions while abdominal lifting is being done. If decelerations occur, abdominal lifting should be discontinued. Also, if the fetus becomes noticeably active during the abdominal lift, the mother should discontinue it. See Chapter 9, pages 318–320, for complete instructions on abdominal lifting.

(a) (b)

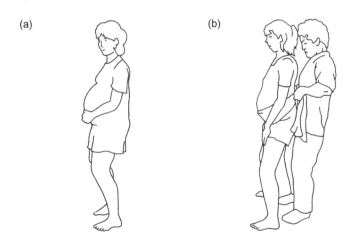

Fig. 5.14. (a) Abdominal lifting. (b) Abdominal lifting with a shawl.

An uncontrollable premature urge to push

Many women feel a mild or moderate urge to push before complete dilation. This can be handled with a change of position or by allowing her to satisfy the urge with "grunt pushes" (brief grunts). However, an uncontrollable, almost convulsive urge to push during active labor sometimes accompanies an OP position, especially when the fetus is engaged. The caregiver is faced with the question of whether the woman should push (Chart 5.3). On the one hand, with a prolonged active phase and an OP fetus, her pushing might lead to a swollen cervix or even a torn cervix and no further progress. On the other hand, it is sometimes impossible for the woman to control this urge.

A change of position to hands and knees (Fig. 5.15), semiprone (exaggerated Sims, Fig. 5.16), or open knee–chest (Fig. 5.17) may

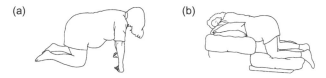

Fig. 5.15. (**a**) Hands and knees. (**b**) Kneeling on foot of bed.

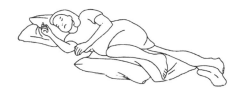

Fig. 5.16. Semiprone (exaggerated Sims' position).

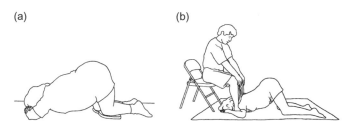

Fig. 5.17. (**a**) Open knee–chest position. (**b**) Open knee–chest position, shoulders resting on partner's padded shins.

relieve the urge to push by using gravity to move the head away from the cervix and ease pressure on the posterior vaginal wall (which seems to be the factor responsible for the urge to push). Manually repositioning of the fetal head (see Chapter 8, pages 246–250) may also help.

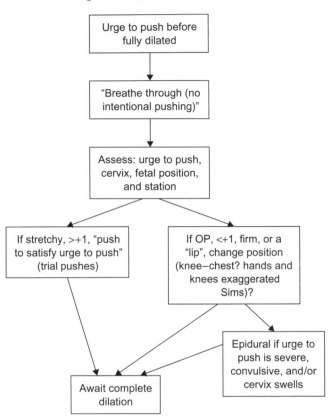

Chart 5.3. Premature urge to push.

IF CONTRACTIONS ARE INADEQUATE

If contractions seem to be of inadequate intensity, consider whether immobility, medication, dehydration, or emotional factors could be contributing factors.

Immobility

Has the woman been in one position for longer than 30 minutes? Changing her position may trigger stronger contractions, either by shifting the fetus's weight or by improving circulation to the uterus. Upright positions and movements, including walking, may intensify contractions. The supine position, by contrast, is correlated with weaker contractions, compared with other positions.[39,40] The supine position also a contributes to supine hypotension (low maternal blood pressure and decreased placental blood flow).

Women who are restricted to bed (e.g., for hypertension, analgesia or anesthesia, nonreassuring fetal heart rate responses, or institutional custom) may still be able to use position changes to improve labor progress. If the woman has back pain or other indicators of malposition, see *Side-lying Positions* (pages 279–281) for suggestions as to which side the mother should lie on.

If the mother does not have indicators of malposition or if it is difficult to determine which side the fetal back is on, it is appropriate to try the "rollover." In the "rollover," shown in Figure 5.18, the bedridden woman spends 20 to 30 minutes in each of the following positions: semisitting, left side-lying, left semiprone, hands and knees, right semiprone, right side-lying, and back to semisitting. She should, however, avoid any positions that she or her fetus does not tolerate well (see page 282).

Unfortunately, few trials have been conducted on the effects of walking or position changes as an intervention to correct labor dystocia. However, a recent Cochrane review found that walking and upright positions reduce the length of the first stage of normal labor by an average of 1 hour and do not seem to be associated with increased intervention or negative effects on mothers or babies.[41] Therefore, women should be encouraged to use any positions they prefer. It is interesting that walking shortens labor by about as much as AROM and oxytocin.[28] See Chapter 9, page 315, for an explanation of how walking or stair-climbing may enhance labor progress. There may also be a psychological benefit of upright positions in that a horizontal position may reinforce feelings of helplessness or powerlessness when laboring women are surrounded by people who are standing and looking down at them. By sitting or standing upright, the women may feel more powerful and become more optimistic.

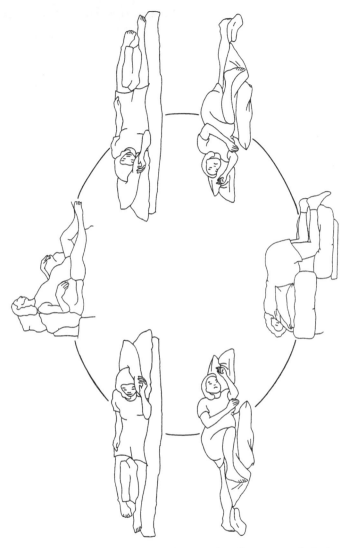

Fig. 5.18. The "rollover sequence" for use when there are no indicators of malposition, or when it is difficult to determine the location of the fetal back.

Medication

Narcotic analgesia received early in labor may temporarily weaken the woman's contractions. Simply allowing medications to wear off may lead to stronger contractions, although the woman may find this intolerable.

Does the epidural interfere with labor progress? Although epidural and combined spinal epidural analgesia provide the most effective pain relief and fewest maternal mental effects, two literature reviews concluded that epidural use, compared to no epidural use, is associated with longer labors, fewer spontaneous vaginal births, more instrumental deliveries, and other undesirable side effects unrelated to labor progress.[42,43] Having an epidural on request seems to influence the rate of malpositions at delivery. A large prospective study compared outcomes of 1562 nulliparas (1437, or 92% with an epidural, and 125 without).[14] Before receiving their epidurals, the women had no greater labor pain, no more pain specifically in the back, and no more fetal malpositions than did those who did not use epidurals. At delivery, however, there were 4 times more OPs in the epidural group (12.9% versus 3.3%). The incidence of OTs was similar (8.1% versus 7.3%). The authors reported that surgical delivery rates (including instrumental deliveries and cesareans) were extremely high among women with a malpositioned fetus—82% for OP and 86.5% for OT fetuses, compared with 23.8% for OA fetuses. This study indicates that elective epidurals may contribute indirectly to cesarean and instrumental delivery rates by increasing the incidence of OP.

Recent surveys in the United States, Canada, and the United Kingdom found the epidural rates to be 76%, 57%, and 37% (the U.K. 37% rate included spinal and general anesthesia), respectively.[44–46] Because of the variety of management protocols with epidurals, it is difficult, if not impossible, to establish positive or negative associations between epidural duration and undesirable effects, except for intrapartum fever, which increases with duration of the epidural.[42] Some low-intervention caregivers and their clients plan to use a variety of nonpharmacologic pain-coping measures first, to avoid or postpone the epidural, with a goal of minimizing any possible undesirable side effects.

Dehydration

Most laboring women prefer to drink liquids to satisfy thirst and alleviate dryness in their mouths. If they are allowed to drink as desired and offered a beverage frequently, they will hydrate themselves adequately during labor. The "nothing by mouth" order for healthy women in normal labor is rare, although the practice of limiting the amount and choice of fluids (for example, sips or ice chips only, water only) is still widespread,[44,47,48] especially with caregivers who perceive all laboring women as presurgical patients. These providers prefer intravenous hydration, even though this carries its own set of potential risks and drawbacks (neonatal hypoglycemia, maternal and fetal hyponatremia, maternal psychological stress, fluid overload, postpartum swelling, and breast engorgement).[47] The simplest practice to prevent dehydration is to encourage the woman to drink to thirst (water, electrolyte balanced beverages, broth, or fruit juice) and to note whether and approximately how much she is drinking.

Some women vomit frequently throughout labor and are at higher risk of dehydration. Contrary to widely held opinion, withholding oral fluids under such circumstances does not decrease the likelihood of vomiting, although it may decrease the volume. In fact, sips of water or juice may make the woman feel better, even if she continues to vomit, but she may require intravenous fluids for adequate hydration.

Taking in too much fluid orally or intravenously

On the other hand, there is evidence that forcing oral fluids beyond the amount a woman needs to quench her thirst—similar to an overload with hypotonic intravenous fluids—can cause overhydration and hyponatremia, with some of the same sequelac: prolonged second stage and associated interventions.[49] See Chapters 2 and 5, pages 34, 150–151, for more explanation.

Note regarding oral food and fluids in labor

A policy of withholding food and fluids from laboring women became widespread in North America and the United Kingdom in the 1940s and 1950s and remained until the 1980s. The policy was based on concerns over the dangers of general anesthesia for laboring women who had food in their stomachs, because they were more likely to vomit and aspirate the vomitus (food particles and gastric acid) while under general anesthesia. Fasting has not been proved to solve such problems; in fact, gastric secretions are actually more acidic and thus more damaging if aspirated than when the woman is not fasting. Safe anesthesia techniques appear to be the best safeguard against aspiration. Furthermore, the use of general anesthesia has been almost entirely replaced by epidural and spinal anesthesia (for cesareans).

The risks of withholding nourishment, especially during a long labor (ketosis, hypoglycemia, maternal hunger, and thirst), may be greater than the risks of general anesthesia for the low-risk woman. Digestion usually slows down by active labor and the woman has little appetite for food, although she will probably want to continue to drink fluids. For all these reasons, therefore, policies of "nothing by mouth," at least in early labor (and even for some oral fluids with epidural analgesia), have been relaxed, with some practitioners being more open than others to letting hunger and thirst guide the woman's intake throughout labor.

Caution *regarding overhydration with oral fluids:* Urging women to drink more than they voluntarily take may result in overhydration and subnormal sodium levels. Beverages should be provided when the woman requests and offered frequently during labor, but whether and how much she drinks should be regulated by the woman.[49]

5

Exhaustion

Fatigue or exhaustion, especially if the woman is upset or afraid, is a major concern for women experiencing long labors. Massage, music, dim light, aromatherapy, guided imagery, a bath, or whatever she finds soothing may relax her and help her accept the slow pace of her labor. Reassurance from a patient and empathic caregiver and/or doula can ease the woman's worry. Positions for tired women, shown in Figure 5.19, are more restful than others and may provide a welcome change.

Uterine lactic acidosis as a cause of inadequate contractions

Recent research studies indicate that in some women, occlusion of myometrial blood vessels during contractions may decrease tissue

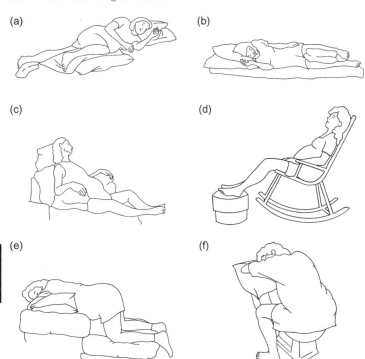

Fig. 5.19. Positions for tired women: (a) Semiprone. (b) Side–lying.
(c) Semi–sitting. (d) Sitting in a rocking chair. (e) Kneeling on foot of bed.
(f) Straddling a toilet.

oxygen levels and cause an accumulation of lactic acid in the myometrium. This local lactic acidosis (lowered pH in myometrial capil-
lary blood) and decreased oxygen saturation can decrease the intensity
and frequency of uterine contractions.[50] In such cases, augmentation
with oxytocin may exacerbate the lactic acidosis, and resting the
uterus (and the woman) may be more appropriate. Allowing the
contractions to space out temporarily may hasten the clearance of
lactic acid and the return of an efficient labor pattern. Further
research on the pathophysiology, prevention, and treatment of myometrial lactic acidosis is needed to clarify the contribution of this
condition to the cesarean rate. The potential benefits of identifying

women with lactic acidosis during dysfunctional labor and developing methods to reverse the condition should be investigated.

When the cause of inadequate contractions is unknown

Besides the techniques described in Chapter 2 (*Techniques to Elicit Stronger Contractions*), the following measures may lead to stronger contractions:

Breast stimulation

Used for centuries to start or augment labor, breast stimulation is frequently used by midwives and other low-intervention caregivers, especially in out-of-hospital settings. The caregiver asks the woman or her partner to lightly stroke one or both nipples or massage her breasts to increase oxytocin release, thus augmenting contractions. Other regimens include using a breast pump.[51] When nipple stimulation is used, it is important to monitor for fetal well-being and the possibility of excessive contractions. Only one small trial has compared breast stimulation to oxytocin for labor augmentation.[52] Because of methodologic problems, reliable conclusions regarding effectiveness could not be drawn. The other studies of breast stimulation investigated it as a method of conducting the Contraction Stress Test and as a method of inducing labor.[53] Case reports of nipple stimulation by high-risk women as part of a contraction stress test have described tetanic contractions. A Cochrane review comparing breast stimulation with no treatment for labor induction found that breast stimulation increased the chances that women would go into labor within 3 days if they had a favorable cervix when they initiated it.[53] Compared with oxytocin, breast stimulation had similar success rates for starting labor. Uterine hyperstimulation did not occur in the low-risk women in the reviewed trials. Breast stimulation for labor augmentation, as opposed to induction, has not been effectively studied, although it seems promising as a useful technique for slow labor progress.[51]

Walking and changes in position

Walking and position changes, including upright positions, improve the effectiveness of contractions and reduce the length of the first stage of labor by an average of 1 hour, without increasing intervention use or negative effects on either mother or baby. The freedom to move improves women's satisfaction with the birth experience.[39–41] Although the benefits of free movement seem modest and its effectiveness in speeding a slow labor is not established, for some women this apparently harmless practice improves their comfort and sense of control.

Acupressure or acupuncture

These traditional Eastern healing approaches may be used to stimulate more frequent contractions. Acupressure has been studied scientifically for its effects on labor pain and for its effects on labor progress. The trials indicated that acupressure lowers women's assessments of their pain, compared to control groups of women who received light skin stroking or no treatment except conversation.[54,55] Two trials reported significant decreases in the duration of first stage.[55,56] No harmful effects have been reported when it was used properly (see Chapter 10, pages 345–346, for instructions).

The use of acupuncture during labor requires specialized training for the midwife or consultation with a qualified acupuncturist. See Chapter 8 for specific information on acupuncture.

Hydrotherapy (baths and showers: Fig. 5.20)

Buoyancy, hydrostatic pressure, warmth, skin stimulation, and other factors induce relaxation, temporarily reduce pain awareness, and may reduce catecholamine production[57,58] and/or speed progress in active labor. Some of these benefits may be due to the relief of stress, tension, anxiety, or pain. For guidelines on the use of hydrotherapy, see Chapter 10, pages 332–337.

One randomized controlled trial compared usual labor augmentation procedures (amniotomy and/or oxytocin) with immersion in water for women diagnosed with dystocia. After up to 4 hours of immersion, the women in the bath group were reassessed for progress and, if there was no improvement in progress, they then were given the usual augmentation procedures. In the bath group, 29% needed no further augmentation, a significant reduction compared to the usual care group (96% of whom received usual augmentation).[59]

Timing of the bath may be important. As stated in Chapter 4, using the bath in early labor may slow the contractions, whereas using it in the active phase often speeds dilation.[57]

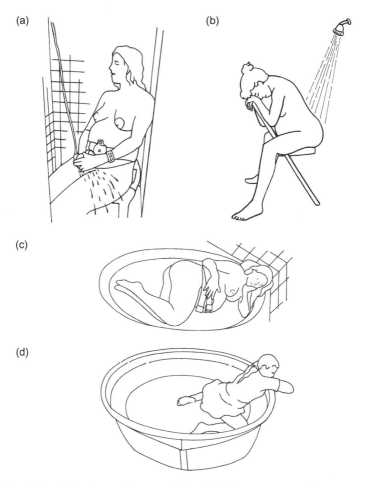

Fig. 5.20. Hydrotherapy to speed labor: (**a**) Shower on woman's abdomen. (**b**) Shower on woman's back. (**c**) Laboring in bath. (**d**) Laboring in birthing pool.

A recent Cochrane review reported that baths during the first stage of labor significantly reduce the use of epidural/spinal analgesia. Other proposed benefits from bathing during labor cannot be confirmed because of limited information for other outcomes. However, the reviewers found no evidence of increased adverse effects to the fetus/neonate or woman from laboring in water or waterbirth.[60]

In summary, contractions may be slowed or weakened by policies that restrict movement, withhold food or drink, raise maternal anxiety, overmedicate the woman, or medicate her too early in labor. A policy of prevention by avoiding such policies seems desirable, since the adverse effects are difficult to reverse with physiologic interventions. By giving priority to less risky comfort and labor progress measures, normality may be maintained; if not, then AROM and/or intravenous oxytocin and other obstetric interventions may become necessary.

IF THERE IS A PERSISTENT ANTERIOR CERVICAL LIP OR A SWOLLEN CERVIX

5

Position changes can often be used to reduce a persistent cervical lip (that is, a cervix that is fully dilated except for an anterior lip) or to reduce a swollen cervix, which may become increasingly edematous without treatment. A cervical lip is thought to be formed either by uneven pressure by the presenting part on the cervix or by the anterior cervix becoming caught between the fetal head and pubic arch. The following approaches may correct the problem.

Positions to reduce an anterior cervical lip or a swollen cervix

Often the woman seems to know what to do. When free to seek more comfortable positions, she is likely to choose a position that helps reduce the anterior lip or swelling. If that does not succeed, time and positions that reduce the pressure of the fetal head or pubic arch on the cervix seem to be the best methods to use. Gravity-neutral or anti-gravity positions, such as hands and knees, kneeling on a ball, or the open knee–chest position (Fig. 5.21), may move the fetal head away from the cervix and take off some of the pressure. Side-lying, semiprone, or standing positions (Fig. 5.22) redistribute the pressure on the cervix and may reduce a lip.

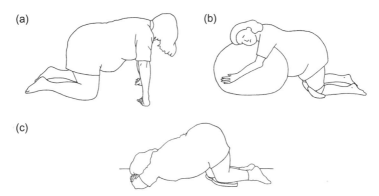

Fig. 5.21. (**a**) Hands and knees. (**b**) Kneeling with a ball and knee pads. (**c**) Open knee–chest position.

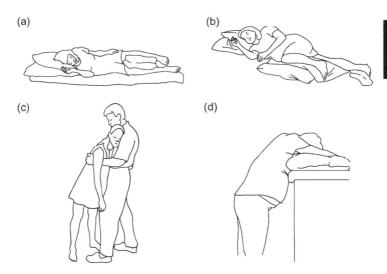

Fig. 5.22. (**a**) Side–lying. (**b**) Semiprone, lower arm forward. (**c**) Standing, leaning on partner. (**d**) Standing, leaning on counter.

Other methods

By immersion in deep water, the "weightlessness" and buoyancy reduce the effects of gravity and may relieve pressure on the cervix.

We are intrigued by suggestions in a holistic midwifery text for reducing swelling of the cervix by applying ice, evening primrose oil, or arnica directly on the cervix.[61] As is common with many complementary healing techniques, there are no published trials of these techniques. They merit scientific evaluation.

Manual reduction of a persistent cervical lip

Sometimes, if patience, position changes, or the bath do not succeed in reducing the lip, manual reduction may be warranted. The technique, used by many midwives, nurses, and physicians, is explained in Chapter 8 (pages 250–251).

IF EMOTIONAL DYSTOCIA IS SUSPECTED

The term "emotional dystocia" refers to dysfunctional labor caused by emotional distress and the resulting excessive production of catecholamines. High catecholamine levels can reduce the circulation to the uterus and placenta during labor, causing inefficient contractions and reduced fetal oxygenation. In addition, according to Michel Odent,[62,63] constant disturbance in a busy, strange environment, including noise, bright lights, conversation and questions to the mother, may make it difficult or impossible for the woman to relax mentally or physically. Such disturbances overly stimulate the neocortex, which prevents the woman from laboring instinctually. If the neocortex is calmed, the more "primitive" parts of the brain guide the labor process, as explained in Chapter 2. Chapter 2 also explains the psychobiological basis of emotional dystocia.

Assessing the woman's coping

Western cultural attitudes on coping with labor

Childbirth education programs first emerged in the 1940s, when much less was known about the powerful, multisensory ways in which women spontaneously cope with labor. Much has been learned since then, but older ideas have left their stamp on Western culture and seem to be reiterated endlessly by popular media. Many people still think that "coping well" means that the woman remains silent and does not move during contractions. Often, caregivers, partners, and the women themselves believe that women who are physically active and vocal are coping poorly, and they may strive to help these women to be quiet. However, we know now that women with kinesthetic and auditory coping styles often derive much more effective relief from pain and stress when they move and make sounds than when they try to use the quiet, still techniques of the early childbirth methods.

The essence of "coping" during the first stage of labor

When we look closely at active vocal women, we notice that some follow a rhythm and others vocalize irregularly and move jerkily, without rhythm. The women whose activities are rhythmic and repetitious are actually coping well, even though they may be loud and active.

Rhythm is the common element in coping during the first stage of labor, just as it is the key to success in physical endurance events and some kinds of meditation, yoga, and self-calming techniques. Rhythmic breathing, vocalizing, swaying, tapping, self-stroking—even rhythmic mental activities, such as counting breaths through a contraction, repeating a mantra or verse, or singing a song aloud or to herself—are all are examples of ways women use rhythm as a coping technique. Usually, by the time a woman is in active labor, she is no longer using techniques she was taught in prenatal classes, although these may have been helpful earlier. Rhythmic activities in active labor are unique and unplanned. They emerge spontaneously when women are not afraid and are not disturbed or restricted in their behavior. When women begin to develop these spontaneous rhythmic behaviors, the cognitive parts of their brains are less active and their behavior becomes more instinctual. In fact, women often express surprise later at the repetitive rhythmic behaviors they discovered during labor and at how effective they were.

Other spontaneous coping behaviors exhibited by these women include relaxation during and/or between contractions and routines, or "rituals," which are the repetition of the same rhythmic activities for many contractions in a row. Coping rituals often involve other people (the partner, doula, or someone else); the mother wants them to continue doing the same comforting behaviors with each contraction. They may hold her, stroke or sway with her, speak to her or moan softly in her rhythm, and help her regain her rhythm if she loses it. These three coping mechanisms—relaxation, rhythm, and ritual—are referred to as the 3 Rs. They constitute the essence of coping during the first stage of labor.

The caregiver, in assessing the woman's well-being during labor, should observe her coping behavior. If she has rhythm in whatever she is doing, she is coping; if she has lost her rhythm, she needs help to regain it. See also pages 166–167, *If the source of the woman's anxiety cannot be identified,* for more on assessing the woman's emotional state.

In summary, "coping well" during labor and birth often includes instinctive vocalization, movement, and self-comforting behavior. During the first stage, relaxation, rhythm, and ritual (the 3 Rs) represent good signs of coping.

5   Indicators of emotional dystocia during active labor

A woman experiencing emotional dystocia may do some of the following:

- express or display fear, anxiety, or exhaustion
- lack rhythm and ritual in her responses to contractions
- ask many questions, or remain very alert to her surroundings
- exhibit very "needy" behavior
- display extreme modesty
- exhibit strong reactions to mild contractions or to examinations
- show a high degree of muscle tension
- appear demanding, distrustful, angry, or resentful toward staff
- seem hypervigilant, highly alert, "jumpy," or easily startled
- exhibit a strong need for control over caregivers' actions
- seem "out of control" in labor (in extreme pain, writhing, panicked, screaming, unresponsive to suggestions or questions intended to help)
- express fear that she will lose control as labor becomes more intense

Alternately, she may not exhibit any external behaviors that would lead one to consider emotional dystocia. (See Chapter 4, pages 112–113, and Chapter 10, pages 350–354, for ways to discover whether fear or anxiety may be contributing to the dystocia.)

Predisposing factors for emotional dystocia

Whatever are the woman's fears or anxieties, she probably cannot simply "snap out of it." Her emotional state results partly from pre-existing factors, which may include:

- previous difficult births
- previous traumatic hospitalizations
- childhood abuse or neglect: physical, sexual, or emotional (see page 164 on the impact of sexual abuse on childbearing women)
- dysfunctional family of origin (mental illness, substance abuse, fighting by parents, or other family problems)
- fears about current serious health problems for herself or her baby
- domestic violence (previous or present)
- cultural factors, including beliefs leading to extreme shame when viewed nude or when viewed in labor by men or when behaving in a way that is contrary to cultural expectations
- language barriers, or inability to hear or understand what is happening or being done
- substance abuse by the woman
- death of her own mother (especially in childbirth or at a young age)
- beliefs resulting from what she has been told about labor (for example, the woman whose sibling was handicapped by a "birth injury" or whose mother had a "terrible time" giving birth to her)

Helping the woman state her fears

Of course, maternity professionals are not expected to provide psychotherapy. On the other hand, addressing the woman's concerns by asking a few sensitive questions between contractions may help the woman state her fears and allow those around her to give more effective care: "What was going through your mind during that contraction?" or "How are you feeling right now?" or "Do you have any idea why your labor is slowing down?" She may indicate any of the following common fears or others, which could interfere with labor progress:

- exhaustion
- dread of increasing pain
- fear of damage or disfigurement to her own body, including stretching, episiotomy, tears, stitching, or a cesarean, and "never being the same again"
- fear of uterine rupture, if she has had a cesarean before
- fear that labor will harm her baby (a belief that a cesarean is safer and easier for the baby)
- fear of loss of control, of modesty, or of dignity; "acting like a fool" or "losing face" (shame)
- fear of invasive procedures, such as vaginal exams, injections, blood tests, or others
- fear of her caregivers, many or all of whom may be unknown to her (She may perceive them as strangers who have power and authority over her.)
- fear of being unable to care for her baby adequately, of being a "terrible mother"
- fear of abandonment by the baby's father, her caregiver, or others
- fear of dying [*Note*: A brief transient period of fear of dying in the late first stage, associated with a surge of catecholamines and the "fetal ejection reflex" (see page 30) is not unusual, and it is not associated with dystocia.[63] A deep prolonged persistent fear throughout pregnancy and labor is what we are referring to here.

It is important to acknowledge that most women have some fear or anxiety about labor, birth, and the impact of a new child on their lives. This does not mean that all those women will have labor dystocia. For some women, however, emotional issues are powerful enough to interfere with an efficient labor pattern. Being able to recognize and help those women may reduce the negative impact of emotional distress. In any case, your sensitivity and attentiveness will contribute to a woman's sense of being cared for and cared about.

How to help a laboring woman in distress

After having identified (or having guessed) the woman's fears, it may be helpful to do some or all of the following:

- Provide language interpreters and culturally competent or culturally sensitive caregivers, if needed.
- Restate what she has said to check that you understand ("It sounds as if you're afraid of what the labor might do to your baby. Is that right?"). If the woman confirms this, then:
  - Validate her fear, rather than dismissing it. "Yes, other women have told me they worried about that, too" or "That must be frightening. We're also concerned about babies during labor and that's why we check your baby's heartbeat frequently."
  - Provide reassuring information (but not empty promises). "As I listen to his heartbeat, he sounds just fine right now. Would you like to know how babies adapt to contractions during labor? They have some really amazing coping mechanisms."

- Observe her affect and behavior during conversations and elicit further concerns or needs.
- Between contractions, let her know that after the baby is born, there are helpful resources available to her (and follow up with this information later). For example, if the woman is worried about being an inadequate mother, she might be relieved to know there are parenting classes and support groups and a hotline she can call for help at any time, day or night. Helping her recognize that labor is not the time to address her fears about parenthood, while also reassuring her that she will not be alone with her concerns, may ease her anxiety enough that labor progress will resume. Perhaps calming her conscious fears will help her enter a more relaxed state in which the "primitive" parts of her brain will predominate and promote the labor process.
- Provide ideas (nonjudgmentally) that the woman can use to alter the situation. If the woman feels "helpless" lying down, she might feel stronger if she is standing up and active.
- Visualization and reframing can be powerful tools to help a woman overcome her fear. For example, if she expresses concern about her "poor baby's head being forced through that tiny tight opening," she can be helped to imagine her "little baby nuzzling his head down in that soft stretchy place" (describing her ripe cervix and vagina as being as soft and stretchy, like the inside of her cheek when she presses inside it with her tongue).

- If the woman is unable to cope with overwhelming physical sensations, she may benefit from massage, hydrotherapy, or pain medication.

Chart 5.4 summarizes ways to help women when emotional distress is a likely cause of dystocia. See the following for a summary of the special needs of childhood abuse survivors.

Special needs of childhood abuse survivors[64]

A woman who was sexually or physically abused as a child may have great anxieties in labor, especially related to:

- invasive procedures that remind her of the abuse, such as: vaginal exams, instruments and fingers placed in the vagina, blood draws, or intravenous lines
- lack of control: as a child she was hurt when she was out of control and vulnerable. She may have learned never to lose control
- modesty, nakedness, exposure issues
- powerful authority figures (midwives, nurses, doctors) who know more than she and who do painful things to her: as a child she was a victim of those with authority over her.
- being asked to "relax, surrender, or yield to the contractions" with the promise that it will not hurt so much: she may have been told similar things during the abuse
- pushing her baby out of her vagina: the pain and prospect of damage may remind her of sexual abuse

Sometimes an abuse survivor seems difficult or demanding when she responds very emotionally or angrily in the above situations. It is important that the caregiver does not take her reaction personally and keeps in mind that the woman has very good reason to react the way she does but also that the caregiver is not the reason. If a caregiver observes some of the behaviors listed above, she or he should suspect a history of sexual or another type of abuse and try to be patient and kind, to listen to her, and to meet her special needs to the extent possible, even if they seem unusual or unreasonable. If she feels emotionally safe, her labor may progress more normally, and she may reap other psychological benefits as well.

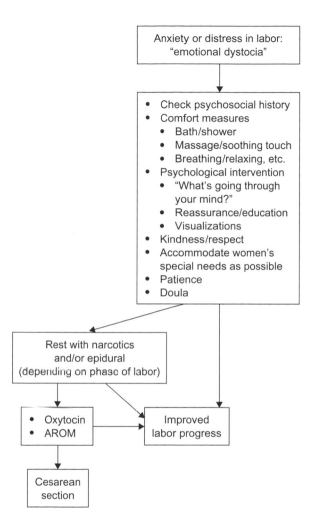

Chart 5.4. Anxiety or distress in labor.

Incompatibility or poor relationship with staff

If the woman has developed a poor relationship with any staff member, it will help to have a discussion with the staff member or with that person's superior regarding the specific concerns or differences of opinion. Sometimes all the woman needs is to be listened to, respected, and taken seriously, so that she may be more able to trust the people around her. Perhaps the staff will be able to make some compromises in their usual routines in order to meet her needs, while still accomplishing those clinical tasks that are essential to basic safety.

Sometimes the simplest solution, once the woman discovers that she and her assigned nurse or midwife are incompatible, is to change to someone else to provide a fresh start in the relationship. There is no need to lay blame, only to recognize the incompatibility and to do something about it. (*Note:* This is less likely to be a problem where a policy of "continuity of caregiver" is in place, as it is in some parts of the United Kingdom.)

If it is possible to anticipate these difficulties before labor, it makes sense to suggest that this patient be assigned to a particularly diplomatic or understanding midwife or nurse and that the woman bring a doula (professional labor support person) with her in labor. The doula can provide extra psychological support to relieve the burden on the caregiver.

If the source of the woman's anxiety cannot be identified

Sometimes a caregiver cannot understand why the labor is not going well. All the physical factors seem normal, and the woman does not exhibit any particular psychosocial problems. It sometimes helps to wait until after a contraction and ask her, "Could you tell me what was going through your mind during that contraction?" If necessary, ask, "Anything else?" The answer she gives may be a clue to her emotional state. For example, if she responds, "I am just trying to do the breathing and relaxation I learned in childbirth class," it is clear that she is coping and should be encouraged to continue the self-comforting measures. If, however, she says she is afraid or feels helpless or that it hurts terribly or that she cannot do it much longer, she is obviously in distress and needs more emotional support. The caregiver can help (in culturally appropriate ways) by acknowledging her distress, reassuring her, addressing her fear, holding her hand, and helping her and her partner with some self-comforting measures (see Chapter 2). One notable study found that women who expressed distress in early labor were more likely to have longer labors, more fetal distress, and all the interventions that go along with these problems.[65] If emotional distress can be identified and alleviated early in labor with extra support, reassurance, encouragement, and assistance, these damaging effects of distress may be prevented.

In summary, the psychoemotional factors that influence labor progress are less well understood than the physical factors, but they may be as important. Try to remain sensitive to this aspect of childbirth. Your influence on the mind–body connection in labor may be greater than you think.

CONCLUSION

Labor progress may slow in active labor for a variety of reasons. We have provided guidelines for determining the possible cause. When mother and fetus are faring well, interventions or actions specific to the cause may be used to address the problem. Sometimes more than one cause exists for a problem, and several measures are appropriate.

REFERENCES

1. O'Driscoll K, Meagher D, Boylan P. (1993). Active Management of Labour (Vol. 2). London, Mosby–Year Book Europe.
2. Friedman E. (1995). Dystocia and "failure to progress" in labor. In Flamm BL, Quilligan EJ, editors. Cesarean Section: Guidelines for Appropriate Utilization. New York, Springer-Verlag.
3. Sweet B, Tiran D, editors. (2009). Mayes' Midwifery: A Textbook for Midwives, 13th edition. London, Bailliere Tindall.
4. Enkin M, Keirse M, Neilsen J, Crowther C, Dulet L, Hodnett E, et al. (2000). Monitoring the progress of labour. In A Guide to Effective Care in Pregnancy and Childbirth, 3rd edition. New York, Oxford University Press.
5. Zhang J, Troendle J, Yancey M. (2002). Reassessing the labor curve in nulliparous women. Am J Obstet Gynecol 187(4), 824–828.
6. Satin A. (2009). Abnormal labor protraction and arrest disorders. In Basow D, editor. Waltham, MA, UpToDate.

7. Albers L, Schiff M, Gorwoda J. (1996). The length of active labor in normal pregnancies. Obstet Gynecol 87(3), 355–359.
8. Page L, editor. (2000). The New Midwifery: Science and Sensitivity in Practice. Edinburgh, Churchill Livingstone.
9. Foley M, Alarab M, Daly L, Keane D, Rath A, O'Herlihy C. (2004). The continuing effectiveness of active management of first labor, despite a doubling in overall nulliparous cesarean delivery. Am J Obstet Gynecol 191(3), 891–895.
10. Sinclair C. (2004). A Midwife's Handbook. St. Louis: Saunders.
11. Sutton J. (2001). Let Birth Be Born Again: Rediscovering and Reclaiming Our Midwifery Heritage. Bedfont, Middlesex, UK, Birth Concepts.
12. King J. (1993). Back Labor No More!! What Every Woman Should Know before Labor. Dallas, TX, Plenary Systems.
13. Simkin P. (2010). The fetal occiput posterior position: State of the science and a new perspective. Birth 37(1), 61–71.
14. Lieberman E, Davidson K, Lee-Parritz A, Shearer E. (2005). Changes in fetal position during labor and their association with epidural analgesia. Obstet Gynecol 105(5 pt 1), 974–982.
15. Gardberg MEL, Salevaara M. (1998). Intrapartum sonography and persistent occiput posterior position: A study of 408 deliveries. Obstet Gynecol 91(5 pt 1), 746–749.
16. Ponkey S, Cohen A, Heffner L, Liberman E. (2003). Persistent fetal occiput posterior position: Obstetric outcomes. Obstet Gynecol 101(5 pt 1), 915–920.
17. Varney H. (2003). Varney's Midwifery, 4th edition. Boston, Jones Bartlett.
18. Hofmeyr G. (2004). Obstructed labor: Using better technologies to reduce mortality. Int J Gynecol Obstet 85(Suppl 1), S62–S72.
19. Sherer D, Miodovnik M, Bradley K, Langer O. (2002) Intrapartum fetal head position, I: Comparison between transvaginal digital examination and transabdominal ultrasound assessment during the active stage of labor. Ultrasound Obstet Gynecol 19(3), 258–263.
20. Akmal S, Tsoi E, Kametas N, et al. (2002). Intrapartum sonography to determine fetal head position. J Matern Fetal Neonat Med 12(3), 172–177.
21. Souka A, Haritos T, Basayiannis K, et al. (2003). Intrapartum ultrasound for the examination of the fetal head position in normal and obstructed labor. J Matern Fetal Neonat Med 13(1), 59–63.
22. Nizard J, Haberman S, Paltieli Y, et al. (2009). Determination of fetal head station and position during labor: A new technique that combines

ultrasound and position-tracking system. Am J Obstet Gynecol 404.e401–e405.

23. Sherer D, Miodovnik M, Bradley K, Langer O. Intrapartum fetal head position, II: comparison between transvaginal digital examination and transabdominal ultrasound assessment during the second stage of labor. Ultrasound Obstet Gynecol 19, 264–268.

24. Dupuis O, Ruimark S, Corinne D, et al. (2005). Fetal head position during the second stage of labor: Comparison of digital vaginal examination and transabdominal ultrasonographic examination. Eur J Obstet Gynecol Reprod Biol 123(2), 193–197.

25. Akmal S, Kametas N, Tsoi E, et al. (2003). Comparison of transvaginal digital examination with intrapartum sonography to determine fetal head position before instrumental delivery. Ultrasound Obstet Gynecol 21(5), 437–440.

26. Kreiser, D, Schiff E, Lipitz S, et al. (2001). Determination of fetal occiput position by ultrasound during the second stage of labor. J Matern Fetal Med 10(4), 283–286.

27. Chou M, Kreiser D, Taslimi M, et al. (2004). Vaginal versus ultrasound examination of fetal occiput position during the second stage of labor. Am J Obstet Gynecol 191(2), 521–524.

28. Wei S, Wo B, Xu H, Luo Z, Roy C, Fraser W. (2009). Early amniotomy and early oxytocin for prevention of, or therapy for, delay in first stage spontaneous labour compared with routine care. Cochrane Database Syst Rev (2)CD006794. doi: 006710.001002/14651858.CD14006794.pub2.

29. Schwarcz R, Diaz A, Belizan J, Fescina R, Caldeyro-Barcia R. (1976). Gynecology and Obstetrics, Proceedings of the VIII World Congress of Gynecology and Obstetrics, Mexico City, October 17–22, 1976. New York, Amsterdam Excerpta Medica.

30. Cheng Y, Shaffer B, Caughey A. (2006). Associated factors and outcomes of persistent occiput posterior position: A retrospective cohort study from 1976 to 2001. J Matern Fetal Neonat Med 19(9), 563–568.

31. Fraser W, Vendittelli F, Krauss I, Breart G. (1998). Effects of early augmentation of labour with amniotomy and oxytocin in nulliparous women: A meta-analysis. Br J Obstet Gynaecol 105, 189–194.

32. Hofmeyr G. (2004) Obstructed labor: Using better technologies to reduce mortality. Int J Gynecol Obstet 85(Suppl 1):S62–S72.

33. Michel S, Rake A, Treiber K, Seifert B, Chaoui R, Huch R, et al. (2002). MR obstetric pelvimetry: Effect of birthing position on pelvic bony dimensions. AJR Am J Roentgenol, 179, 1063–1067.

5

34. Simkin P. (2003). Maternal positions and pelves revisited. Birth 30(2), 130–132.

35. Stremler R, Hodnet E, Petryshen P, Stevens B, Weston J, Willan A. (2005). Randomized controlled trial of hands-and-knees positioning for occiput posterior position in labor. Birth 32(4), 243–251.

36. Scott P. (2003). Sit Up and Take Notice! Positioning Yourself for a Better Birth. Tauranga, New Zealand: Great Scott Publications.

37. Tully G. (2010) Belly Mapping. (Condensed by author from Belly Mapping: How Kicks and Wiggles Reveal Fetal Position.) Bloomington, MN, Maternity House Publishing. www.spinningbabies.com/baby-positions/belly-mapping.

38. Fenwick L, Simkin P. (1987). Maternal position to prevent or alleviate dystocia in labor. Clin Obstet Gynecol 30(1), 83–89.

39. Roberts J. (1989). Maternal position during the first stage of labour. In Chalmers I, Enkin M, Keirse M, editors. Effective Care in Pregnancy and Childbirth (Vol. 2). Oxford, Oxford University Press.

40. Simkin P, O'Hara M. (2002). Nonpharmacologic relief of pain during labor: Systematic reviews of five methods. Am J Obstet Gynecol 186(5 Suppl Nat), S131–S159.

41. Lawrence A, Lewis Hofmeyr G, Dowswell T, Styles C. (2009). Maternal positions and mobility during first stage labour. Cochrane Database Syst Rev (2)CD003934. doi: 003910.001002/14651858.CD14003934.pub14651852

42. Lieberman E, O'Donoghue C. (2002). Unintended effects of epidural analgesia during labor: A systematic review. Am J Obstet Gynecol 186(5 Suppl Nat), S31–S68.

43. Leighton B, Halpern S. (2002). The effects of epidural analgesia on labor, maternal, and neonatal outcomes: A systematic review. Am J Obstet Gynecol 186(5 Suppl Nat), S69–S77.

44. DeClerq E, Sakala C, Corry M, Applebaum S, Risher P. (2002). Listening to Mothers: Report of the First National U.S. Survey of Women's Childbearing Experiences. New York, Maternity Center Association, Harris Interactive.

45. Chalmers B, Dzakpasu S, Heaman M, Kaczorowski J. (2008). The Canadian maternity experiences survey: An overview of findings. J Obstet Gynaecol Can 30(3), 217–228.

46. The Information Centre for Health and Social Care. (2009). NHS Maternity Statistics, 2008–2009. Retrieved February 13, 2010, from http://www.ic.nhs.uk/pubs/maternity0809

47. Smith L. (2010). Impact of Birthing Practices on Breastfeeding, 2nd edition. Boston, Jones Bartlett.

48. Enkin M, Keirse M, Neilsen J, Crowther C, Dulet L, Hodnett E, et al. (2000). Monitoring the progress of labour. In A Guide to Effective Care in Pregnancy and Childbirth, 3rd edition. New York, Oxford University Press.

49. Moen V, Brudin L, Rundgren M, Irestedt L. (2009). Hyponatremia complicating labour—rare or unrecognised? A prospective observational study. Br J Obstet Gynaecol 116(4), 552–561.

50. Quenby S, Pierce S, Brigham S, Wray S. (2004). Dysfunctional labor and myometrial lactic acidosis. Obstet Gynecol 103(4), 718–723.

51. Razgaitis E, Lyvers A. (2009). Management of protracted active labor with nipple stimulation: A viable tool for midwives? J Womens Health 55(1), 65–69.

52. Curtis P, Resnick J, Evens S, Thompson C. (1999). A comparison of breast stimulation and intravenous oxytocin for the augmentation of labor. Birth 26(2), 115–122.

53. Kavanaugh J, Kelly A, Thomas J. (2005). Breast stimulation for cervical ripening and induction of labour. Cochrane Database Syst Rev (3) CD003392. doi:003310.001002/14651858.CD14003392.pub14651852 (assessed as up to date in September 2009).

54. Chung U, Hung L, Kuo S, Huang C. (2003). Effects of LI4 and BL 67 acupressure on labor pain and uterine contractions in the first stage of labor. J Nurs Res 11(4), 251–260.

55. Lee M, Chang S, Kang D. (2004). Effects of SP6 acupressure on labor pain and length of delivery time in women during labor. J Altern Complement Med 10(6), 959–965.

56. Kashanian M, Shahali S. (2009). Effects of acupressure at the Sanyinjiao point (SP6) on the process of active phase of labor in nulliparas women. J Matern Fetal Neonat Med (Sep 15), 1–4 [Epub ahead of print].

57. Odent M. (1997). Can water immersion stop labor? J Nurs Midwif 42(5), 414–416.

58. Grossman E, Goldstein D, Hoffman S, Wacks I, Epstein M. (1992). Effects of water immersion on sympathoadrenal and dopamine systems in humans. Am J Physiol 262(6), R993–R999.

59. Cluett E, Pickering R, Getliffe K, Saunders N. (2004). Randomized controlled trial of labouring in water compared with standard of augmentation of dystocia in first stage of labour. BMJ 328(314), doi:10.1136/bmj.37963.606412.EE.

5

60. Cluett E, Burns E. (2009). Immersion in water in labour and birth. Cochrane Database of Syst Rev (2)CD000111. doi:000110.001002/14651858.CD14000111pub14651853.

61. Frye A. (2004) Holistic Midwifery: A Comprehensive Textbook for Midwives in Homebirth Practice. Volume 2, Care During Labor and Birth. Portland, OR, Labrys Press.

62. Odent M. (1999). Birth reborn, Chapter 6. In The Scientification of Love. London, Free Association Books.

63. Odent M. (1992). The Nature of Birth and Breastfeeding. Westport, CT, Bergin Garvey.

64. Simkin P, Klaus P. (2004). When Survivors Give Birth: Understanding and Healing the Effects of Early Sexual Abuse on Childbearing Women. Seattle, Classic Day Publishing.

65. Wuitchik M, Bakal D, Lipshitz J. (1989). The clinical significance of pain and cognitive activity in latent labor. Obstet Gynecol 73(1), 35–41.

5

Chapter 6

Prolonged Second Stage of Labor

Penny Simkin, BA, PT, CCE, CD(DONA),
and Ruth Ancheta, BA, ICCE, CD(DONA)

Definitions of the second stage of labor, 174
Phases of the second stage of labor, 174
The latent phase of the second stage, 174
The active phase of the second stage, 177
Physiologic effects of prolonged breath-holding and straining, 178
If the woman has an epidural, 182
How long an active phase of second stage is too long? 186
Possible etiologies and solutions for second-stage dystocia, 188
Maternal positions and other strategies for suspected occiput posterior or
    persistent occiput transverse fetuses, 188
Manual interventions to reposition the occiput posterior fetus, 200
Early interventions for suspected persistent asynclitism, 200
If cephalopelvic disproportion or macrosomia ("poor fit") is suspected, 205
Positions for "possible cephalopelvic disproportion" in second stage, 206
Shoulder dystocia, 214
If contractions are inadequate, 215
If emotional dystocia is suspected, 215
The essence of coping during the second stage of labor, 215
Conclusion, 219
References, 219

6

The Labor Progress Handbook: Early Interventions to Prevent and Treat Dystocia.
Edited by Penny Simkin, Ruth Ancheta
© 2011 by Penny Simkin and Ruth Ancheta; illustrations copyright Ruth Ancheta

DEFINITIONS OF THE SECOND STAGE OF LABOR

By definition, the second stage of labor begins with complete dilation of the cervix and ends with the birth of the baby. The clinical significance of complete dilation is controversial. There are two basic schools of thought regarding the conduct of the second stage. One, which has dominated North American obstetrics for many years, is based on a desire for a speedy delivery and calls for the woman to commence maximal breath-holding and bearing-down (pushing) efforts when she is discovered to be fully dilated, even though her urge to push may occur before or after complete dilation. If the urge to push occurs before complete dilation, the woman is told to resist pushing by panting throughout each contraction (see pages 144–146 for further discussion of what to do with a premature urge to push). If the urge to push is not present when the woman is completely dilated, the desire for a speedy delivery may lead the caregiver to exhort her to begin pushing.

This approach has largely given way to a less hurried approach, in which being completely dilated, in itself, is not believed to be sufficient reason to begin pushing. Rather, the conduct of second stage is based on complete dilation plus involuntary expulsive efforts (an urge to push). This approach has a basis in physiology since, in the normal course of events, contractions sometimes decrease temporarily around the time of full dilation. This approach has always been followed in Europe and other parts of the world. With this less-hurried approach, the woman begins actively pushing later and pushes less than with the former approach.

PHASES OF THE SECOND STAGE OF LABOR

The second stage of labor can be divided into phases (the latent phase and the active phase), just as is the first stage. Each phase represents different maternal behaviors and different physiologic accomplishments.

The latent phase of the second stage

An apparent lull in uterine activity around the time of complete dilation is frequently observed and is sometimes referred to as the "latent phase of the second stage"[1] or the "resting phase."[2] There are no reports of the frequency with which a noticeable lull actually occurs, although it is a phenomenon widely recognized by maternity professionals. How and why it occurs are not fully understood, but there are interesting hypotheses.

Let us review what happens to the uterus during the first stage of labor (Fig. 6.1). During most of the first stage, the uterus is tightly wrapped around the fetus. Uterine contractions in the first stage not only dilate the cervix but also shorten the uterine muscle fibers, and these actions gradually reduce the intrauterine space and press the fetus down.

The last 2 cm of dilation are accompanied by cervical retraction around the head (or presenting part) and the beginnings of descent of the head into the vaginal canal.[3,4]

The fetal head represents 25% to 30% of its entire body. Simkin's hypothesis suggests that when the head (representing one fourth of the contents of the uterus) slips through the cervix, the uterine muscle slackens because it is no longer tightly stretched around the entire fetus, and the intrauterine space must now shrink to "catch up" with the fetus.[1]

(a)   (b)   (c)

6

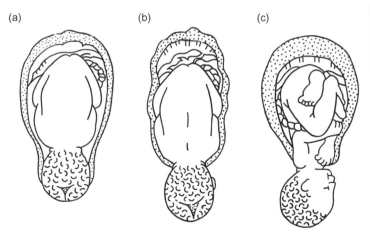

Fig. 6.1. Latent phase of second stage. Fetal head slips through cervix, and uterine muscle slackens. Uterine muscle fibers shorten until the uterus is once again tightly wrapped around fetal trunk. (**a**) Fetus in uterus at full dilation. (**b**) Head out of uterus, which slackens. (**c**) Uterus shortened and thickened around fetal torso.

This "catching up" consists of shortening of the uterine muscle fibers (as happened gradually in the first stage), further reducing the intrauterine space until once again the uterine muscle is tightly wrapped around the fetal trunk. This may take minutes or longer, during which the woman's contractions are weak or unnoticeable, and the woman may doze. The contractions resume and the woman experiences an increasingly powerful urge to push, accompanied by a documented spurt in oxytocin release.[5-7] Only some women, however, experience such a lull. Fetal position and station may be two of the factors that determine whether, when, and how long the woman will experience a resting phase.

This hypothesis is consistent with our knowledge of uterine physiology in labor, with Friedman's classic observations of normal labor progress, and with the numerous observational studies of maternal spontaneous bearing-down efforts that document an increasing urge to push and greater spontaneous bearing-down efforts with time and descent of the presenting part.[8,9]

A second hypothesis to explain the rest early in the second stage is offered by Roberts as follows.[10] During the latent phase, contractions continue and are measurable by electronic monitoring, although they may be below the threshold of the woman's awareness. These cause fetal rotation, alignment, and descent. Women exhibit less pain and distress than earlier in labor because of the retraction of the cervix around the descending fetal head, as described by Friedman.[3] Women begin to experience involuntary bearing-down efforts once the fetal head is at a +1 station and has rotated to occiput anterior and the contractions have achieved and maintained an intensity of 30 mm Hg.

Asking women to push during the latent phase of the second stage

During the latent phase, when uterine activity is markedly reduced, the fetal heart tones usually remain reassuring. With no interventions at all, powerful pushing contractions usually resume within 5 to 30 minutes. During the latent phase, the woman gets some rest, her spirits rise, and she begins to look forward to delivering her child.

Caregivers who subscribe to the approach of speeding the delivery sometimes misinterpret the latent phase to mean labor has slowed down and make efforts to speed the second stage, by enlisting the woman's maximal bearing-down efforts, which are exhausting and nonproductive because of the absence of adequate contractions or an urge to push, or by ordering intravenous Oxytocin (Pitocin) to augment uterine contractions. Although widely used to augment labor, Oxytocin is not free from potential adverse effects, such as tetanic contractions and fetal intolerance of labor, leading to increased reliance on cesarean deliveries.[11,12]

These unnecessary interventions are less likely to be used by those who recognize and are patient with the distinct phases of the second stage. In an unanesthetized woman with an uncomplicated labor, her uncontrollable urge to push is usually the best indicator of when she should begin bearing down spontaneously.[13,14]

What if the latent phase of the second stage persists?

If the lull in uterine activity persists for more than 20 or 30 minutes, the caregiver may continue monitoring and waiting or may initiate measures to bring on contractions and an urge to push. See page 180. These measures may include a change in the woman's position to sitting upright (in bed or on the toilet, pages 284–289), squatting (pages 297–299), or walking (page 315); "trial" expulsive efforts (breath-holding and bearing down) by the woman; acupressure (pages 345–346); and nipple stimulation (pages 15, 153, 244–245).

Many professionals now await evidence of an urge to push before checking the woman's cervix. By doing so, they are less likely to perceive second stage as prolonged. They prefer the two-fold definition of second stage: complete dilation plus spontaneous expulsive efforts.

The active phase of the second stage

The active phase of the second stage is characterized by an involuntary urge to push and descent of the fetus. It is sometimes referred to as the "pelvic division" of labor,[3] the "press period,"[15] or the descent phase.[1] The woman's contractions, her expulsive efforts, her body positions, and fetal efforts are the forces that combine to bring about the delivery. Recent research regarding expulsive efforts (positions, breathing, bearing down) for second stage has resulted in some new thinking about how women should push and the role of clinical personnel in assisting the woman at this time.

Directed expulsive efforts

Just how a woman should "push" is the subject of some disagreement among caregivers. According to one school of thought, the woman should remain horizontal, that is, flat on her back, in a semireclining position or lying on her side. When the contraction begins, she is to draw her legs up and curl her body, take a deep breath, hold it, and strain (bear down) maximally for at least 10 seconds. Then she is to release her breath, quickly take another, and repeat this routine until the contraction ends. The caregiver actively, enthusiastically, and sometimes loudly directs these efforts.

This technique of maximal maternal effort was devised by natural childbirth advocates in the 1950s as a way to overcome the antigravity effects of the mandatory lithotomy position and to deliver the baby quickly enough to avoid forceps.[16] It was incorporated into obstetric, nursing, and midwifery practices and continues to be a widespread practice today. There are problems with this approach, however.

Physiologic effects of prolonged breath-holding and straining

6

Physiologic effects of prolonged breath-holding and straining on the woman

Prolonged breath-holding and straining lead to a closed pressure system in her chest, which leads to the following chain of events:

- decreases in venous return, cardiac output
- lowering of maternal arterial blood pressure
- an increase in peripheral stasis of blood in her head, face, arms, and legs. Her face reddens, and if an intravenous line is in place, blood often backs up in the intravenous catheter
- a decrease in maternal blood oxygen levels and blood flow to the placenta
- an increase in maternal carbon dioxide levels until she gasps for air
- a sudden increase in her blood pressure as she gasps for air, causing bursting of tiny blood vessels in the whites of her eyes, face, neck, and eyes (petechial hemorrhages)

- rapid distention of the vaginal canal and pelvic musculature, along with stretching of supportive ligaments, leading to perineal trauma and possible urinary stress incontinence
- maternal exhaustion
- lactic acidosis
- longer pushing time[15]

These effects are well tolerated by young healthy women but may present risks for older or high-risk women and those with residual pelvic floor weakness, especially if such efforts are required for several hours. Perineal damage is increased (denervation, muscle damage, later incontinence) when women bear down forcefully in unfavorable positions.[15,17]

Physiologic effects of prolonged breath-holding and straining on the fetus

Nonreassuring fetal heart rate patterns sometimes occur when the woman holds her breath for prolonged periods and her straining may increase fetal head compression. If such bearing-down efforts are combined with a dorsal position, supine hypotension may exacerbate the nonreassuring heart rate patterns. The decreases in maternal blood pressure, blood oxygen content, and placental blood flow cause a decrease in the oxygen available to the fetus (fetal hypoxia and acidosis).[18,19] These effects are well tolerated by a healthy, well-nourished term fetus but may distress the fetus who is pre-term, small for gestational age, or already compromised earlier in labor or is experiencing cord compression.

Furthermore, such a bearing-down technique, while it may slightly shorten the second stage compared with spontaneous bearing-down efforts, is not associated with better neonatal outcomes.[18,19]

Spontaneous expulsive efforts

Observational studies of women's behavior in the second stage reveal that women who are not directed in pushing will breathe more and bear down less during second stage contractions than will women who are directed to use prolonged maximal bearing-down efforts.[8,9] Also, undirected women change positions more.[15,20] With spontaneous bearing down in various positions, the undesirable side effects of both prolonged maximal breath-holding and the supine position do not occur.

If a woman is not required to push in a prescribed manner or in a prescribed position, she may use a number of positions (side-lying, semireclining, standing, a supported squat, hands and knees, kneeling on one or both knees, or squatting). She may hold her breath, moan, or even bellow during the contractions.[21]

Most women experience an involuntary urge to push that comes and goes several times during each contraction. Their spontaneous bearing-down efforts last approximately 5 to 7 seconds, with several breaths between bearing-down efforts.[1,8–10,13–15,22] As the second stage progresses and the fetus descends, the woman's spontaneous bearing-down efforts usually become more forceful and more frequent.[8]

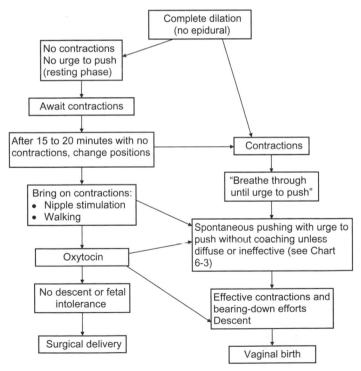

Chart 6.1.   Spontaneous bearing down.

The caregiver's role is different when the woman is pushing spontaneously in physiologic positions than when she is expected to push maximally in a supine position. In the former, the caregiver encourages and praises the woman's efforts and reassures her that her sensations are normal. The caregiver emphasizes the value of relaxing her perineum rather than holding her breath or pushing to a count of 10. Chart 6.1 illustrates the caregiver's step-by-step approach to bearing-down (pushing) efforts once dilation is complete.

Diffuse pushing

Sometimes the woman's spontaneous pushing is unfocused, or "diffuse," and may result in little progress (Chart 6.2). It is almost as if all her effort has no single direction. Such diffuse pushing seems to occur when the woman's eyes are tightly closed, and there may be little or no apparent progress after 20 or 30 minutes. If she is making progress with diffuse pushing, there is no reason to intervene, unless she seems distressed. If she is not making progress, the caregiver should first encourage the woman to change positions (see Toolkit, Chapter 9, for positions for second stage)—perhaps to a gravity-enhancing position. This often helps her to focus and push more effectively. If not, the caregiver should instruct the woman to open her eyes and direct her gaze (and her bearing down efforts) toward her vagina, and think about pressing the baby down and out. The woman may need frequent reminders to keep her eyes open. It may also help to remind her of her baby, that her baby is bringing her pain out of her body. We call this "self-directed pushing," because the caregiver is helping the woman to direct her own bearing-down efforts.

These simple measures, opening her eyes and focusing on her baby moving down, usually result in progress without fetal distress or serious perineal damage. In those rare cases when these measures do not succeed, the caregiver may need to resort to encouraging her to do the prolonged breath-holding and maximal bearing down described earlier. If so, the caregiver should remember that the fetus usually tolerates the second stage better when the woman holds her breath and strains for less than 7 seconds at a time.[10,13,14,18,22] If these measures do not succeed, consider emotional distress as a possible underlying cause; see pages 162–167 for measures to alleviate emotional dystocia.

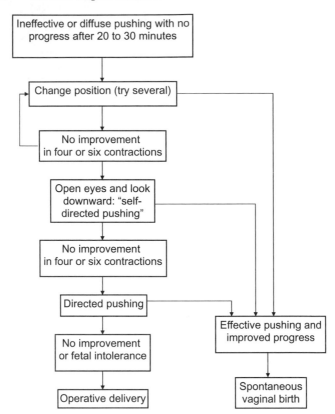

Chart 6.2. Diffuse pushing without progress.

If the woman has an epidural

Although epidural analgesia confers excellent pain relief most of the time, there are tradeoffs involved that may increase both the length of the second stage and the need for instrumental delivery.[23] The search for the safest and most effective management of both the first and second stages with an epidural is a subject of great interest and

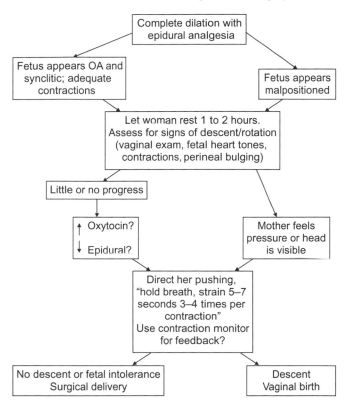

Chart 6.3. Delayed pushing with an epidural.

some controversy for caregivers as well as for childbearing women, especially in areas where epidural use is extremely prevalent.[24–26]

Certainly, epidurals change the second stage for both the woman and her caregivers (Chart 6.3).

Consider the following:

• Normally, the woman's pelvic floor provides a resilient platform on which the fetal head can rotate, and the muscles lining the pelvis also provide a resilient cushion that encourages rotation. Pressure on these muscles elicits a stretch response that plays an important role in the cardinal movements of descent (flexion, internal rotation, extension, and external rotation). With epidural analgesia, however, the pelvic floor muscles are anesthetized, resulting in a reduction of muscle tone, which may inhibit rotation of the fetal head.[27] This inhibition of the cardinal movements may help explain the increased need for instrumental deliveries with epidural analgesia.[23] When combined with maximal breath-holding and straining by the woman from the onset of the second stage, the likelihood of a difficult delivery due to a persistent malposition or a deep transverse arrest may be increased. Delaying pushing until the head is visible at the introitus or until the woman feels pressure or an urge to push decreases the instrumental delivery rate,[28,29] possibly by allowing more time for the fetus to gradually rotate and follow the path of least resistance down the birth canal.

(Delayed pushing may provide little benefit if the fetus is already occiput anterior.) With anesthesia, the woman also lacks kinesthetic feedback to help her discover how to push effectively.

- An anesthetized woman is restricted to the few positions that she can assume without full sensation or use of her legs. These are usually limited to side-lying, supine, semisitting, sitting upright, or—in some cases with light anesthesia and good physical support—squatting and hands and knees. Changing position usually requires assistance.

  Few studies of maternal positioning with an epidural exist, but it is an important area for investigation. One recent randomized controlled trial of women with an epidural in which passive descent (i.e., delaying pushing until the woman felt an urge to push or the fetal head was visible) was being used compared outcomes with the lateral position versus supported sitting during the second stage.[30] The likelihood of instrumental delivery was more than twice as great in the women in the sitting position. This is the first trial to investigate position without prolonged bearing-down efforts.

- Anesthesia may interfere with the usual spurt of endogenous oxytocin that is associated with pressure of the presenting part within the lower vagina.[5-7] Normally, the pressure on the posterior vaginal wall or the pelvic floor signals the pituitary gland to release more oxytocin, resulting in stronger contractions, a greater urge to push, and more pressure on the pelvic floor. Anesthesia blocks this oxytocin-producing feedback loop, and progress is often impaired. Because of the reduced urge to push associated with an epidural, pushing requires a greater voluntary effort than pushing in response to an urge.

Some caregivers have tried to remedy the above problems by the following approaches to epidural management. The evidence for each is summarized:

- Use of lower concentrations of the anesthetic when the epidural is first placed, possibly combining it with low-dose narcotics, or using a combined spinal-epidural (CSE) technique in hopes of allowing the woman more awareness and more motor control. A systematic review of 19 randomized controlled trials comparing the CSE with the standard epidural or the low-dose epidural found no difference in mobility or obstetric or neonatal outcomes, including operative deliveries, maternal hypotension, maternal satisfaction, or other outcomes. In fact, the CSE was associated with more urinary retention and pruritis. The authors concluded that the review favored the low-dose epidurals.[24]
- Discontinuing or decreasing the dose of the epidural at the end of the first stage of labor is sometimes done, with the purpose of improving pelvic floor muscle tone, encouraging rotation, and reducing the need for instrumental delivery. A systematic review of trials of this technique found insufficient evidence of benefit and inadequate pain relief. The numbers of women in the trials were quite small, and a large trial would provide stronger evidence on the real effect of discontinuing the epidural.[25]
- As described above, delaying pushing for up to 2 hours, or until the fetal head is occiput anterior or becomes visible at the vaginal outlet (when the labia are parted), may reduce the need for forceps rotation without risk to the newborn.[28,29] Evidence indicates that when pushing is delayed, thus avoiding forcing descent, the malpositioned fetus will often rotate and align well in the pelvis, rather than becoming stuck in an unfavorable position.
- Removing the time limit for second stage with an epidural improves the chances of a spontaneous delivery without risk to the neonate. The evidence supports this approach. Even if rotation and descent are slow, as long as fetus and woman are tolerating it well, many caregivers see no medical reason to intervene.[15]

6

Pushing effectively with an epidural

Pushing with an epidural is often frustrating and ineffective, especially if the woman is unaware of an urge to push. The caregiver's urgent pleas for her to "Push! Push!" along with a count to 10 may make her feel that she cannot do it right. One way to help the woman push well and feel good about it is to use the electronic fetal monitor as a biofeedback device to encourage her efforts. By positioning himself or herself with both the monitor and the woman in view, the partner, doula, or nurse can watch the digital contraction indicator and instruct the woman when to begin bearing down (when the intensity rises about 30 mm Hg above baseline). He or she calls out the numbers as the contraction builds, then instructs her to bear down, and continues to call out the numbers, which will increase rapidly with her bearing-down effort and should last for 5 to 7 seconds. Then the partner tells her to breathe "for the baby" several times and to bear down again, repeating the numbers. ("Now bear down. ... That's it, 70, 73, 77, 84, 90! Go for 100! Great! You did it! Now breathe for the baby!")

This approach to bearing down emulates spontaneous bearing down, which results in better fetal oxygenation than prolonged and constant breath-holding and straining.[8,10,15] Chart 6.3, page 183, summarizes the instructions for delayed pushing with an epidural.

If progress is slow, changing positions every 20 to 30 minutes often improves progress. Figure 6.2 illustrates pushing positions that may be used when women have epidurals, depending on the density of the epidural block.

How long an active phase of second stage is too long?

Although some doctors and midwives limit the duration of second stage labor to 2 hours from complete dilation to birth, there is no scientific rationale for such an approach. The length of the second stage is not as important to a good outcome as the status of mother and baby during that time. Individualized care and careful assessment often allow more time for second stage with no compromise in the well-being of mother or baby.[15,31]

An extensive review of the scientific literature on this issue concludes, "There is no evidence to suggest that, when the second stage of labor is progressing and the condition of both woman and fetus is

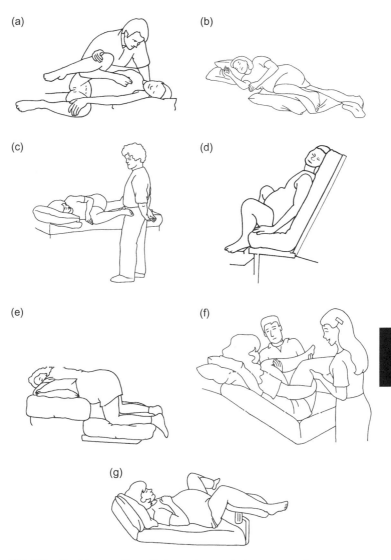

Fig. 6.2. Pushing positions that may be used when women have epidurals. (**a**) Side-lying to push. (**b**) Semiprone. (**c**) Side-lying lunge; (**d**) Semisitting. (**e**) Kneeling on foot of bed. (**f**) Semisitting, with people supporting the woman's legs. (**g**) Supine with leg supports.

satisfactory, the imposition of any upper arbitrary limit on its duration is justified. Such limits should be discarded."[32] A recent retrospective review of the effect of duration of second stage on fetal heart tones and maternal perinatal morbidity concluded that duration alone should not form the basis for decisions to intervene.[33–35] If pushing is delayed, and the woman's efforts mimic spontaneous bearing down as seen in unanesthetized women, she will tolerate a long second stage better than if she bears down forcefully for most of each contraction from complete dilation on.[36]

POSSIBLE ETIOLOGIES AND SOLUTIONS FOR SECOND-STAGE DYSTOCIA

The challenge for caregivers in a long second stage is to identify reasons for the slow progress and institute appropriate corrective measures. The choice of early interventions depends, to an extent, on the presumed etiology, although a trial-and-error approach is sometimes warranted.

Maternal positions and other strategies for suspected occiput posterior or persistent occiput transverse fetuses

Figure 6.3 illustrates abdominal and vaginal views of the OP and OT positions. As long as the woman is well supported and she has no musculoskeletal or medical problems and her fetus is monitored, a wide variety of positions may be used to promote descent.

Why not the dorsal position?

Dorsal maternal positions tend to exacerbate fetal malpositions and deny the effects of gravity. See pages 211–213 and Chapter 9 for information on the disadvantages of supine positions. In some specific situations, however, the advantages of exaggerated lithotomy may outweigh the risks (see, pages 213–214, 262–263, 309–310)). For most women, the positions shown in Figure 6.4 on page 190 are more effective in promoting fetal rotation and descent and may be more comfortable for the woman than the dorsal positions. Changing positions every 20 minutes (every five or six contractions) when progress is slow may help solve the problem. Even if the fetus cannot be rotated, these same measures may make a vaginal birth possible in a persistent OP or OT position.

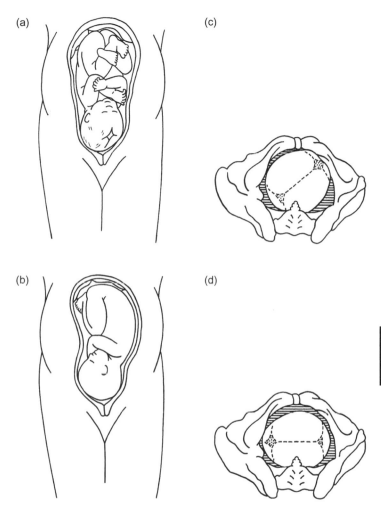

Fig. 6.3. (a) Right occiput posterior fetus, abdominal view. (b) Left occiput transverse fetus, abdominal view. (c) Right occiput posterior, fetus in synclitism, vaginal view. (d) Left occiput transverse fetus, vaginal view.

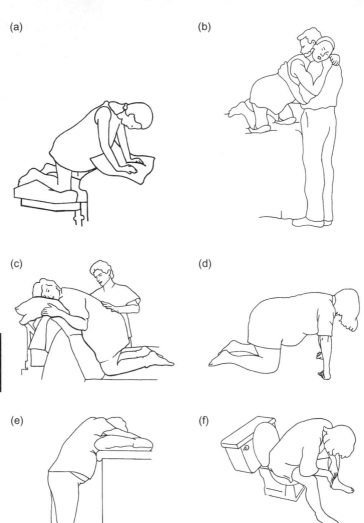

Fig. 6.4. a–f Pushing positions to promote rotation and descent
(**a**) Kneeling on foot of bed. (**b**) Kneeling, leaning on partner to push.
(**c**) Kneeling, leaning on the raised head of the bed. (**d**) Hands and knees.
(**e**) Standing, leaning on counter. (**f**) Sitting forward on toilet.

Differentiating between pushing positions and birth positions

Many maternal positions used to enhance progress would be awkward or uncomfortable for the caregiver during the actual birth. It may help to think of these as "pushing positions" and to distinguish them from "birth positions." The woman may use a variety of pushing positions to bring the baby down and, then when the birth is imminent, assume a position that allows the attendant to see adequately, support the perineum, and "catch" the baby without awkwardness or back strain.

Leaning forward while kneeling, standing, or sitting

These positions (see Fig. 6.4) take advantage of gravity to encourage rotation of the fetal trunk from posterior to anterior. Back pain, common with OP, is also relieved because the pressure of the fetal head on the sacrum is relieved. See the Toolkit 1, Chapter 9, for more information.

Squatting positions

Squatting positions use weight-bearing with hip abduction to widen the pelvic outlet, which may enlarge the space in the pelvic basin enough to promote rotation and descent. See Figure 6.5 and Chapter 9 for more information on squatting.

6

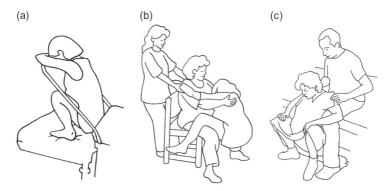

(a)   (b)   (c)

Fig. 6.5. (**a**) Squatting with bar. (**b**) Lap squatting. (**c**) Squatting, supported by seated partner's legs.

Asymmetric positions

In asymmetric positions, the woman's legs are in different positions (for example, one knee up and one knee down). This changes the shape of the pelvis in ways that are different from "symmetric" positions such as squatting, and hands and knees. The pelvic joints on one side of the pelvis widen more than the joints on the other side. Sometimes the fetus is more likely to rotate with asymmetric positions. See Figure 6.6 and page 141 for more information on asymmetric positions. If the fetal position is known with a degree of certainty, then the woman should be in a position to widen the side of her pelvis toward which the occiput is directed. If the position is uncertain, the woman should alternate knees, raising one during several contractions and then the other. If raising one knee clearly feels better than the other, we think it makes sense for her to remain longer on that side. Our rationale, supported by clinical experience, is that when the woman's position provides space for the fetus to rotate or descend, the woman is likely to feel less pain. This is an area where further study would be useful. See pages 76–79, 129, 133–134 for discussion about the difficulty of accurately determining fetal position.

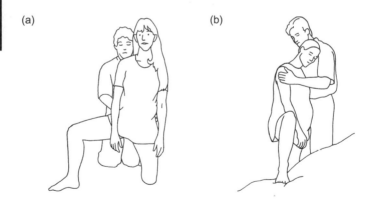

Fig. 6.6. (**a**) Asymmetric kneeling. (**b**) Asymmetric standing.

Lateral positions

For the woman who is exhausted or restricted to bed, side-lying (Fig. 6.7a) and the semiprone (exaggerated Sims', Fig.6.7b) positions

(a)

(b)

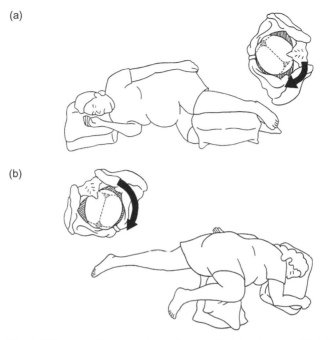

Fig. 6.7. (a) Woman with suspected or known OP fetus in pure side-lying on the "correct" side, with fetal back "toward the bed." If fetus is ROP, woman lies on her right side. Gravity pulls fetal occiput and trunk toward ROT. (**b**) Woman with suspected or known OP fetus semiprone on the "correct" side, with fetal back "toward the ceiling." If fetus is ROP, the semiprone woman lies on her left side. Gravity pulls fetal occiput and trunk toward ROT, then ROA. If position is uncertain, woman should alternate sides after a few contractions.

are good alternatives to the dorsal or semisitting positions. If the fetus is known with some certainty to be OP, the woman should lie on:

- the same side as the posterior occiput if side-lying, and
- the side *opposite* the posterior or transverse occiput if in semiprone (exaggerated Sims') (Fig. 6.7b).

See the explanation of the different effects of the side-lying and semiprone positions in Chapter 5.

6

If the position is uncertain (see the discussion of reliability of determining fetal position on pages 133–134, Chapter 5), then it is best to alternate between the two sides on a trial-and-error basis, since theoretically, at least, the woman could do more harm than good if she spends all her time in the "wrong" position.

Supported squat or "dangle" positions

In a "dangle position," the woman is supported under her arms, with minimal or no weight-bearing by her legs or feet (Fig. 6.8). These unique positions are the only ones in which the woman is supported

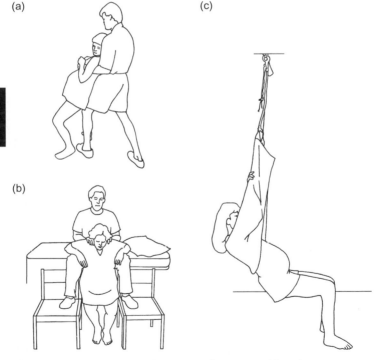

Fig. 6.8. Positions in which the woman is supported from her upper body. (**a**) Supported squat. (**b**) Dangle. (**c**) Dangle with birth sling.

from her upper body. We propose the following mechanisms to explain how the dangle positions enhance the fetus's position.

The woman's own body weight lengthens her trunk by providing traction to her spinal column. This provides more vertical space for the fetus to maneuver. Most second-stage positions require that the woman flex her trunk and neck, to add pressure to the fundus and promote descent of the fetus. However, this added pressure may not help if the head will not fit because it is asynclitic or deflexed. The dangle positions offer room for the head to reposition itself.

Furthermore, the dangle positions are free from external pressures on the pelvis, such as those that occur when the woman is sitting or lying down, or when her joints are stretched (for example, when she squats or pulls her legs back). An absence of such external pressures, in cases where the fetal head appears to be "stuck," may allow the pressure from the descending fetal head (and, presumably, fetal head movements) to change the shape of the pelvic basin as needed for the fetus to find the path of least resistance through the pelvis.

Other strategies for malposition and back pain

The pelvic press may help in cases of deep transverse arrest, occiput posterior, or a "tight fit" in the second stage, to increase midpelvic and outlet dimensions and make room for fetal rotation and descent.[37] (See Fig. 6.9 and the Toolkit, Chapter 9, pages 321–323, for a description of the pelvic press.) Please note that the pelvic press is not the same as the "double hip squeeze" (Fig. 6.10). The main difference between the two is the placement of the hands. In the pelvic press, the helper's hands are placed on the iliac crests; in the double hip squeeze, they are placed over the gluteal muscles on the buttocks. The pelvic press is used to enlarge the pelvic outlet in the second stage; the double hip squeeze is used to relieve back pain at any time in labor.

A variety of movements may help reposition the fetus. See Chapter 9 for descriptions of the following: pelvic rocking (Fig. 6.11 and pages 311–313), lunging (Fig. 6.12 and pages 313–314), the kneeling lunge (Fig. 6.13), and slow dancing (Fig. 6.14 and pages 316–317). Because severe back pain often accompanies some fetal positions, such as OP or OT, asynclitism (see later Fig. 6.22 and 6.23, pages 201–202), nuchal hand (see later Fig. 6.24 on pages 204–205) or hands, and some maternal spinal or pelvic variations, measures to relieve this

Table 6.1. Difference between Pelvic Press and the Double Hip Squeeze

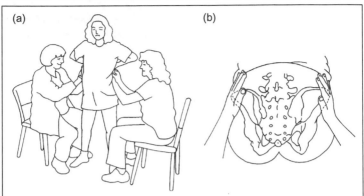

Fig. 6.9. (**a**) Pelvic press. (**b**) Pelvic press (detail, seen from rear)

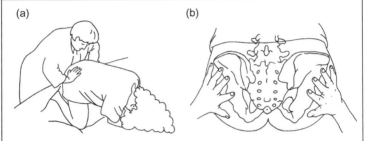

Fig. 6.10. (**a**) Double hip squeeze. (**b**) Double hip squeeze (detail, seen from rear).

Fig. 6.11. Pelvic rocking, back rounded in flexion.

Fig. 6.12. Standing lunge.

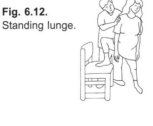

Fig. 6.13. Kneeling lunge.

Fig. 6.14. Slow dancing.

pain should be used as needed (Figs. 6.15 through 6.21). If the back pain remains tolerable, the woman may have more patience to await fetal repositioning and descent.

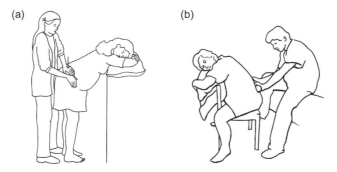

Fig. 6.15. (**a**) Counterpressure. (**b**) Counterpressure with tennis balls.

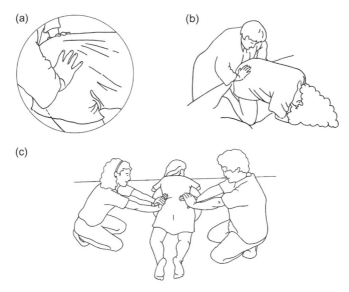

Fig. 6.16. More strategies for malposition and back pain. (**a**) Detail of double hip squeeze. (**b**) Double hip squeeze. (**c**) Double hip squeeze with two support people.

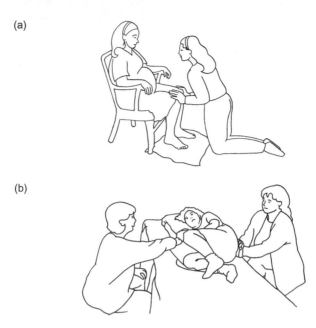

Fig. 6.17. (**a**) Knee press, woman seated. (**b**) Knee press, woman on her side.

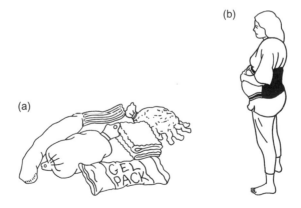

Fig. 6.18. (**a**) Objects for heat and cold. (**b**) Strap-on cold pack.

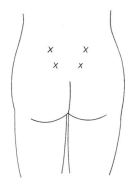

Fig. 6.19. Intradermal sterile water injection sites for back pain.

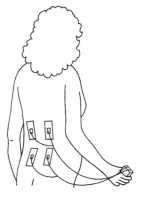

Fig. 6.20. TENS in use.

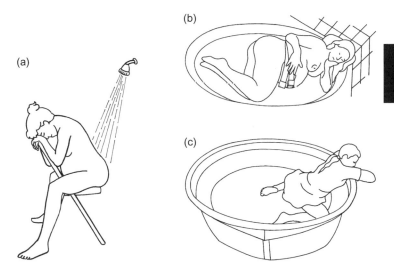

Fig. 6.21. Hydrotherapy for back pain: (**a**) Shower on woman's back to relieve back pain. (**b**) Side-lying in bath to relieve back pain. (**c**) Kneeling, leaning forward in birthing pool to relieve back pain.

Manual interventions to reposition the occiput posterior fetus

Manual rotation of a persistent occiput posterior head is a technique that has been used for years and described in many obstetrics and midwifery textbooks.[37,38] Chapter 8 (pages 246–250) describes techniques for manual and digital rotation of a malpositioned fetus.

Early interventions for suspected persistent asynclitism

Normally, at the onset of labor the fetal head is asynclitic (angled so that one parietal bone—located above the ear—is presenting), which facilitates entry of the head into the pelvic basin. This usually resolves spontaneously to synclitism as the fetus moves lower in the pelvis. (Figure 6.22 shows vaginal views of asynclitic and synclitic fetuses in OA, OP, and OT.) However, persistent asynclitism (Fig. 6.23) in the second stage may interfere with flexion, rotation, molding, and descent of the fetal head. A caput (swelling of soft tissue) often forms over one parietal bone.

Extra time, a variety of measures to alter the space within the pelvis, and some specific movements are thought to encourage the fetus to shift into a more synclitic position. Chart 6.4 provides an overview of measures to help in cases of occiput posterior and asynclitism in second stage. If the caregiver suspects persistent asynclitism, changing the woman's position may assist labor progress in three ways:

1. Shifting the woman may shift the fetus's weight so its position resolves.
2. Changing the woman's position may alter the shape of her pelvis slightly, allowing more room for the angle of the fetal head to shift.
3. Having the woman take a position that elongates her torso and relieves pressure on the pelvis (i.e. , the dangle and supported squat) may give the fetus room enough to "wiggle" out of asynclitism or mold the pelvis for a better fit. See pages 299–302 for a complete explanation.

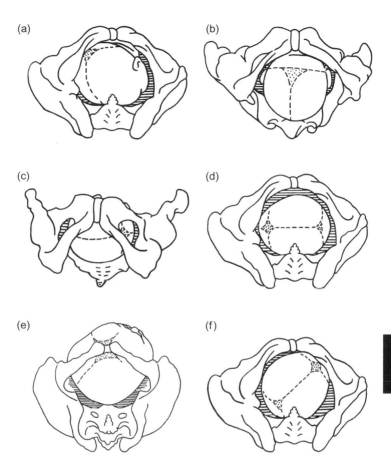

Fig. 6.22. (a) Asynclitic fetus in occiput anterior. (b) Occiput anterior in synclitism. (c) Asynclitic fetus in occiput transverse. (d) Occiput transverse in synclitism. (e) Asynclitic fetus in right occiput posterior. (f) Right occiput posterior in synclitism.

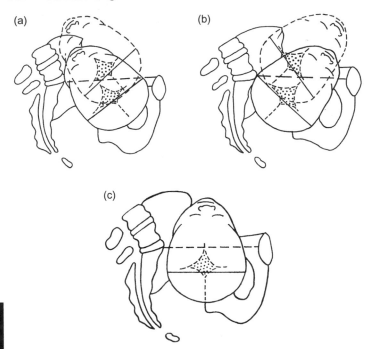

Fig. 6.23. (**a**) Posterior asynclitism (*dotted lines*) and persistent posterior asynclitism, which indicates that the fetus is at a low station and asynclitic (*solid lines*). (**b**) Anterior asynclitism (*dotted lines*) and persistent anterior asynclitism (*solid lines*) (**c**) Synclitism at a low station.

Positions and movements for persistent asynclitism in second stage

In general, the same positions and movements and back pain relief techniques discussed on pages 136–141, 144 for persistent OP/OT are useful when the fetus seems to be in a persistent asynclitic position. (See the Toolkit, Chapter 9, for specific information.) Specifically, pelvic press and the dangle and supported squat positions may be especially helpful when the fetus is thought to be asynclitic during

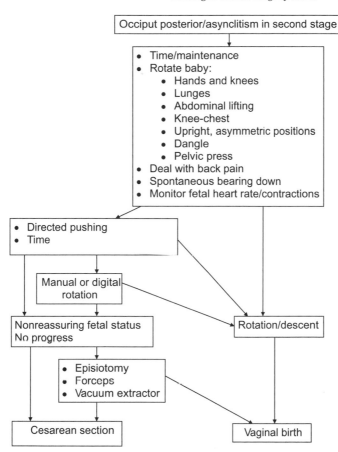

Chart 6.4. Occiput posterior/asynclitism in second stage.

the second stage. Success with these positions will be influenced by the degree of engagement of the fetal head and the fit between fetal head and woman's pelvis. These techniques merit further study, since the advantages ascribed to them are theoretical and observational.[39]

Nuchal hand or hands at vertex delivery

A search of the obstetric and midwifery literature on nuchal hands (that is, one or both of the baby's hands at the baby's neck or face) at birth retrieved only scanty anecdotal advice, yet a nuchal hand is a well-known and troublesome deterrent to spontaneous vaginal birth (Fig. 6.24). Mothers' personal reports of their own "hand-by-face" deliveries abound on the Internet, with a common theme of difficult painful births and perineal lacerations. The authors have observed that some women who have intractable unrelenting back pain during labor give birth to babies with one or both nuchal hands tucked beneath their chins or alongside their heads. Yet this situation is not easily diagnosed during labor. Therefore, the same measures used for other conditions causing back pain and slow progress should also be used when a nuchal hand is suspected.

The nuchal hand is a condition worthy of detailed study.

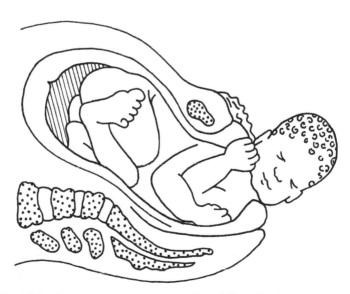

Fig. 6.24. Fetus emerging with a nuchal hand ("hand by face").

If cephalopelvic disproportion or macrosomia ("poor fit") is suspected

A variety of factors may contribute to a slow second stage and create doubt whether the baby will fit through the woman's pelvis. These include the size and shape of the fetal head, the size and shape of the woman's pelvis, the position of the fetus, and the woman's ability to move around during labor.

Note: Ultrasound Predictions of Fetal Size

Ultrasound measurements of fetal weight and head size are not always reliable. For babies weighing over 4000 g (8 lb 13 oz), ultrasound estimates can err by up to 10% (almost a pound) or more in either direction. Furthermore, even accurate estimates of fetal head size and weight do not predict the capacity of the fetal head or the pelvis to mold to accommodate safe passage of the fetus.[40,41]

The influence of time on cephalopelvic disproportion

Many suspected cases of cephalopelvic disproportion actually involve fetuses who are subtly malpositioned (asynclitic, deflexed, occiput transverse or posterior), who will fit well through the pelvis once the malposition has been resolved. The shape of the woman's pelvis is also a consideration. The woman may need to try pushing in a variety of positions to find the ones that optimize descent. Resolving problems of position or fit often requires extra time.

Many large fetal heads will mold and fit safely through the pelvis, but molding takes time. When heart tones are reassuring and the woman's condition is good, time can be an ally, not an enemy, in allowing labor progress to take place.

Some high-intervention caregivers have strict expectations for an acceptable rate of progress in descent. If progress falls behind the expected rate, they initiate interventions such as oxytocin, episiotomy, forceps, vacuum extraction, or cesarean delivery. Low-intervention caregivers, however, who prefer to exercise patience use less aggressive interventions as long as the fetus appears to be doing well and the woman is willing and able to continue.

Positions for "possible cephalopelvic disproportion" in second stage

Because "suspected CPD" often results from fetal malpositions, rather than from a true excess of the diameters of the fetal head over the diameters of the pelvic basin, it makes sense to encourage the woman to try positions and movements that might resolve an OP, OT, or asynclitic position (Figs. 6.25 through 6.30). See also Chapter 9 for a discussion of these positions and movements.

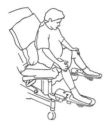

Fig. 6.25. Sitting upright to push.

6

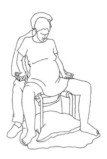

Fig. 6.26. Pushing on a birthing stool (adapted from a photograph of the DeBY Birth Support).

(a)

(b)

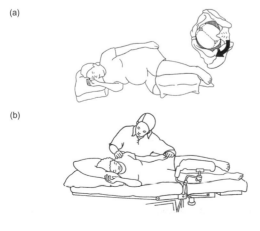

Fig. 6.27. (a) and (b) Woman with a known or suspected ROP fetus in pure **side-lying** on the "correct" side, with fetal back "toward the bed." With an ROP fetus, woman lies on her right side. Gravity pulls fetal head and trunk toward OT.

Positions for 'possible CPD' second stage, cont'd

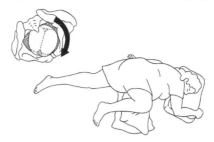

Fig. 6.28. Woman with a known or suspected ROP fetus lies **semiprone** on the "correct" side, with fetal back "toward the ceiling." If fetus is ROP, the semiprone woman lies on her left side. Gravity pulls fetal head and trunk toward ROT, then ROA.

(a)

(b)

6

(c)

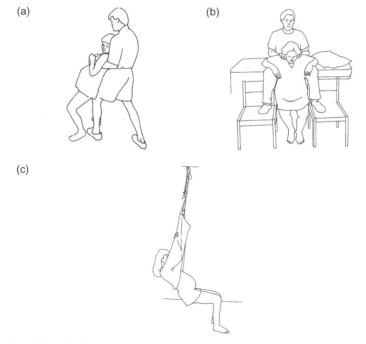

Fig. 6.29. (**a**) Supported squat. (**b**) Dangle. (**c**) Dangle with a birth sling.

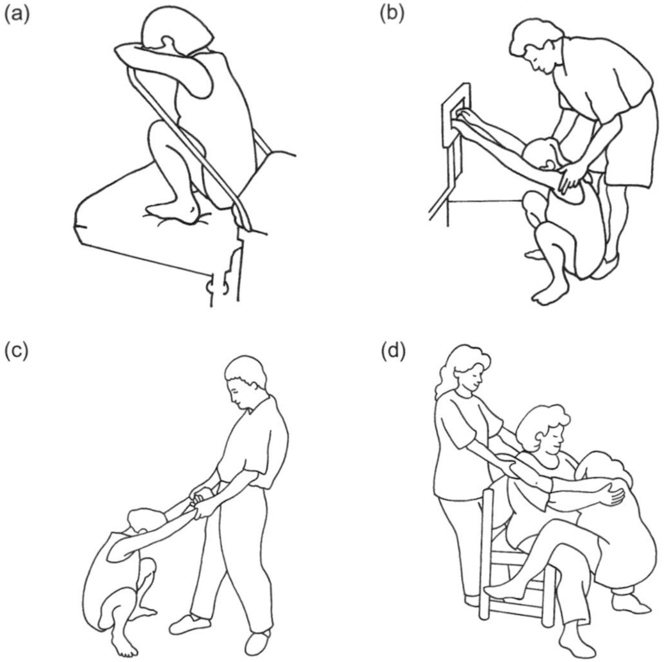

(a)

(b)

(c)

(d)

Fig. 6.30. (a) Squatting with a bar. (b) Squatting with bed rail. (c) Partner squat. (d) Lap squat, with three people.

Toilet-sitting and hydrotherapy may also enhance progress (Figs. 6.31 and 6.32).

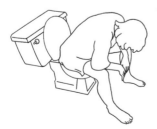

Fig. 6.31. Sitting, leaning forward on toilet.

(a)

(b)

(c)

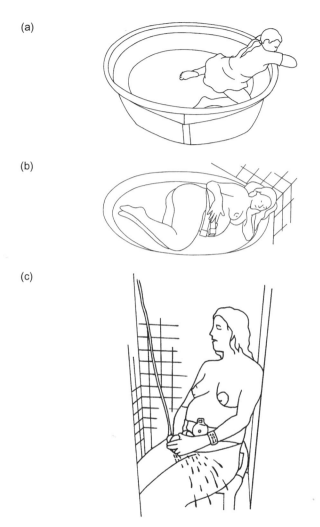

Fig. 6.32. (**a**) Woman in a birth pool. (**b**) Woman in bath, with telemetry monitors. (**c**) Woman in shower, with telemetry monitors.

Encourage movements that alter pelvic size and shape and encourage fetal descent (Figs. 6.33 and 6.34). See pages 311, 323–324 for notes on movement and why it helps.

Note: To master the technique of the lunge, see the instructions on pages 313–314 before teaching it to the woman in labor.

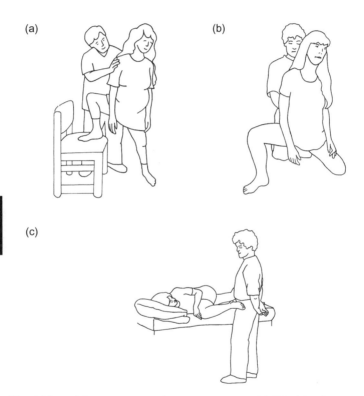

6

Fig. 6.33. (**a**) Standing lunge. (**b**) Kneeling lunge. (**c**) Side-lying lunge to view the perineum easily and to perform vaginal exams.

(a) (b)

(c)

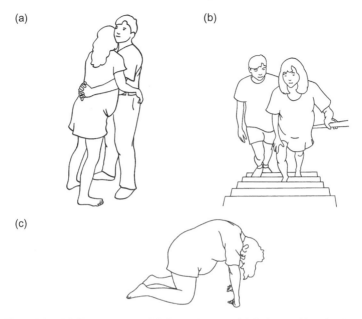

Fig. 6.34. (a) Slow dancing. (b) Stair climbing. (c) Pelvic rocking, back rounded in flexion.

6

The use of dorsal positions

Dorsal positions are the most commonly suggested positions for the second stage in North America today. According to two North American surveys of women's birth experiences, 57% of American women laid on their backs and another 35% were in semisitting,[42] while 48% of Canadian women laid on their backs and 46% were propped up or sitting; 57% had their legs in stirrups.[43] In fact, many women spend the entire second stage in dorsal or semisitting positions (Fig. 6.35), even though they would probably use a variety of positions, including upright ones, if they were free to move as they choose.[20] Although dorsal positions are convenient for caregivers to view the perineum and to perform vaginal examinations, episiotomy, vacuum extraction, and forceps, there are some problems associated with these positions. The woman's body weight on the bed creates

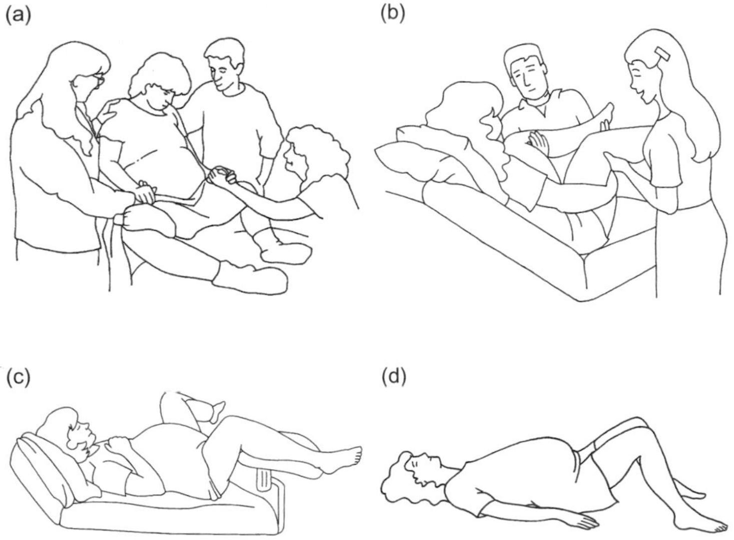

(a)

(b)

(c)

(d)

Fig. 6.35. (a) Semisitting to push. (b) Semisitting with people supporting the woman's legs. (c) Supine with leg supports. (d) Supine, hips and knees flexed.

6

pressure on her sacrum and coccyx, which reduces the anteroposterior diameter of the pelvic outlet.[44,45] Compare Figure 6.36a and Figure 6.36b. The effects of gravity in promoting descent are lost with supine or any recumbent positions. Maternal supine hypotension is caused by the weight of the uterus on the inferior vena cava and aorta, which leads to a reduction in venous return and cardiac output. The fetus may then experience hypoxia due to the concomitant decrease in blood flow to the placenta and resulting reduction in oxygen supply to the fetus, especially if combined with prolonged breath-holding and maximal straining.[10,15,17]

Besides supine hypotension, the weight of the uterus along the spinal column reduces the angle of the uterus with the spine, resulting in poor alignment of the fetus with the pelvis[44] (Fig. 6.36a).

With persistent OP, persistent asynclitism, or other malpositions, the woman should be encouraged to do most of her pushing in positions other than supine or semisitting. It is ironic that two widely

(a)   (b)

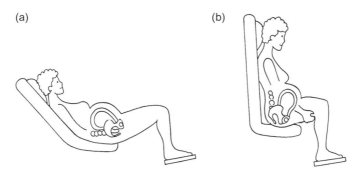

Fig. 6.36. Drive angle. (**a**) supine, (**b**) standing. [Adapted from Fenwick L, Simkin P. (1987). Maternal position to prevent or alleviate dystocia in labor. Clin Obstet Gynecol 30(1), 83–89.]

prescribed practices for second stage— prolonged breath-holding and straining, and the supine position—are at least partly responsible for the frequently observed fetal bradycardias and prolonged second stage that have led caregivers to believe that the duration of the second stage must be curtailed. The further irony is that if laboring women were encouraged to behave instinctually, they would rarely lie on their backs, nor would they use prolonged breath-holding and straining. They could avoid some nonreassuring fetal heart rate tracings in the second stage. Last, the long-term pelvic floor damage, widely attributed to vaginal birth, is likely to be largely caused by these two entrenched practices and the widespread use of episiotomy.[15,17] Misguided efforts to improve birth outcomes have not only made outcomes worse, but the harmful practices have been extremely difficult to change, so the problems persist.

Use of the exaggerated lithotomy position

Notwithstanding what was stated earlier, there are occasions when one particular dorsal position—the exaggerated lithotomy (McRoberts') position—may succeed in promoting descent when other positions do not. When the woman has been unable to bring her baby beneath the pubic symphysis in any other position, this problem may in some cases be resolved by having the woman lie flat on her back with her knees drawn back (by herself or others) so that

(a)   (b)

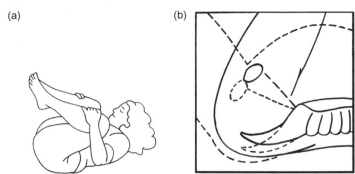

Fig. 6.37. (a) Exaggerated lithotomy position. (b) Exaggerated lithotomy (detail). Dotted line shows pelvic position when woman's feet are on bed; solid line, when the woman's legs are drawn up.

her buttocks are lifted slightly off the bed and her hips are in a very flexed, abducted position (Fig. 6.37). This position passively rotates the pubic arch upward toward the mother's head and brings the pelvic inlet perpendicular to the maximum expulsive force.[44–47]

Such a position may facilitate the passage of the fetal head beneath the pubic arch. In persistent delays in descent, this benefit may outweigh the disadvantages of supine hypotension and loss of any gravity advantage. Such a position is combined with maximal breath-holding and straining. It is worth trying when operative delivery is anticipated. This position is also used along with other procedures for shoulder dystocia (see Chapter 8, pages 258–265).

A note of caution: Those who are supporting the woman's legs in the exaggerated lithotomy position must exercise particular caution not to pull her legs into extreme abduction and/or flexion. This can cause damage to her pubic symphysis, sacroiliac joints, or hip joints or it may cause nerve damage.[48]This is of particular concern if the mother cannot feel these joints, as occurs with use of an epidural.

Shoulder dystocia

Shoulder dystocia is defined as a birth requiring extra maneuvers to deliver the fetus after the head is born.[49] One shoulder is caught on the mother's pubic symphysis, and internal rotation and descent are delayed. Shoulder dystocia can become a true emergency and requires quick thinking and calm, effective management, at a time when the caregiver may be anxious. The specific maneuvers to free the baby and deliver him or her require knowledge and skill. Most cases resolve quickly with appropriate actions. See Chapter 8, pages 258–265, for a discussion of these clinical skills.

If contractions are inadequate

If contraction intensity and frequency decrease during the second stage, the possible causes should be considered. They are likely to be the same as those discussed in Chapter 5. Immobility, medications, dehydration, and maternal exhaustion are all possible causes. Contractions might be improved by such measures as changing positions, allowing the medications or epidural to wear off (if the woman can tolerate it), breast stimulation, hydration, allowing the woman to avoid voluntary or forceful pushing for a number of contractions, or immersion in water. These are almost the same measures as those suggested for inadequate contractions during the active phase of first stage. Please read pages 146–156 for detailed explanations of these possible causes and solutions for inadequate contractions.

IF EMOTIONAL DYSTOCIA IS SUSPECTED

6

Emotional distress sometimes underlies a lack of progress in the second stage. Much of the information in Chapters 2 and 5 on the physiology of emotional dystocia and on measures to alleviate it during the first stage of labor also applies to the second stage.

The essence of coping during the second stage of labor

Before discussing other factors that may trigger emotional distress, let us review what "coping well" during the second stage means.

When the second stage begins, the woman, if undisturbed and unrestricted, often becomes more aware of her surroundings, alert, and energetic.[50] Then, as her reflexive urge to push intensifies, it guides her to bear down and find a position that feels right. As the baby moves down the vaginal canal, she may temporarily "hold back" (that is, tense her perineum, fearing the stretching feeling). Then her body's strong urges take over and she lets go, releasing her pelvic floor and her attempts to control the process. The woman may grunt, moan, or even bellow with her contractions as she instinctively moves into different positions. The 3 Rs (relaxation, rhythm, and ritual; see pages 159–160) no longer apply.

The caregiver's role when a woman is coping in this way is to monitor the fetus's and mother's well-being as unobtrusively as possible, provide encouragement and reassurance as needed, and accommodate and support her instinctive behaviors as much as possible. There are many safe and effective positions and ways of bearing down. As long as mother and baby are tolerating the second stage and some progress is being made, there is no reason to intervene. (When it is clear that the baby will be born soon, it may be necessary to ask the mother to adopt a position in which the clinical caregiver has adequate access.)

In summary, "coping well" during the second stage includes grunting and bearing down reflexively with the urge to push (even bellowing at times), breathing as desired between bearing down efforts, and moving into positions that feel right. These behaviors are signs of normal coping, not signs of distress.

Signs of emotional distress in second stage:

- verbal or facial expressions of fear
- crying or panic
- inability to get beyond holding back to releasing the pelvic floor
- holding her legs together
- diffuse bearing down (pages 181–182)
- begging the caregiver to take the baby out or to "knock" her out with drugs
- desperation, inability to follow caregiver's suggestions

Triggers of emotional distress unique to the second stage

These factors might trigger emotional distress and interfere with the woman's ability to cope during the second stage:

- fatigue or exhaustion, which can lead to hopelessness or anxiety
- the intense sensations of second stage or of manual stretching of the vagina. These sensations may be especially frightening if the woman has been sexually abused or otherwise traumatized in the genital region in the past, as they may trigger flashbacks.

- fear of behaving inappropriately or offensively (making noise, passing stool while pushing)
- the immediacy of the birth and the responsibility of parenting the child, especially if her own parents were dysfunctional or she has relinquished a child for adoption or had a child removed from her care
- fear for the baby's well-being, especially if a sibling or a previous child died around birth or had another adverse outcome
- the loss of privacy, sense of modesty when surrounded by strangers watching her perineum
- previous cesarean during second stage
- thoughtless or unkind treatment by loved ones or caregiver during labor

One common response to such fears in the second stage is extreme tension in the pelvic floor as if to deter the fetus's descent, while pushing. The woman may be pushing hard but not effectively. Sometimes she unintentionally and unconsciously contracts her pelvic floor muscles and buttocks as she pushes with her diaphragm and abdominal muscles. Tension in the perineum and constriction of the anus while pushing indicate that the woman is holding back.

(It is important not to confuse this excessive and prolonged pelvic tension with the normal confusion many women have when they first begin to push. It is normal for women to need to experiment a bit in order to discover how to push effectively. This is particularly true for women who do not initially have a strong urge to push. In such cases, it may be best for them to rest and await a stronger urge to push.)

If a woman exhibits "diffuse pushing" (see Chart 6.2 and pages 181–182) and does not benefit from the measures to improve her bearing down efforts (see page 181), consider the possibility of emotional dystocia.

Whatever fears or anxieties cause the woman to hold back, she probably cannot simply "snap out of it." However, those around her may be able to address and alleviate her fears. The measures described in Chapter 4 may help, along with the following:

- Encourage the woman to express her feelings. Ask her, "What was going through your mind during that last contraction?" Listen to her, acknowledge and validate her concerns, and try to give appropriate reassurance, encouragement, or information and suggestions. Often, all the woman needs is a chance to express her concerns. She needs to know that she is being heard, that her fears are normal, and that she will get through this event. Even normal events can be very troublesome to an anxious woman.

- Sometimes, when it is clear to everyone including the woman, that there is a delay, asking her why she thinks labor has slowed down, reveals useful information. Answers such as, "I can't push right" or "The baby doesn't want to come out" might indicate emotional dystocia.

- Provide appropriate information. For example, if the woman is afraid of having a bowel movement as she pushes (and it is too late for her to go to the bathroom), she can be reassured that passing stool indicates that she is pushing effectively, that this is a common event, that any fecal material will be quickly wiped away and disposed of. In fact, this is one of many good reasons to apply warm compresses to the perineum at this time—to be able to unobtrusively remove any stool.

- If she is afraid she will "rip" or split apart while pushing, reassure her that, by relaxing her perineum or letting the baby come, her perineum will actually stretch better and a tear is less likely. Also, unless there is a good reason not to do so, let her try a few contractions without pushing. "Let's try breathing through this next one," so that she feels she has some options during this frightening time.

- Give the woman time to adjust to the intense sensations and emotions of second stage. Avoid creating a sense of rushing. There is usually no need for the caregiver to raise his or her voice.

- Encourage the woman to relax her perineum between contractions and let it bulge during contractions. The application of hot compresses (washcloths soaked in warm water, wrung out) to the perineum often feels good and promotes relaxation. The compresses should not be too hot for the person applying them to hold comfortably in her hand. Encourage the woman to push as if she is blowing up an imaginary balloon, or as if she were trying to urinate rapidly. Give her positive reinforcement whenever she bears down effectively. Pushing in this manner sometimes causes the pelvic floor to bulge, which the caregiver can see. If she seems reluctant to sustain a bearing-down effort and she is not making progress, advise her to "push to the pain, and right through it. It will feel better when you push through it."

- Have the woman try pushing while sitting on the toilet. If she is worried about passing stool, the toilet is a reassuring place to be. Toilet-sitting also elicits the conditioned response of releasing the pelvic floor. Whoever is responsible for the woman's care can monitor what the woman is feeling. If the woman feels that the baby is coming, she will need to move to a more appropriate delivery site.

If the woman is pushing in a "diffuse" manner, see Chart 6.2 and pages 181–182.

CONCLUSION

The conduct of second stage of labor has long been guided by principles of speed and convenience for the care provider. Many practices, such as early maximal bearing down, immobility, the dorsal position, and a time limit, actually interfere with progress and frequently necessitate such interventions as intravenous oxytocin, forceps, vacuum extractor, episiotomy, or cesarean delivery. In this chapter, we present an approach designed to foster optimal progress, and implement simple interventions in order to prevent serious cases of failed progress.

6

REFERENCES

1. Simkin P. (1984). Active and physiologic management of second stage: A review and hypothesis. In Kitzinger S, Simkin P, editors. Episiotomy and the Second Stage of Labor. Minneapolis, MN, ICEA.
2. Simkin P. (2008). The Birth Partner, 3rd edition. Boston, Harvard Common Press.
3. Friedman E. (1978). Normal labor. In Labor: Clinical Evaluation and Management, 2nd edition. New York, Appleton-Century-Crofts.
4. Cohen W, Friedman E. (1983). Dysfunctional labor. In Management of Labor. Baltimore, MD, University Park Press.
5. Vasicka A, Kumaresan P, Han G, Kumaresan M. (1978). Plasma oxytocin in initiation of labor. Am J Obstet Gynecol 130(3), 263–273.
6. Fuchs A, Romero R, Keefe D, Parra M, Oyarzun E, Behnke E. (1991). Oxytocin secretion and human parturition: Pulse frequency and duration increase during spontaneous labor in women. Am J Obstet Gynecol 165(5 pt 1), 1515–1523.

7. Rahm V, Hallgren A, Hogberg H, Hurtig I, Odlind V. (2002). Plasma oxytocin levels in women during labor with or without epidural analgesia: A prospective study. Acta Obstet Gynecol Scand 81(11), 1033–1039.

8. Beynon C. (1957). The normal second stage of labour: A plea for reform in its conduct. J Obstet Gynaecol Br Commonw 64(6), 815–820.

9. Enkin M, Keirse M, Neilsen J, Crowther C, Dulet L, Hodnett E, et al. (2000). Monitoring the progress of labour. In A Guide to Effective Care in Pregnancy and Childbirth, 3rd edition. Oxford, Oxford University Press.

10. Roberts J. (2002). The "push" for evidence: Management of the second stage. J Midwif Womens Health 47(1), 2–15.

11. Clark S, Simpson K, Knox G, Garite T. (2009). Oxytocin: New perspectives on an old drug. Am J Obstet Gynecol 200(1), 35.e31–e36.

12. Rooks J. (2009). Oxytocin as a "high alert medication": A multilayered challenge to the status quo. Birth 36(4), 345–348.

13. Rosevear S, Stirrat G. (1996). The Handbook of Obstetric Management. Oxford, Blackwell Scientific.

14. Fraser D, Cooper B. (2009). Myles' Textbook for Midwives, 15th edition. Oxford, Churchill Livingstone Elsevier.

15. Roberts J, Hanson L. (2007). Best practices in second stage labor care: maternal bearing down and positioning. J Midwif Women's Health 52(3), 238–245.

16. Bing E. (1994). Personal communication.

17. Schaffer J, Bloom S, Casey B, McIntire D, Nihira M, Leveno K. (2006). A randomized trial of coached versus uncoached maternal pushing during the second stage of labor. Am J Obstet Gynecol 194(1), 10–13.

18. Aldrich C, D'Antona D, Spencer J, Wyatt J, Peebles D, Delpy D, et al. (1995). The effect of maternal pushing on fetal cerebral oxygenation and blood volume during the second stage of labour. Br J Obstet Gynaecol 102(6), 448–453.

19. Simpson K, James D. (2005). Effects of immediate versus delayed pushing during second-stage labor on fetal well-being. Nurs Res 54(3), 149–157.

20. Carlson J, Diehl J, Sachtleben-Murray M, McRae M, Fenwick L, Friedman E. A. (1986). Maternal position during parturition in normal labor. Obstet Gynecol 68(4), 443–447.

21. Fuller B, Roberts J, McKay S. (1993). Acoustical analysis of maternal sounds during the second stage of labor. Appl Nurs Res 6(1), 8–12.

22. Caldeyro-Barcia R. (1986). Influence of maternal bearing-down efforts during second stage on fetal well-being. In Kitzinger S, Simkin P,

6

editors. Episiotomy and the Second Stage of Labor. Minneapolis, MN, ICEA.

23. Anim-Somuah M, Smyth R, Howell C. (2005). Epidural versus non-epidural or no analgesia in labour. Cochrane Database Syst Rev (4):CD000331. doi:000310.001002/14651858.CD14000331.pub2

24. Simmons S, Cyna A, Dennis A, Hughes D. (2007). Combined spinal-epidural versus epidural analgesia in labour. Cochrane Database Syst Rev (3):CD003401. doi:003410.001002/14651858.CD14003401.pub2

25. Torvaldsen S, Roberts C, Bell J, Raynes-Greenow C. (2004). Discontinuation of epidural analgesia late in labour for reducing the adverse delivery outcomes associated with epidural analgesia. Cochrane Database Syst Rev (4):CD00457.pub00452. doi:00410.01002/14651858. CD14004457.pub2

26. Kotaska A, Klein M, Liston R. (2006). Epidural analgesia associated with low-dose oxytocin augmentation increases cesarean births: A critical look at the external validity of randomized trials. Am J Obstet Gynecol 194(3), 809–814.

27. Bonica J, Miller F, Parmley T. (1995). Anatomy and physiology of the forces of parturition. In Bonica J, McDonald J, editors. Principles and Practice of Obstetric Analgesia and Anesthesia, 2nd edition. Philadelphia, Williams & Wilkins.

28. Fraser W, Marcoux S, Krauss I, Douglas J, Goulet C, Boulvain M. (2000). Multicenter, randomized, controlled trial of delayed pushing for nulliparous women in the second stage of labor with continuous epidural analgesia. The PEOPLE (Pushing Early or Pushing Late with Epidural) Study Group. Am J Obstet Gynecol 182(5), 1165–1172.

29. Brancato R, Church S, Stone P. (2008). A meta-analysis of passive descent versus immediate pushing in nulliparous women with epidural analgesia in the second stage of labor. JOGNN 37(1), 4–12.

30. Downe S, Gerrett D, Renfrew M. (2004). A prospective randomized trial on the effect of position in the passive second stage of labour on birth outcome in nulliparous women using epidural analgesia. Midwifery 20(2), 157–168.

31. Yildirim G, Beji N. (2008). Effects of pushing techniques in birth on mother and fetus: A randomized study. Birth 35(1), 31–32.

32. Enkin M, Keirse M, Neilsen J, Crowther C, Dulet L, Hodnett E, et al. (2000). The second stage of labour. In A Guide to Effective Care in Pregnancy and Childbirth, 3rd edition. Oxford, Oxford University Press, p 298.

33. Rouse D, Weiner S, Bloom S, Varner M, Spong C, Ramin S, et al. (2009). Second-stage labor duration in nulliparous women: Relationship to

6

maternal and perinatal outcomes. Am J Obstet Gynecol 201(357), e1–e7.

34. Allen V, Baskett T, O'Connell C, McKeen D, Allen A. (2009). Maternal and perinatal outcomes with increasing duration of the second stage of labor. Obstet Gynecol 113(6), 1248–1258.

35. Altman M, Lydon-Rochelle M. (2006). Prolonged second stage of labor and risk of adverse maternal and perinatal outcomes: A systematic review. Birth 33(4), 315–322.

36. Lai M, Lin K, Li H, Shey K, Gau M. (2009). Effects of delayed pushing during the second stage of labor on postpartum fatigue and birth outcomes in nulliparous women. J Nurs Res 17(1), 62–72.

37. Davis E. (2004). Heart and Hands: A Caregiver's Guide to Pregnancy and Birth, 4th edition. Berkeley, CA, Celestial Arts.

38. Hamlin RHJ. (1959). Stepping Stones to Labour Ward Diagnosis. Adelaide, Rigby Ltd.

39. Simkin P. (2003). Maternal Positions and Pelves Revisited. Birth 30(2), 130–132.

40. Dudley N. (2005). A systematic review of the ultrasound estimation of fetal weight. Ultrasound Obstet Gynecol 25(1), 80–89.

41. Coomarasamy A, Connock M, Thornton J, Khan K. (2005). Accuracy of ultrasound biometry in the prediction of macrosomia: A systematic quantitative review. Br J Obstet Gynaecol 112(11), 1461–1466.

42. Declercq E, Sakala C, Corry M, Applebaum S, Risher P. (2002). Listening to Mothers: Report of the First National U.S. Survey of Women's Childbearing Experiences. New York, Maternity Center Association.

43. Chalmers B, Dzakpasu S, Heaman M, Kaczorowski J. (2008). The Canadian Maternity Experiences Survey: An overview of findings. J Obstet Gynaecol Can 30(3), 217–228.

44. Fenwick L, Simkin P. (1987). Maternal position to prevent or alleviate dystocia in labor. Clin Obstet Gynecol 30(1), 83–89.

45. Michel S, Rake A, Treiber K, Burkhardt S, Chaoui R, Huch R, et al. (2002). MR obstetric pelvimetry: Effect of birthing position on pelvic bony dimensions. AJR Am J Roentgenol 179(4), 1063–1067.

46. Gherman R, Tramont J, Muffley P, Goodwin T. (2000). Analysis of McRoberts' maneuver by x-ray pelvimetry. Obstet Gynecol 95(1), 43–47.

47. Henderson C, MacDonald S, editors. (2004). Mayes' Midwifery, 13th edition. London, Bailliere Tindall.

48. Health T, Gherman R. (1999). Symphyseal separation, sacroiliac joint dislocation transient lateral femoral cutaneous neuropathy associated with McRoberts' maneuver. A case report. J Reprod Med 44(10), 902–904.

49. Baxley E, Gobbo R. (2004). Shoulder dystocia. Am Fam Physician 69(7):1707–1714.

50. Odent M. (1999). The Scientification of Love. London, Free Association Books.

6

Chapter 7

Optimal Newborn Transition and Third and Fourth Stage Labor Management

Lisa Hanson, PhD, CNM, FACNM, and
Penny Simkin, BA, PT, CCE, CD(DONA)

Overview of the normal third and fourth stages of labor for baby and unmedicated mother, 225
Third stage management: care of the baby, 227
Oral and nasopharynx suctioning, 227
Delayed clamping and cutting of the umbilical cord, 228
Third stage management: the placenta, 229
Expectant physiologic management of the third stage of labor, 229
Active management of the third stage of labor, 230
The fourth stage of labor, 234
Keeping the mother and baby together, 234
Baby-friendly (breastfeeding) practices, 236
Ten steps to successful breastfeeding, 237
Routine newborn assessments, 237
Conclusion, 238
References, 238

7

The Labor Progress Handbook: Early Interventions to Prevent and Treat Dystocia.
Edited by Penny Simkin, Ruth Ancheta
© 2011 by Penny Simkin and Ruth Ancheta; illustrations copyright Ruth Ancheta

OVERVIEW OF THE NORMAL THIRD AND FOURTH STAGES OF LABOR FOR UNMEDICATED MOTHER AND BABY

The third stage of labor encompasses both the delivery of the placenta and the baby's enormous physiologic shift from complete in utero dependence on her placenta to dependence on herself. She takes over the tasks of taking in and using oxygen and food, adapting to her new surroundings, and regulating her own temperature and all life functions. A compelling drama that began with the stimulation and beneficial stress caused by labor contractions continues to unfold with her first breath and first cry. The transition from fetus to neonate is under way and completed in a few minutes, much to everyone's relief and joy. During those first minutes after birth, she inflates her lungs, and they will never deflate for the rest of her life. Now that her lungs have taken over as her organs of respiration, her circulation is rerouted and her heart is restructured so that soon all her blood will circulate through her lungs to pick up the oxygen needed throughout her body. Her skin tones become ruddy due to the increased oxygenation of her blood. She is soaking wet and streaked with blood, mucus, amniotic fluid, and vernix. Her body, at first very warm to the touch, begins to lose heat, which challenges her underdeveloped temperature-regulating system and, with help from the person who wipes her dry and the warmth from her mother's body where she is lain, she stays warm. All her senses, well developed in the womb, inform her about her new world. She sees, smells, hears, feels, and tastes her mother. She calms down, stares alertly and intently at her mother, squirms on her mother's abdomen, and sputters and rids her airway of mucus and fluid.

After 15 to 30 minutes, she becomes active, crawling in a rudimentary way, bringing her hands to her mouth, bobbing her head up and down and side to side, and showing her interest in finding the breast. Guided by the scent of her mother's breast and other mysterious knowledge, she works her way slowly and steadily, but erratically, toward one breast. She knows when she has reached her destination, and she opens her mouth and bobs her way onto her mother's nipple. She may have to adjust a bit, and then, finding the perfect target, zeroes in and draws deep on her mother's nipple, stunning and impressing her mother with her power.

For the mother, the third stage of labor represents the final act of pregnancy—giving birth to her placenta—and an enormous shift within her body and psyche from the task of maintaining the pregnancy to taking on the complex new role of motherhood. As her uterus contracts to expel the placenta, a cocktail of hormones floods her body to give her what she needs to make the shift. The fourth stage, beginning after the birth of the placenta, and lasting for 1 to 2 hours, is sometimes referred to as the "recovery" or "stabilization" stage for the mother. However, Rising, thinking of fourth stage in terms of the mother–baby dyad or family triad, referred to it as the stage of "family integration."[1] It is inappropriate to discuss the fourth stage in terms of only the mother or baby, because mothers and babies, as with all other mammals, are so entwined and mutually dependent. With today's customary involvement in birth by the father or significant other, the fourth stage also includes other family members.

The mother's first emotions, once her baby appears, may be relief and some disbelief that "it's over!" Labor, which had consumed her entire being for hours, is now in the past. It may take some time to absorb that reality. Or she may focus immediately on her baby—with curiosity, disappointment, engrossment, or rapture. Oxytocin, which began to surge during the baby's journey down the birth canal, is at high levels, endorphins are flowing, and these combine to give the mother "high" spirits and feelings of love and gratefulness. These hormones also help override the fatigue, pain, and discouragement that she may have felt earlier.

With her baby in her arms, not only is she providing everything the baby needs at this time, but the baby is reciprocating—that is, giving her much that she needs for involution, successful breastfeeding, and bonding with her baby. The baby's squirming on her abdomen stimulates her uterus to contract and expel the placenta. Once the baby begins nuzzling and suckling at her breast, oxytocin flows and helps her uterus contract and stimulates the pituitary gland to secrete prolactin, the key to the production of breastmilk.

This ideal scenario for third and fourth stages, however, presents a challenge for the midwife or physician—to try to preserve a calm, peaceful private environment, while remaining vigilant. The caregiver and nurse can assess and monitor mother and baby calmly and unobtrusively, but they cannot be swept up completely in the emotions of joy and relief. They know the importance of the third and fourth stages to the well-being of mother and baby and must remain vigilant to events that may require quick action. These concerns sometimes dominate and lead to practices that interrupt the normal maternal–infant tasks of third and fourth stages, which are discussed in this chapter.

If the delicate hormonal interaction and mutual regulation between baby and mother are postponed, rushed, disturbed, altered with medications, or interrupted by surgery, they may not resume as smoothly later, when the delay is over. The chances increase for emotional stress for mother and baby, more crying by the baby, temperature drops in the baby, poorer uterine muscle tone, challenges in the initiation of breastfeeding, and increased need for medical interventions.[2]

In this chapter, we describe common third and fourth stage labor care practices, with a critical examination of usual practices and suggestions for alternative approaches that help to foster the mother–infant and family interactions described above. Topics to be discussed include routine intrapartum oral and nasal suctioning, management of the umbilical cord, evidence-based third stage management approaches, and fostering uninterrupted maternal–newborn contact and breastfeeding.

THIRD STAGE MANAGEMENT: CARE OF THE BABY

Oral and nasopharynx suctioning

Over millennia, during the birth process, the fetal chest has been compressed tightly as it passes through the vagina, providing pressure that helps to clear amniotic fluid and mucus from the respiratory passages. For decades, babies have had their noses and mouths suctioned during the birth process in order to clear them of amniotic fluid and secretions. However, there is no evidence that routine suctioning the oral cavity and nasopharynx of the neonate prior to delivery of the shoulders is necessary or improves neonatal outcomes.[3,4] In fact, routine intrapartum suctioning may lead to instability in neonatal breathing, heart rate, and oxygen saturation.[4] Just as suctioning prior to birth is unnecessary and potentially harmful, the routine of bulb suctioning the normal newborn's nose and mouth immediately following birth has no known benefits, since healthy newborns can usually clear their own airways. Potential hazards of bulb suctioning include laryngospasm and pulmonary artery vasospasm.[5] A policy of no bulb suctioning unless indicated will ensure an airway free of amniotic fluid.

Historically, birth attendants around the world used elaborate strategies to suction babies when the amniotic fluid was meconium stained. However, routine intrapartum oral and nasopharynx suctioning of babies who have meconium-stained amniotic fluid is also not supported by scientific evidence.[3,4] Currently, it is up to the birth attendant to quickly evaluate the infant to decide the best plan of action. Babies born with thick meconium-stained amniotic fluid who are *vigorous* at birth require only routine care and observation.[6] Infants who are *not vigorous* are immediately placed in the radiant warmer, and endotracheal intubation is performed by a trained professional to assess for the presence of meconium below the vocal cords.[6] When this rather brief intubation is necessary, the woman and her family should be educated to understand the need for this procedure and the observation period that follows. Further, parents need reassurance that once the baby is stable, they will be able to hold the baby and initiate breastfeeding.

Delayed clamping and cutting of the umbilical cord

The routine practice of immediate clamping of the umbilical cord at birth has been challenged by a growing body of scientific evidence indicating that both term and preterm neonates benefit significantly from delayed cord clamping.[7–9] When cord clamping is delayed, the newborn gains 30% to 60% more red blood cells (RBCs) as the cord pulses, delivering placental blood to the baby. These additional RBCs transfused from the placenta to the infant are associated with reduced neonatal anemia and improved heart and lung transitioning to the extrauterine environment. Delayed cord clamping has not been associated with adverse outcomes such as jaundice or polycythemia.[7] While delayed cord clamping may slightly elongate the third stage of labor, it is not associated with an increased risk of postpartum hemorrhage.[10]

Several factors impact the amount and speed of RBC transfer. When the healthy neonate is placed on the mother's abdomen immediately following birth and cord clamping is delayed for 3 or more minutes, an increase in the blood volume can be expected. When a newborn is pale or slightly cyanotic following a tight nuchal cord, the baby can held at a level lower than the placenta for 30 seconds to 1 minute (in order to maximize the blood that is transfused), then placed on the mother's abdomen while cord clamping is delayed for a least a total of 3 minutes.[7] This strategy promotes optimal transition to extrauterine life and can improve the color and the tone of neonates who are otherwise healthy at birth.

In the situation of a tight nuchal cord, it is possible to avoid cutting it by using the "somersault maneuver" to deliver the baby. By holding the baby's head against the woman's thigh while the baby's trunk is born, the cord is not overstretched and remains intact. (See Chapter 8, pages 265–267, for a complete description and illustrations.)

THIRD STAGE MANAGEMENT: THE PLACENTA

The third stage of labor begins following the birth of the baby and ends with delivery of the placenta. Placental separation follows a predictable pattern. Initially strong contractions lead to thickening of the uterus, which results in shearing off, eventual separation, and then finally expulsion of the placenta.[11] The signs of placental separation include (a) the uterus rising in the maternal abdomen, (b) the uterus changing shape from discoid to globular, (c) the umbilical cord lengthening, and (d) a small gush of blood flowing from the mother's vagina. Recognition of placental separation is important to appropriate management. The average duration of the third stage of labor is 5 to 10 minutes with the risk of postpartum hemorrhage increasing beyond 30 minutes.[10]

During the third stage of labor, most birth attendants use one of two approaches to provide care—active management or expectant management. However, some practitioners use a combination of both of these approaches.[12]

Expectant physiologic management of the third stage of labor

Expectant management, also referred to as physiologic management of the third stage of labor, is an approach in which the placenta is allowed to deliver spontaneously without the routine administration of oxytoxic medications. However, there are variations in definitions between sources.[12] Birth attendants who use expectant management await the signs of placental separation. Once these signs have occurred, some birth attendants will guard the uterus and use gentle traction to deliver the placenta; others await completely spontaneous placental delivery aided by gravity. Although physiologic management is congruent with the noninterference philosophy held by most midwives and some low-intervention physicians,[13] it has not been adequately studied with a population of women at low risk for postpartum hemorrhage, as defined by midwives.[12] Fahy[12] lists these criteria, all of which are necessary for the midwifery designation of low risk: good maternal health and nutrition; single baby at term; maternal desires for spontaneous placental birth, active participation in the process, prolonged skin-to-skin contact (SSC), and early breastfeeding; trusting relationship with her midwife; an informed and supportive birth team; an environment where the woman feels safe; a midwife who is skilled in physiologic management; normal pregnancy, first and second stage; a healthy infant; and maternal willingness to accept oxytocics if indicated.[12] The midwifery criteria (coined as "psychophysiologic management"[14]) for women at low risk for postpartum hemorrhage are more stringent than accepted obstetric risk factors, because they add psychological and environmental factors. The trials comparing expectant management with active management of third stage have included women who are high risk according to the midwifery criteria just listed. Findings of most existing randomized trials are that expectant management is associated with greater blood loss and a higher incidence of immediate postpartum hemorrhage than is an active management approach to third stage care.[12] Because scientific evidence supporting expectant management for low-risk laboring women is limited,[12,15] all birth attendants have been encouraged to adopt active third stage management.[16,17] This topic will remain controversial among midwives and low-intervention physicians until further evidence becomes available.

Active management of the third stage of labor

Active management of the third stage has been promoted worldwide for decades as a means to shorten the third stage and prevent maternal hemorrhage, a leading cause of maternal death. Active management originally included the following for all women, regardless of risk status: immediate administration of oxytoxic drugs, early clamping and cutting of the umbilical cord, controlled cord traction (*without massage*) during contractions while guarding the uterus (Fig. 7.1), and uterine massage only after placental delivery.[18]

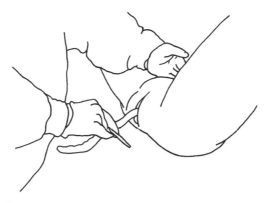

Fig. 7.1. Guarding the uterus.

This approach, however, has resulted in mismanagement by some due to overemphasis on a rapid delivery of the placenta, which may actually increase the risk of postpartum hemorrhage.[19] For example, impatient birth attendants commonly massage the uterus when the placenta is still attached in order to promote a rapid delivery of the placenta. This hurried approach may lead to partial separation of the placenta and *increase* the risk of hemorrhage. Further, attempts to deliver a placenta that is unseparated may lead to uterine inversion that can be life-threatening for the woman.[19]

While uterine massage before delivery of the placenta is a dangerous practice, the value of uterine massage *afterward* is clearly beneficial and its value cannot be overemphasized. As a part of a controlled trial, 200 Egyptian women were randomized to either uterine massage or no uterine massage following the administration of 10 units of oxytocin.[20] Uterine massage was performed every 10 minutes for 60 minutes in the experimental group. Blood loss was measured and compared between the two groups. The women in the massage group had a significantly lower than average blood loss at both 30 and 60 minutes. Further, the need for additional uterotonic medications was significantly reduced in the uterine massage group. These findings support the recommendation that the uterus should be massaged following delivery of the placenta.

Although other features of active management are often omitted, the one critical feature that has consistently been promoted is the prophylactic administration of the oxytoxic medication.[18] Drugs commonly used routinely in active management of the third stage include oxytocin (Pitocin), methylergonovine maleate (Methergine), and misoprostol (Cytotec). Each of these agents stimulates contractions of the uterus via a unique mechanism. Several studies indicate that misoprostol is equally effective as Pitocin[21] and Methergine[22] with the added benefits of low cost and administration that requires no needles and no refrigeration. However, misoprostol has side effects including shivering and the development of a transient fever found to be unacceptable to women who had received it.[23] While misoprostol has potential to reduce postpartum hemorrhage in developing countries,[21] the World Health Organization[16] guideline for hemorrhage preventions contains a recommendation that oxytocin be administered by skilled birth attendants prophylactically and in preference to misoprostol. Therefore, careful selection of appropriate uterotonics requires continuing critical evaluation of the current literature as well as weighing the risks and benefits of the available options.

The timing of the administration of uterotonics as a part of active management is controversial.[24] Most sources on active third stage management indicate that one of these drugs should be administered within 1 minute of the birth.[17,18] However, birth attendants who delay cord clamping also delay the administration of medication until the cord is clamped and cut. Jackson and colleagues conducted a controlled trial where 1,486 women were randomized to receive oxytocin before placental delivery (n = 745) or following birth of the placenta (n = 741). There was no significant difference in the incidence of postpartum hemorrhage (indicated by estimated blood loss, lowering of hemoglobin levels, or the need for additional uterotonic medications), third stage duration, or retained placenta between the two groups. The authors concluded that the prophylactic administration of uterotonics as a part of active management of the third stage could safely be done either before or after the delivery of the placenta.[24]

Research studies on the active management approach used early cord clamping ranging from immediate to within 1 minute of birth.[12] However, early cord clamping robs the baby of 20% of its blood volume.[7] This practice has been removed from the recommended components of active third stage management because of the growing evidence that delayed cord clamping benefits the neonate.[12] This change may encourage more birth attendants to adopt active third stage management.

All well-educated birth attendants are prepared to manage postpartum hemorrhage. Women who have large babies, long labors, a history of postpartum hemorrhage, multiple gestation, or a history of five or more births are at higher risk.[10] However, risk factors do not adequately predict those women who will actually experience postpartum hemorrhages.[10,17] Uterine atony accounts for approximately 70% of postpartum hemorrhages, followed by lacerations and trauma (20%), retained placental tissue (10%), and coagulopathies (1%).[17]

While any of the uterotonic agents can be used for the initial prophylactic administration, during a postpartum hemorrhage the birth attendant will ask for the following: help, a large-bore intravenous line if one is not in place, and use of vigorous uterine massage. If these strategies do not succeed in contracting the uterus, the birth attendant will compress the uterus between both hands (bimanual compression; Fig. 7.2). Careful examination of the placenta for completeness and of the cervix, vagina, and perineum for lacerations are essential components of the management of postpartum hemorrhage. The "Four T's" mnemonic (Tone, Trauma, Tissue, and Thrombin) is used to assist birth attendants to find the cause of the hemorrhage in order to direct appropriate management.[17,p.876] Some or all of the uterotonic medications previously described may be used in sequence, including

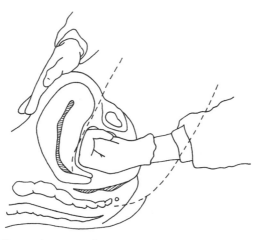

Fig. 7.2. Bimanual compression.

the final addition of another prostaglandin agent (carboprost [Hemabate]) to stop the bleeding.[17] While this agent has unpleasant side effects for the woman, such as nausea and vomiting; administration can be a lifesaving measure.

The management of a hemorrhage can be frightening to the woman and her family. The doula can support the woman during the sometimes painful procedures required to achieve resolution. The doula can also be prepared to keep an eye on the baby if all staff members are focused on the mother. If the baby seems to have difficulty breathing, seems cyanotic, or becomes limp, the doula will need to summon help for the baby.

THE FOURTH STAGE OF LABOR

The "fourth stage of labor" has been used as a term to describe the time from birth of the placenta through the first 1 or 2 postpartum hours. Most definitions focus on the mother—stabilization of her vital signs, control of bleeding, repair of any lacerations, and evidence of the beginnings of involution. However, in keeping with the description of fourth stage that introduces this chapter, our definition includes family integration.[1] The fourth stage is not complete until mother and baby are together, preferably skin to skin and breastfeeding, and "ready to adjust together to their new roles in continuing the lifecycle of the woman and the family."[25,p.424] In other words, rather than stating a specific time period for fourth stage, we suggest specific processes of mother and baby as defining criteria.

Keeping the mother and baby together

Klaus and colleagues (1972)[26] suggested that mothers and their infants need to be kept together during a sensitive period of bonding during the first hour after birth, and that if this process is interrupted there may be serious consequences in attachment between mother and baby. Over the next decades, Klaus and Kennell[27] further developed the concept of the "sensitive period" lasting about 1 hour after birth. These researchers modified this concept, acknowledging that the outcomes of disruption of this sensitive period did not appear to be as long lasting or irrevocable as previously hypothesized. Their work was pivotal in highlighting the third and fourth stages as times when a great deal of physiologic and interpersonal interactions take place that foster other outcomes such as neonatal adaptation, breastfeeding, and maternal recovery, as described later and in the first few pages of this chapter. Today, a Cochrane systematic review of 30 randomized controlled trials of early skin-to-skin contact (SSC) confirm numerous benefits on both mother and baby.[28] Yet, even though many hospitals have established protocols that allow or encourage early maternal–infant contact immediately and for hours afterward, a large American survey of new mothers' experiences during birth found that only 34% reported having their babies in their arms during the first hour after birth.[29] A Canadian survey found better rates of mother–infant contact: 72% had their babies in their arms within 5 minutes after birth (but only one-third of those had SSC). Also, 22% of Canadian women put their babies to their breast within 5 minutes after birth, and by 30 minutes, 45% of babies were at their mothers' breasts.[30]

Currently, in hospitals that are committed to keeping the mother and infant together, initial third and fourth stage management practices used by health providers set the stage. For example, many birth attendants place the baby directly on the mother's abdomen with the umbilical cord still attached and pulsating. The baby is dried and placed on the bare skin of the mother's chest, and both the mother and baby are covered with a prewarmed blanket. This SSC is considered an important component of the initiation of breastfeeding. The specific benefits of early SSC found in the Cochrane systematic review mentioned earlier are positive effects on the following: newborn temperature, early initiation and duration of breastfeeding, maternal loving and attachment behaviors, less neonatal crying, and improved transition to extrauterine life in late preterm infants.[28] SSC was not associated with any negative outcomes. The baby's temperature is stabilized by SSC with the mother in a manner that is superior to that of the electronic radiant warmers.[3] Based on the evidence, there appears to be no rationale for using the radiant warmer instead of SSC.

The term "kangaroo care" (KC) refers to a practice where low-birth-weight neonates are given early and prolonged SSC between the breasts of their mothers. KC was associated with improved outcomes in some studies, such as better weight gain and reduced risk of infections. However, a meta-analysis demonstrated that the level of evidence is insufficient to recommend routine KC for all low-birth-weight infants.[31] This is an example of a situation where a harmless procedure that does not result in the outcomes measured may still have great appeal to worried helpless parents of premature babies. Holding their babies skin to skin may be important to their attachment and a sense of being able to nurture their babies. The involvement they feel and the opportunity to know their babies well are worth making the practice commonplace. In fact, many believe that KC should be the standard method of care for all newborn babies, both premature and full term.[32]

BABY-FRIENDLY (BREASTFEEDING) PRACTICES

The World Health Organization's Baby Friendly Initiative encourages that women be assisted to breastfeed within 30 minutes of birth.[16] Instinctual infant suckling behaviors manifest in a predictable pattern within the first hour of life.[33] The initiation of breastfeeding promotes uterine contractility and therefore placental separation and expulsion. Specifically, breastfeeding stimulates the release of oxytocin from the posterior pituitary gland in the mother's brain. This hormone is also strongly associated with maternal love.[27,34] Breastfeeding is a synergy between mother and baby where both benefit physically and emotionally. Table 7.1 contains the 10 steps to successful breastfeeding that are a part of the Baby Friendly Initiative. These principles can guide healthcare providers and doulas while they support breastfeeding.

Newborns, placed in the middle of their mother's abdomen (nose at the level of the nipples), have the ability to move to find the nipple and initiate breastfeeding rather independently.[35] This has been called the "breast crawl" and is being promoted internationally as a strategy to initiate and to encourage breastfeeding.[32] Infants born following unmedicated births have more coordinated suckling activity during the breast crawl than those born to mothers who have received analgesics.[36] The Breast Crawl benefits the mother by enhancing placental expulsion and reducing postpartum blood loss.[37] This occurs mechanically, as the newborn kicks his legs and stimulates uterine contractions, and also hormonally, as the stimulation to the nipples releases oxytocin into the maternal circulation. Therefore, this instinctual breastfeeding behavior benefits both the mother and the newborn and ultimately assures the mother that breastfeeding can be successful.

Ten steps to successful breastfeeding

Table 7.1.   Ten Steps to Successful Breastfeeding

Every facility providing maternity sevices and care for newborn infants should:

1. Have a written breastfeeding policy that is routinely communicated to all healthcare staff.
2. Train all healthcare staff in skills necessary to implement this policy.
3. Inform all pregnant women about the benefits and management of breastfeeding.
4. Help mothers initiate breastfeeding within a half-hour of birth.
5. Show mothers how to breastfeed, and how to maintain lactation even if they should be separated from their infants.
6. Give newborn infants no food or drink other than breastmilk unless *medically* indicated.
7. Practice rooming in—allow mothers and infants to remain together—24 hours a day.
8. Encourage breastfeeding on demand.
9. Give no artificial teats or pacifiers (also called dummies or soothers) to breastfeeding infants.
10. Foster the establishment of breastfeeding support groups and refer mothers to them on discharge from the hospital or clinic.

From the Ten Steps to Successful Breastfeeding, a summary of the guidelines for maternity care facilities presented in the Joint WHO/UNICEF Statement Protecting, Promoting, and Supporting Breastfeeding: The Special Role of Maternity Services, (WHO, 1989), which have been accepted as the minimum global criteria for attaining the status of a Baby-Friendly Hospital. From: http://whqlibdoc.who.int/publications/2009/9789241594967_eng.pdf. Reprinted with permission from WHO/UNICEF.

7

ROUTINE NEWBORN ASSESSMENTS

In many hospitals, a high priority is placed on efficiently completing a checklist of routine newborn assessments and procedures before uniting mother and baby for extended time together. It is not necessary to separate them during this time. The nurse can observe the baby's initial transition with assessments of the baby's color, respirations, muscle tone, and pulse while the baby is in the mother's arms and without the need for equipment. For example, the pulse of the baby is readily palpable on the umbilical cord or the stump of the cord if it was already clamped and cut. While this approach is appealing to most mothers, some mothers find it disagreeable when the baby is unwashed.

Therefore, it is optimal if the approach to immediate care of the newborn is discussed with the woman and her family prior to the birth.

Following this initial transition period, the series of routine assessments and required procedures interfere with parent–infant interactions when they take place in the radiant warmer, several feet away from the mother and her significant others. The nurse observes the infant's transition to extrauterine life by careful monitoring of vital signs (temperature, heart rate, respiratory rate, and blood pressure). The nurse also administers the erythromycin opthalmic ointment to the infant to prevent neonatal conjunctivitis and vitamin K injections to prevent hemorrhagic disease of the newborn. Last, the careful documentation of the baby's identification through the use of matching bands on both the mother and the infant requires significant nursing time. Creative nurses who are committed to SSC accomplish these tasks with the baby in the parent's arms and with minimal interference with parental interaction. Alternatively, they may postpone whatever tasks can be delayed to allow for SSC and the initiation of breastfeeding. Parents who wish to remain in constant contact with their newborn need to clearly communicate this to the nursing staff. If there is no other option, the radiant warmers have wheels that allow them to be rolled next to the mother's birthing bed. A doula can help parents with their desires regarding SSC and minimal separation from their babies by learning their preferences in advance and encouraging them to voice them early in a birth plan, during labor and again after the birth.

7

CONCLUSION

The third and fourth stages of labor are busy times in terms of care and observation of mother and baby, yet they are also times of mutual mother–baby regulation. Continuous SSC between mother and baby fosters newborn adaptation, maternal recovery, and deep emotional connections within the family. Sensitive care at this time includes respect for the benefits of SSC and a belief by the staff in the importance of minimal disturbance combined with vigilant oversight.

REFERENCES

1. Rising SS. (1974). The fourth stage of labor: Family integration. Am J Nursing 74(5), 870–874.

2. Buckley SJ. (2005). Leaving well alone—Perspectives on a natural third stage. Chapter 15, In: Gentle Birth, Gentle Mothering: The Wisdom and Science of Gentle Choices in Pregnancy, Birth, and Parenting (pp. 184–213). Brisbane, Australia, One Moon Press.

3. Mercer JS, Erickson-Owens DA, Graves B, Haley MM. (2007). Evidence-based practices for the fetal to newborn transition. J Midwif Women's Health 52(3), 262–272. doi:10.1016/j.jmwh.2007.01.005.

4. Velaphi S, Vidyasagar D. (2008). The pros and cons of suctioning at the perineum (intrapartum) and post-delivery with and without meconium. Semin Fetal Neonat Med 13, 375–382. doi:10.1016/j.siny.2008.04.001.

5. Enkin M, Keirse MJNC, Neilson J, et al. (2000). A Guide to Effective Care in Pregnancy and Childbirth, 3rd edition. Oxford, UK, Oxford University Press.

6. American Heart Association and American Academy of Pediatrics. (2006). 2005 American Heart Association (AHA) guidelines for cardiopulmonary resuscitation (CPR) and emergency cardiovascular care (ECC) of pediatric and neonatal patients: Neonatal resuscitation guidelines. Pediatrics 117, e1029–e1038. doi:10.1542/peds.2006-0349.

7. Mercer JS. (2001). Current best evidence: A review of the literature on umbilical cord clamping. J Midwif Womens Health 46(6), 402–414.

8. Mercer JS, Skovgaard RL, Peareara-Eaves J, Bowman TA. (2005). Nuchal cord management and nurse-midwifery practice. J Midwif Womens Health, 50(5), 373–379. doi:10.1016/j.jmwh.2005.04.023

9. Hutton EK, Hassan ES. (2007). Late vs early clamping of the umbilical cord in full term neonates: Systematic review and meta-analysis of controlled trials. JAMA 297, 1241–1252. doi:10.1001/jama.297.11.1241.

10. Bair ME, Williams J. (2007). Management of the third stage of labor. J Midwif Womens Health 52(4), 412–414.

11. Herman A, Zimerman A, Arieli S, et al. (2002). Down-up sequential separation of the placenta. Ultrasound Obstet Gynecol 19, 278–281.

12. Fahy KM. (2009). Third stage labour care for women at low risk of postpartum hemorrhage. J Midwif Womens Health 54, 380–386. doi:10.1016/j.jmwh.2008.12.016.

13. Tan WM, Klein MC, Saxell L, Shirkoohy SE, Asrat G. (2008). How do physicians and midwives manage the third stage of labor? Birth 35(3), 220–229.

14. Hastie C, Fahy K. (2009). Optimising psychophysiology in the third stage of labour: Theory applied to practice. Women Birth, 22, 89–96.

15. Fahy K, Hastie C, Bisits A, Marsh C, Smith L, Saxton A. (2010). Holistic physiological care compared with active management of the third stage

of labour for women at low risk of postpartum haemorrhage: A cohort study. Women Birth 23(4), 146–152.

16. World Health Organization. (2007). WHO Recommendations for the Prevention of Postpartum Haemorrhage. Geneva, Switzerland, World Health Organization.

17. Anderson, J. M, Etches, D. (2007). Prevention and management of postpartum hemorrhage. American Family Physician, 75, 875–882.

18. International Confederation of Midwives (ICM) & International Federation of Gynaecologists and Obstetricians (FIGO). (2004). Joint statement: Management of the third stage of labour to prevent postpartum haemorrhage. Journal of Midwifery & Women's Health, 49(1), 76–77. doi:10.1016/j.jmwh.2003.11.005

19. Varney H, Kriebs JM, Gegor CL, eds. (2004). The normal third stage of labor. In Varney's Midwifery, 4th edition (pp. 905–911). Sudbury, MA, Jones & Bartlett.

20. Hofmeyr G, Abdel-Aleem H, Abdel-Aleem M. (2008) Uterine massage for preventing postpartum haemorrhage. Cochrane Database Syst Rev (3):CD006431.

21. Kundodyiwa TW, Majoko F, Rusakaniko S. (2001). Misoprostol versus oxytocin in the third stage of labor. Int J Gynecol Obstet, 75, 235–241.

22. Garg P, Batra S, Gandhi G. (2005). Oral misoprostol versus injectable methylergometrine in management of the third stage of labor. Int J Gynecol Obstet 91, 160–161.

23. McDonald S. (2007). Management of the third stage of labor. J Midwif Womens Health 52, 254–261.

24. Jackson KW, Allbert JR, Schemmer GK, Elliot M, Humphrey A, Taylor J. (2001). A randomized controlled trial comparing oxytocin administration before and after placental delivery in the prevention of postpartum hemorrhage. Am J Obstet Gynecol 185, 873–877.

25. Gould D. (2000). Normal labour: A concept analysis. J Adv Nursing 31, 418–427.

26. Klaus MH, Jerauld R, Kreger NC, McAlpine W, Steffa M, Kennell JH. (1972). Maternal attachment: Importance of the first post-partum days. N Engl J Med 286, 460–463.

27. Klaus MH, Kennell JH. (2001). Care of the parents. In Klaus MH, Fanaroff AA, eds. Care of the High-Risk Neonate, 5th edition (pp. 195–222). Philadelphia, Saunders.

28. Moore ER, Anderson GC, Bergman N. (2007). Early skin-to-skin contact for mothers and their healthy newborn infants. Cochrane Database Syst Rev (3):CD003519. doi:10.1002/14651858.CD003519.pub2.

7

29. Declerq E, Sakala C, Corry M, Appelbaum S. (2006). Listening to Mothers, II: Report of the Second National U.S. Survey of Women's Childbearing Experiences. New York, Childbirth Connection.
30. Chalmers B, Dzakpasu S, Heaman M, Kaczorowski J. (2008). The Canadian Maternity Experiences Survey: An overview of findings. J Obstet Gynaecol Can 30, 217–228.
31. Conde-Agudelo A, Belizán JM. (2003). Kangaroo mother care to reduce morbidity and mortality in low birthweight infants. Cochrane Database Syst Rev (2)CD002771. doi:10.1002/14651858.CD002771.
32. Bergman N. (2010). Kangaroo Mother Care for all. www.kangaroomothercare.com.
33. UNICEF, World Health Organization. (2009). Baby-friendly hospital initiative. http://www.who.int/nutrition/topics/bfhi/en/index.html
34. Uvnas-Moberg K. (2003). The Oxytocin Factor: Tapping the Hormone of Calm, Love and Healing. Cambridge, MA, Da Capa Press.
35. Varendi H, Porter RH, Winberg J. (1994). Does the newborn baby find the nipple by smell? Lancet 344(8928), 989–990.
36. UNICEF, World Health Organization, Worldwide Alliance for Breastfeeding Action. (2009). Initiation of breastfeeding by breast crawl: A scientific overview. http://breastcrawl.org/science.htm
37. Righard L, Alade MO. (1990). Effect of delivery room routines on success of first breast-feed. Lancet 1105(8723), 1105–1107.

7

Chapter 8

Low-Technology Clinical Interventions to Promote Labor Progress

Lisa Hanson, PhD, CNM, FACNM

Intermediate-level interventions for management of problem labors, 243

When progress in prelabor or latent phase remains inadequate, 244

Therapeutic rest, 244

Nipple stimulation, 244

Management of cervical stenosis or the "zipper" cervix, 245

When progress in active phase remains inadequate, 245

Artificial rupture of the membranes (AROM), 246

Digital or manual rotation of the fetal head, 246

Manual reduction of a persistent cervical lip, 250

Reducing swelling of the cervix or anterior lip, 251

Fostering normality in birth, 251

Perineal management, 251

When progress in second stage labor remains inadequate, 257

Duration of second stage labor, 257

Supportive directions for bearing down efforts, 258

Hand maneuvers and anticipatory management of intrapartum problems, 258

Shoulder dystocia, 258

Somersault maneuver, 265

8

The Labor Progress Handbook: Early Interventions to Prevent and Treat Dystocia.
Edited by Penny Simkin, Ruth Ancheta
© 2011 by Penny Simkin and Ruth Ancheta; illustrations copyright Ruth Ancheta

Nonpharmacologic and minimally invasive pharmacologic techniques for intrapartum pain relief, 267
Acupuncture, 267
Sterile water injections, 269
Nitrous oxide, 271
Topical anesthetic applied to the perineum, 271
Conclusion, 271
References, 272

INTERMEDIATE-LEVEL INTERVENTIONS FOR MANAGEMENT OF PROBLEM LABORS

This chapter presents background information, indications, techniques, risks, benefits, and evidence of effectiveness for common interventions used by birth attendants including midwives and doctors. Some of the techniques presented offer alternatives to common higher-technology interventions and are intended to expand the options available for the care of women during labor and birth. While some of these approaches are not widely used, they may be favored by birth attendants who support a lower-technology approach to problems that present during labor. The interventions discussed in this chapter can be considered intermediate steps in a stepwise approach to resolving intrapartum problems. Simpler steps (primary interventions) are presented in earlier chapters. The final, highest level steps in this approach are reserved for the most serious problems that require more complex, invasive or highly technological medical and surgical interventions.

This chapter is not intended to replace professional education concerning birth attendant skills. Professional midwifery, medical, and nursing education should include theory and practice of skills necessary to manage common intrapartum problems. Further, every birth attendant is trained to manage complications within his or her scope of practice and to consult or refer when an intervention is beyond that skill set.

Doulas fulfill an important role in supporting women during intrapartum problems. This chapter also includes suggestions for nonclinical ways in which a doula may help when these birth attendant interventions are needed to manage intrapartum problems.

8

WHEN PROGRESS IN PRELABOR OR LATENT PHASE REMAINS INADEQUATE

If progress seems particularly slow when a woman is in the prelabor or latent phase, there are several strategies that can be used if the situation warrants. The strategies that will be described are therapeutic rest, nipple stimulation, and management of cervical stenosis.

Therapeutic rest

Chapters 2 and 4 present reviews of possible etiologies for a prolonged prelabor or latent phase and offer suggestions for safe low-intervention ways to promote progress. If, after trying these measures, progress has not improved, the woman may be exhausted, discouraged, and frustrated. In most cases, the next appropriate step for the birth attendant is either to augment the labor or to address the exhaustion. Assuming all else is normal, and latent labor is not progressing, the birth attendant may use medications that broadly fit under the term "therapeutic rest" to promote the mother's comfort while enhancing progress.[1] The goal of this therapy is sleep rather than analgesia. However the medication must be carefully selected to enhance benefits and minimize risks.

Nipple stimulation

Nipple stimulation can be used to augment labor when contractions are inadequate as described in Chapters 2 and 5 pages 46, 153. A Cochrane review included five trials with a total of 719 women in whom breast stimulation was compared with no intervention and two trials where breast stimulation was compared to oxytocin.[2] When the cervix was favorable and breast stimulation was compared to no intervention, the number of women not in labor by 72 hours was significantly reduced by the use of nipple stimulation. There was also a significantly lower rate of postpartum hemorrhage. There were no significant differences in the rates of cesarean birth, meconium-stained amniotic fluid, or hyperstimulation of the uterus. When breast stimulation was compared with oxytocin, no significant differences were found on the outcomes of labor initiation by 72 hours, cesarean rate, or meconium-stained fluid. Therefore, nipple stimulation is a viable option to attempt before considering oxytocin augmentation of labor.

Because several fetal deaths were reported in a study that included high-risk laboring women, the authors of the Cochrane review concluded that breast stimulation should not be used in that subgroup until further research verifies the safety of the intervention.[2]

While nipple stimulation appears to be beneficial in initiating labor, protocols vary between sources and a standardized definition is lacking.[3] Several specific protocols have been described as a part of research studies. One approach uses an electric breast pump unilaterally for 15 minutes on each breast.[4] Alternatively, women can use either manual stimulation or an electric breast pump unilaterally (on the lowest setting) for 10 minutes followed by 5 minutes of rest.[5] This pattern is repeated up to four times or until contractions are less than 3 minutes apart. Manual stimulation can be done by the woman herself or by her partner either by gently stroking the nipple directly or indirectly through clothing. Other protocols described by practitioners include instructions for women to stop the nipple stimulation if a contraction occurs or to stimulate the nipples only between contractions.[3] There is no evidence for the efficacy of one protocol over another, and research in this area is needed.[3]

Management of cervical stenosis or the "zipper" cervix

In Chapter 3, page 71, and Chapter 4, pages 111–112, some unusual cervical exam findings were described that slow cervical dilation. When stenosis of the cervical os is encountered, the cause may be adhesions that occurred spontaneously or as a result of prior cervical surgery. When the cervix is completely effaced, the birth attendant can gently massage the cervix in a circular motion to release the adhesions. This will cause less discomfort for the woman if it is done between contractions. Another approach is to insert one or two fingers into the cervical os in order to gently stretch it open. As the adhesions release, the cervical os opens like a zipper, sometimes dilating 1 to 4 cm during a single contraction.

WHEN PROGRESS IN ACTIVE PHASE REMAINS INADEQUATE

If labor progress seems particularly slow during active phase, there are several strategies that can be used if the situation warrants. The strategies that will be described are artificial rupture of the membranes, manual reduction of a persistent cervical lip, and digital or manual rotation of the fetal head.

Artificial rupture of the membranes (AROM)

Low-intervention birth attendants, such as midwives, avoid *routine* interventions because of a philosophy that supports the natural process of labor and birth. Therefore, most midwives do not perform artificial rupture of the membranes (AROM) without a specific indication.[6] Assuming the bag of waters is intact at the onset of labor, if left alone, it remains intact until full dilation in 7 of 10 births.[7] The intact bag of waters appears to provide benefits for fetal head rotation as well as helping prevent ascending infections.[8]

AROM is believed to enhance labor progress by increasing pressure on the cervix and lower uterine segment, thus stimulating the release of prostaglandins and oxytocin,[8] and can be used in active labor to promote progress when other approaches have failed.[7] When AROM is indicated, most midwives wait to use it until the fetal head is engaged in the pelvis and well applied to the cervix during active labor, for reasons of cord safety.[9] For example, a conservative approach is to reserve this intervention until the vaginal exam indicates is at least 4 cm dilation, 100% effacement, and a 0 station. Rupture at higher stations when the fetal head is not well-engaged is associated with an increased risk of umbilical cord prolapse. Even when indicated and when conditions appear optimal, AROM is not without risks. First, it may not have the desired results (i.e., enhanced progress). Second, AROM places the woman at greater risk of infection. Also, severe variable decelerations due to cord compression may occur following AROM.[10] The caregiver should explain to the woman that the next contractions may be quite intense.

The doula's role during AROM is to provide emotional support and help the woman deal with the stronger contractions that may follow AROM.

Digital or manual rotation of the fetal head

When the fetal head persists in an occiput posterior (OP) or occiput transverse (OT) position, the woman is at greater risk of prolonged labor, operative vaginal birth, severe perineal lacerations, and cesarean birth.[11] Half of multiparas and at least one fourth of nulliparas who experience labor with a fetus in a persistent OP or OT position will deliver spontaneously.[12] Therefore, expectant management may be used when the fetal heart tones are reassuring, if pelvic capacity is considered adequate and second stage labor progress continues to be demonstrated.[12] However, when progress does not continue and the interventions suggested in earlier chapters are not successful, the midwife or doctor can attempt to rotate the OP or OT fetus digitally or manually to an occiput anterior (OA) position with only a small risk of complications.[13-15] Complications of both manual and digital rotation are rare but include prolapse of the umbilical cord or fetal small parts, and cervical laceration (with manual rotation only).

It is important to ensure fetal well-being before, during, and after rotation attempts. It has been suggested in the literature that a non-reassuring fetal heart tracing is an indication to attempt manual or digital rotation of an OP fetus, in order to expedite birth. However, the development of category 3 fetal heart tones during the procedure would be an indication to stop the rotation attempt immediately.[13]

While digital and manual rotation are described in obstetric and midwifery text books and have been the subject of recent research studies, they are not mainstream clinical interventions in the United States and elsewhere. However, the Society of Obstetricians and Gynecologists of Canada recommends their use "alone or in conjunction with instrumental birth with little or no increased risk to the pregnant woman or to the fetus."[14,p.749] Therefore, practitioners who would like to attempt these in clinical practice are encouraged to practice with models and then ideally conduct initial rotations under the guidance of a birth attendant who is experienced with the procedure.

In order to accomplish a digital or manual rotation, the midwife or doctor must be skilled in identifying the landmarks on the fetal skull. Further, careful abdominal palpation to fully assess fetal position should be done prior to the attempt. While some birth attendants recommend ultrasound visualization of the fetal head position prior to the procedure, many do not routinely perform ultrasounds prior to digital or manual rotations.[13] With the increasing availability of portable affordable ultrasound units at the bedside, practitioners may become more willing and able to safely attempt these procedures. It has been suggested that digital or manual rotation is best attempted when cervical dilatation is 7 cm or greater.[13] The results of three research studies found approximately two to three times more spontaneous vaginal births when medically indicated digital or manual rotations were done than when they were not done.[13,16,17]

Reichman and colleagues[17)] studied the outcomes of 61 women who entered the second stage of labor with the fetus in an OP position. Half received no intervention and served as controls; half were managed using digital or manual rotation. Digital or manual rotation resulted in a significant increase in the number of women who experienced spontaneous vaginal birth in an OA position and a significant reduction in the length of the second stage of labor, use of episiotomy, incidence of cesarean birth, and length of hospital stay.

The choice of digital versus manual rotation is not discussed in the clinical or scientific literature. Digital rotation may be easier than manual at higher stations because only two fingers are necessary to accomplish the maneuver. Manual rotation may be best accomplished when the station is lower and the fetal head can be more easily reached using the whole hand, during late first or early second stage labor. In either approach, preliminary steps consist of informed consent by the mother, with discussion of the potential benefits, risks, and discomfort associated with the maneuver, as well as alternatives. The woman's bladder should be emptied (via catheter if needed), and she should be assisted to the dorsal recumbent position with adequate physical and emotional support, and possibly pain medications to allow optimal relaxation. Continuous fetal monitoring is recommended during the procedure to monitor fetal tolerance.[13] Both techniques are described and illustrated later.

The doula can assist during this procedure by providing reassurance and coaching the woman to bear down when contractions start, as instructed by her midwife or doctor.

8

Digital rotation

Digital rotation is accomplished by using the tips of the index and middle fingers of one hand. The fingers are inserted into the vagina to palpate the lambdoid sutures located at the posteriormost aspect of the parietal bone at its juncture with the posterior fontanelle where it overlaps the occipital bone.[17] Upward pressure is exerted to rotate the posterior fontanelle toward the symphysis pubis via rotation of the examiner's hand and forearm in a dialing motion.[17] Cargill and

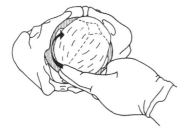

Fig. 8.1. Digital rotation.

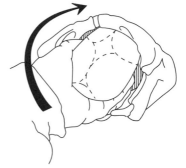

Fig. 8.2. Manual rotation.

colleagues[14] suggested holding the fetal head in the rotated position for several contractions to avoid spontaneous return to the OP (Fig. 8.1).

Manual rotation

There is no specific recommendation that manual rotation requires maternal analgesia; however, since the procedure may be associated with significant discomfort, and maternal relaxation will facilitate manual rotation, epidural analgesia or nitrous oxide may be considered. In fact, many caregivers are unwilling to perform manual rotation without analgesia for the mother.[12]

When performing a manual rotation, the midwife or doctor uses the hand opposite the fetal head position. For example, if the fetus is in the left OP position or left OT position, the birth attendant uses her or his right hand. Following a contraction, the birth attendant places the entire hand (palm up) behind the fetal ear,[13] slightly dislodging the fetal head while encouraging flexion.[14] The fingers are placed under the posterior parietal bone with the thumb positioned on the anterior parietal bone (Fig. 8.2). During the next contraction while the woman bears down, the birth attendant rotates the baby's occiput to an anterior position. Depending on the situation, this may involve rotating one's hand at the wrist or rotating with the entire forearm. As was suggested for digital rotation, the fetal head can be held in the rotated position for several contractions to prevent spontaneous return to the OP position.[14] If this procedure is unsuccessful and the fetal heart rate is reassuring, manual rotation can be reattempted, assuming the mother can tolerate the associated discomfort.[13]

Recently researchers evaluated the outcomes of manual rotation.[13] Multiparity and maternal age less than 35 were associated with successful rotations to the OA position. Rotations done in first stage labor were three times more likely to be unsuccessful than are those done after complete dilation. Prophylactic rotation, not surprisingly, was more successful than rotation done for failure to progress.[13] Following successful rotation, the cesarean rate was 2%, compared with 34% when rotation failed.[16]

Manual and digital rotation procedures offer a lower-technology option to promote progress when the fetus is in an OP or OT position. The use of these rotations may promote successful vaginal birth and should be more widely taught and utilized.

Manual reduction of a persistent cervical lip

The presence of an anterior cervical lip sometimes indicates that the fetus is in an OP or asynclitic position. Sometimes, if patience, position changes, or bathtub immersion do not succeed in reducing the cervical lip, manual reduction may be warranted. This is of particular use if there are concerns about the fetal heart rate or the woman's involuntary bearing-down efforts begin before complete or nearly complete dilation and are strong and uncoordinated. The manual reduction technique, used by midwives and doctors, is explained next:

8

- Explain the procedure, including the discomfort that the woman may experience along with the expected benefit of shortening the time until complete dilation. Emphasize the need for the woman to cooperate with the birth attendant for the procedure to be successful.
- Using water soluble lubricant, place two fingers slightly separated at the 11 and 1 o'clock positions (with the hand palm side down) between the head and the lip of cervix before the onset of a contraction.[9,18]
- Instruct the mother (who may or may not be experiencing a spontaneous urge to push) not to push until you tell her to do so.

- As you feel the contraction begin, push the anterior cervix over the baby's head (as if you were pushing up your upper lip to make your teeth visible). If the cervical lip moves easily, instruct the mother to push to help the head advance, leaving the cervical lip behind it and pushing your fingers out of the vagina.
- Check after the contraction to be sure that the lip has not reappeared.
- Repeat if necessary and if the mother can tolerate it.
- It is prudent to reexamine the woman if, after a few more contractions, progress is not obvious to ensure that the cervix remained completely dilated and is not becoming trapped and swollen.

Reducing swelling of the cervix or anterior lip

Swelling of the cervix or cervical lip is an additional deterrent to continued labor progress. To reduce swelling of the cervix, homeopathic Arnica 12C to 30C can be administered orally, or evening primrose oil or ice can be directly applied and held in place.[18]

FOSTERING NORMALITY IN BIRTH

Perineal management

Prenatal perineal massage

Prenatal perineal massage beginning at 35 weeks is associated with a decrease in perineal damage requiring repair with suture.[19,20] Women's intimate partners can perform antenatal perineal massage using a good-quality water-soluble lubricant, coconut oil, or any vegetable oil for 3 to 10 minutes each day. (Mineral oil and petroleum-based products should be avoided because the vagina cannot clear these oils effectively and they may alter the normal flora and result in an infection from the overgrowth of other organisms.)

To begin, the woman should recline in a semisitting position with her knees bent, using pillows for support. Following good handwashing, the partner applies the oil or lubricant to his or her index finger or fingers and the perineal tissues. The partner places the finger(s) between 1 to 1½ inches into the vagina, and while keeping them inserted and slightly flexed, rubs toward the sides, using a sweeping U-shaped movement, and presses downward (toward the rectum) in the center (Fig. 8.3) .

8

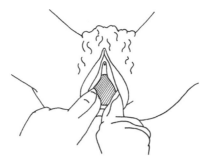

Fig. 8.3. Prenatal perineal massage.

Once the woman experiences a slight burning sensation, her partner maintains one or both fingers in position for 1 to 2 minutes while the woman uses relaxation and breathing techniques. Within a week or less, the woman and her partner will probably notice more elasticity in the tissues, along with a reduction in the burning sensation during perineal massage. In a retrospective study of 368 women, prenatal perineal massage was found to be associated with reduced perineal trauma at birth, especially for women having first babies.[21] Beckman and colleagues[19] reviewed four controlled trials of digital perineal massage that included 2,497 women. Among primigravidas, prenatal massage significantly reduced the incidence of intrapartum perineal damage that required suturing as well as the incidence of episiotomy. Multigravidas did not experience these same benefits. The meta-analysis also revealed that perineal massage did not significantly alter the depth of lacerations when they did occur or the incidence of operative vaginal delivery.[19] No significant differences were found in long-term postpartum pain, sexual satisfaction, or urinary and/or fecal incontinence in women who used perineal massage prenatally. In conclusion, it appears that prenatal perineal massage offers benefits to primigravidas without conferring short- or long-term risks.

Perineal management during second stage

Because scientific evidence does not support routine use of episiotomy,[22] low-intervention birth attendants such as midwives and some family doctors favor strategies that minimize perineal damage. Chief among these is the support of spontaneous bearing down, rather than prolonged forceful pushing.[23,24] Spontaneous maternal bearing down efforts are associated with improved perineal[23,24] and fetal[25] outcomes compared to outcomes of directed Valsalva bearing down.

Verbal support of spontaneous bearing down efforts

The most appropriate verbal support for the woman who is bearing down spontaneously is to offer words of approval and encouragement, along with reminders to relax the legs and perineum. Verbal support and encouragement done in a natural speaking voice can replace the use of outdated, loud directions to "*count to 10*" that are still heard in many birth rooms today.[26] Examples of supportive phrases include:

> "*Let yourself push naturally. Your body knows what to do.*"
> "*That's the way; just like that. There is plenty of room for this baby.*"
> "*Your perineum is starting to stretch. That's a very good sign.*"
> "*Good job.*"
> "*I can see the head.*"
> "*You are moving your baby with every push.*"
> "*Let yourself rest between contractions. Good.*"
> "*That burning you feel is normal. It's your body telling you that the stretching is happening. Feel free to ease off a bit on the push until it starts to go away.*"

Chapter 6 includes extensive discussion of supportive care in the second stage of labor.

Maternal birth positions

8

Laboring women benefit from autonomy in selecting positions that work best for them.[27] During the second stage of labor, the midwife or doctor can create an environment that supports the woman's choices and comfort and may benefit the progress of her labor and birth.[25] Women laboring in upright positions also experience fewer episiotomies, fewer fetal heart rate abnormalities, slight reductions in both the duration of the second stage of labor and the need for operative deliveries, less discomfort, improved satisfaction,[25] and improved ability to participate actively in the birth.

When a woman's legs are separated widely, as in the lithotomy position, there is more tension on the delicate tissue of the perineum,[28] which may result in more tearing with and without an episiotomy. Therefore, positions in which the woman's legs are relaxed may promote better perineal outcomes. A retrospective analysis of 2,756 midwife-attended births supports this hypothesis. The women who gave birth in recumbent positions with their legs spread required significantly more perineal suturing, while women who gave birth in hands-and-knees positions required significantly less.[29] Therefore, if a woman's perineal tissues appear tense in a particular position, a change to another position may reduce that tension. For this reason, periodic position changes during second stage are a good way to protect the perineum from damage, as well as to change pelvic shape and alter gravity effects to aid descent.

When the birth attendant desires to facilitate progress during late second stage labor, positions that allow the sacrum to remain unimpeded by the bed are a good choice. For example, a side-lying position in which only one of the woman's legs is flexed onto her abdomen serves to avoid tension on the perineum and prevents vena caval compression, thereby increasing blood flow to the fetus and maximizing the mobility of the pelvis. This is an example of a position that provides a physiologic alternative to the continued overuse of the exaggerated lithotomy position in some settings. See Chapters 6 and 9 for detailed discussion and illustrations of second stage positions.

Guiding women through crowning of the fetal head

As the baby emerges, the midwife or doctor guides the woman through intense sensations of burning and stretching. She or he may use warm compresses or a topical anesthetic (page 271) to help relieve the pain. It is important that the woman not hear a variety of voices giving conflicting instructions. For this reason, it is helpful when all personnel are familiar with spontaneous bearing down and ways to provide appropriate verbal support, as stated earlier. If other people are speaking, they should provide quiet, unobtrusive encouragement. If the woman appears distracted, the nurse or doula may say quietly in her ear, "*Listen to your midwife (or doctor). She/he will guide you through this part.*" The midwife or doctor can speak to everyone in the room at the same time in a calm assertive voice, using statements like, "*Everything is going well. Both the mother and baby are doing fine.*

There is no need to rush. I need [the woman's name] to hear my voice as I guide her through this part of the process. You don't need to count or tell her how to push. She knows how to give birth and she is doing that beautifully."

Slow delivery of the fetal head over the perineum allows perineal tissues to stretch more gradually.[25] Instead of using prolonged, closed glottis pushing, many midwives encourage women to "breathe" the head out as it crowns. Others prefer to deliver the fetal head between contractions. This usually requires the birth attendant to give the woman specific directions to avoid pushing during contractions when the head is crowning. A recent survey found that a majority of U.S. certified nurse-midwives and certified midwives actively direct maternal pushing during crowning, to prevent perineal damage.[30]

Hand skills to protect the perineum

Methods of managing the delivery of the fetal head appear to impact perineal outcomes. However, this is not well addressed in the current scientific literature. Midwives use a variety of techniques to direct the head as it emerges and vary approaches to meet women's individual needs. If the fetal head is emerging rapidly, gentle counterpressure can be used to slow the birth and protect the perineum for damage. For example, pressure with three fingers on the vertex can offer both support and control. Some midwives gently squeeze the perineum to avoid sudden overstretching of the delicate tissues. The use of a towel can offer mild traction on the moist tissues of the perineum while allowing visualization of crowning.

If the fetus is in an OA position, the midwife may give downward pressure to keep the fetal head flexed (Fig. 8.4). If the fetus is in an

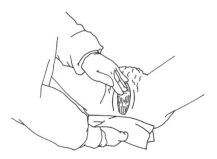

Fig. 8.4. Supported crowning.

OP position, upward pressure is used to maintain flexion.[31] However, the use of this manual flexion technique has been criticized because it counters the extension mechanism of labor that is essential for the fetus to negotiate the curve of the birth canal.[31] More research is needed in this area.

McCandlish and colleagues[32,p.1263] compared "hands-on" to "hand-poised" approaches to delivering the fetus in 5,471 birthing women cared for by midwives. *Hands-on care* was defined as a technique in which the midwife maintained flexion during crowning, while simultaneously supporting the perineum, and then used lateral flexion to deliberately and gently deliver the fetal shoulders. *Hands-poised care* was operationally defined as keeping hands near the perineum (in case of a rapid birth) but otherwise not touching the head or the perineum, and allowing the shoulders to deliver spontaneously. Women in the hands-on group had significantly less postpartum pain than did women in the hands-poised group.

Albers and colleagues studied three techniques commonly used to reduce perineal damage, including:

- Applying warm compresses continuously to the perineum
- Gently massaging the perineum with lubricated fingers in the vagina using gentle side-to-side motions and downward pressure
- Using a "hands-off" approach until the fetal head crowns

These researchers compared these techniques in three randomly selected groups of women cared for by midwives. They found no significant difference in perineal damage among the groups.[33] The authors concluded that midwives should use their clinical judgment to protect the perineum in a way that is comfortable for the specific woman.

Differentiating perineal massage from other interventions

The term "perineal massage" during labor has sometimes been used to describe other more forceful techniques that have *not* been found to reduce perineal damage. These include pressing vigorously against the posterior vaginal wall (to "show the woman where to push"), and they are done in an attempt to hasten the birth. Used along with directed closed glottis (Valsalva) pushing, this may have a detrimental impact on perineal outcomes. This combination of interventions is quite different in technique and outcome than the gentle intrapartum massage described earlier.[33]

WHEN PROGRESS IN SECOND STAGE LABOR REMAINS INADEQUATE

Duration of second stage labor

The support of spontaneous bearing-down efforts does not lead to a clinically significant increase in second stage duration.[25] A reconceptualized approach to second stage labor has been suggested in which the onset is identified by the woman's spontaneous urge to bear down, rather than only the time of complete cervical dilation.[34] Using this approach, as women naturally respond to the sensations they experience, the duration of passive descent will be lengthened and the duration of active spontaneous bearing down will be shortened. This has potential benefits for the fetus because active bearing down is more associated with potentially problematic alterations of fetal hemodynamics.[25]

Women experience the urge to bear down at 9 ± 1 cm with a range of 5 to 10 cm.[35] Some women will not have the urge to bear down when they are completely dilated. Time limits for the duration of second stage labor have been arbitrarily determined and necessitate the use of a large number of intrapartum interventions, such as operative vaginal birth and cesarean.[25] When both mother and fetus are healthy as indicated by assessment data, the birth attendant can continue to support spontaneous bearing down while progress in descent continues to occur.[36]

If the woman is fully dilated but has no spontaneous urge to bear down (sometimes referred to as the latent phase of the second stage [Chapter 6, pages 174–177]), she may be supported to rest and breathe through contractions until there is at least a minimal urge to bear down.[25,37] Alternatively, the use of more upright positions where the sacrum is free of compression (e.g., squatting or standing) may stimulate fetal rotation and descent as well as the fetal ejection (Ferguson) reflex, which can lead to the spontaneous urge to bear down.

When women bear down spontaneously, their efforts vary in duration and strength from one contraction to another.[25] If the mother is becoming fatigued, encouraging her to breathe through contractions may lead to recovery of her energy. Focusing less on time and more on the condition of the mother and baby will allow the birth attendant to acknowledge the variations in spontaneous bearing down efforts, as well as the woman's need to conserve and renew energy.

If the fetal heart rate is nonreassuring, it may be corrected by encouraging the woman to breathe through a few contractions or to bear down with every other contraction. These simple primary intra-uterine resuscitation strategies may lead to resolution.[36,38] During a fetal bradycardia episode, breathing instead of pushing with contractions leads to more rapid resolution to a normal heart rate baseline.[25,36]

Supportive directions for bearing-down efforts

Providers who support spontaneous bearing down occasionally find that they need to provide more direction,[36] such as when the fetal heart rate is nonreassuring or progress in second stage has been less than adequate. Instead of reverting to the outdated "count to 10" instructions, birth attendants can modify their instructions to provide what has been referred to as "supportive direction."[26,30,36] An example of this approach is to instruct the woman to hold the bearing-down efforts for a slightly longer duration. Closed glottis bearing-down efforts of up to 6 seconds' duration will not lead to adverse maternal or fetal hemodynamics.[38] Along with this minor modification in spontaneous bearing-down efforts, position changes can help accomplish progress when it is urgently needed.[36] In situations where significant fetal compromise is suspected, the use of calm, firm statements can elicit the energy and focus of the mother. For example, a statement like, "*Your baby is in trouble and needs to be born. I need you to give birth to the baby,*" signals to woman that she has the power to make the birth happen sooner rather than later.

See Chapter 6 for more discussion of bearing-down efforts.

HAND MANEUVERS AND ANTICIPATORY MANAGEMENT OF INTRAPARTUM PROBLEMS

Shoulder dystocia

During normal mechanisms of second stage labor, the fetal shoulders rotate to an oblique diameter (Fig. 8.5) to align with the

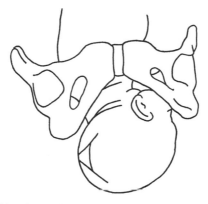

Fig. 8.5. Shoulders in an oblique position.

anterior-posterior diameter of the maternal pelvis. This alignment allows the fetal shoulders to deliver readily following the emergence of the fetal head. If the shoulders do not rotate, spontaneous delivery of the shoulders will not occur. "Shoulder dystocia" is a term used to describe an emergency during which, following the birth of the fetal head, the anterior shoulder becomes wedged behind the symphysis pubis and does not deliver spontaneously. Specifically, the term is used when the birth requires additional hand maneuvers beyond gentle downward traction.[39] Shoulder dystocia happens infrequently, is often unexpected, and may frighten the birth attendant as well as the woman and her family. It requires the health care provider to take rapid action while conveying a sense of calm and reassurance to the woman and her family.

While the risk of shoulder dystocia is higher in large babies, half occur when babies weigh less than 4,000 g.[39] Diabetic mothers are at an increased risk for shoulder dystocia because their babies have a broader than average chest circumference regardless of birth weight and a higher distribution of fat in the upper extremities.[40] There is also a relationship between shoulder dystocia and prolonged labor[41] and prolonged second stage.[42] However, rapid fetal descent is also associated with shoulder dystocia, presumably because the fetal shoulders do not have time to rotate properly.[43] Risks of shoulder dystocia include damage to the fetus such as brachial plexus injury,

8

Erbs palsy, broken clavicle, and anoxia—if the situation is unresolved, even death.[39] Therefore, rapid attention and appropriate interventions are necessary to prevent or minimize these negative outcomes.

Precautionary measures

When a large baby is anticipated, midwives may encourage the use of a side-lying or hands-and-knees position for the birth (Fig. 8.6). In these positions, the woman's weight is off her sacrum. This maximizes the dimensions of her pelvic outlet, allowing more room for both the fetus and the birth attendant to maneuver and for the fetus to be delivered.

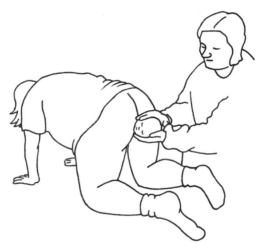

Fig. 8.6. Hands and knees position for birth.

Another preventive strategy that some midwives and doctors use is to allow time for the fetal shoulders to rotate spontaneously. After delivery of the fetal head, the birth attendant waits for another contraction to deliver the shoulders. Those who use this technique believe that rushing the delivery of the anterior shoulder may contribute to its entrapment and increase the risk of shoulder dystocia. Other birth attendants believe that if they wait for a contraction, they have lost valuable minutes that may be needed to resolve a shoulder dystocia if it does occur. This is an example of how a birth attendant's philosophy guides clinical practice.

Anticipating shoulder dystocia is an important strategy that allows the birth attendant to assemble additional health professionals to help in case shoulder dystocia does occur. When a large baby is anticipated, many midwives request an additional nurse to provide suprapubic pressure (see Fig. 8.8) if necessary, and a stool to give the nurse optimal access and maximal downward pressure. The birth attendant should also ensure that the woman's bladder is empty prior to birth, to promote as much room for the baby as possible.

Warning signs

Shoulder dystocia may not be evident until the birth attendant attempts to deliver the anterior shoulder and is not successful using the usual hand maneuvers. However, there are some warning signs that may indicate that a shoulder dystocia is about to occur. They include:

- the need for the birth attendant to "milk the perineum," by pushing perineal tissues manually over the fetal head as it emerges
- the "turtle sign," in which, after the head is born, it recoils against the perineum and turns cyanotic (blue). This signals that a shoulder is caught behind the pubic symphysis

Shoulder dystocia maneuvers

Birth attendants manage shoulder dystocia using a series of maneuvers that are listed in Table 8.1. The key to successful management is for the birth attendant to efficiently continue to try *different* appropriate maneuvers until successful delivery of the baby is achieved. It is important to avoid using the same maneuvers repeatedly without resolution.[44] **HELPERR** is a mnemonic device that can assist providers to remember the management in a series of steps to relieve shoulder dystocia where each letter stands for a step in the process: **H**, call for help; **E**, evaluate for episiotomy; **L**, move legs to McRoberts' position; **P**, suprapubic pressure; **E**, enter maneuvers like internal rotations; **R**, remove the posterior arm; and **R**, roll the woman onto all-fours.[44] Because these steps are so important, providers are encouraged to practice them in simulation drills that include all members of the

Table 8.1. Shoulder Dystocia Maneuvers

Name of Maneuver	Action and Notes
Cut or enlarge episiotomy	Although shoulder dystocia is not a soft tissue problem, some birth attendants cut or enlarge an episiotomy to make more room for their hands to move the fetus.
McRoberts' maneuver	Woman's knees are flexed onto her abdomen, helping to lift the pubic symphysis and free the fetal shoulder.
Gentle downward traction on the fetal head	May be repeated following the use of additional maneuvers to aid the birth.
Suprapubic pressure (not fundal pressure)	An assistant presses down firmly behind the woman's symphysis pubis in an attempt to free the anterior shoulder. Used with downward traction and McRoberts' maneuver.
Hands and knees (Gaskin maneuver)	Woman is quickly moved to the hands-and-knees position. (The birth attendant may attempt to deliver the posterior shoulder first.)
Rubin maneuver	Two fingers are inserted into the vagina behind the uppermost shoulder. Birth attendant attempts to rotate the fetus to an oblique pelvic diameter.
Woods corkscrew	With two fingers positioned as in the Rubin maneuver, birth attendant places two fingers of the opposite hand in front of the lower fetal shoulder. Birth attendant uses both hands to rotate the fetus to an oblique pelvic diameter.
Reverse Woods corkscrew	Similar to the Woods corkscrew, but fetal shoulders are directed in the opposite direction. Used if the Woods corkscrew maneuver is unsuccessful.
Delivery of the posterior arm	The birth attendant reaches in to grasp the fetal hand of the anterior arm and sweeps it across the chest and out through the vagina.

8

healthcare team.[45] As of this writing, there is no requirement to accomplish the shoulder dystocia maneuvers in a particular order. Rather, good clinical judgment should guide the sequence.[44]

The McRoberts' maneuver

The McRoberts' maneuver is most often used first and leads to resolution in 40% to 60% of cases.[39] In this maneuver, the women's legs

(a)

(b)

(c)

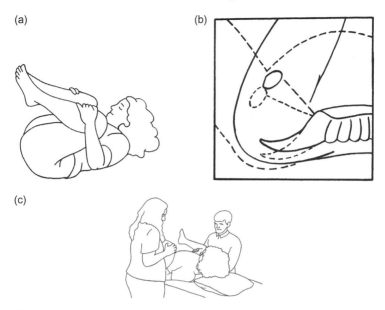

Fig. 8.7. (**a**) Exaggerated lithotomy (McRoberts' position).
(**b**) Exaggerated lithotomy (detail). (**c**) Exaggerated lithotomy (McRoberts')
with people supporting the woman's legs.

are flexed against her abdomen into an exaggerated lithotomy position. The McRoberts' maneuver (Fig. 8.7) appears to increase the
expulsive force of contractions[46] as well as increase the pelvic dimensions.[44] The assistance of several nurses, and even an additional birth
attendant, is optimal for promoting success. However, calling additional personnel into the birth room may frighten the woman and her
family and distract the woman's attention from important instructions given by the birth attendant. Therefore, the birth attendant
should try to maintain a calm but firm tone when she or he requests
assistance and gives instructions. Clinical staff should be ready to
assist with maneuvers as instructed by the midwife or doctor.

The doula's role is to help the woman stay calm, to cooperate with
her birth attendant, and, if the birth attendant requests, to help the
mother change positions rapidly.

8

Suprapubic pressure

Suprapubic pressure (Fig. 8.8) is an essential adjunct to the McRoberts' maneuver. To provide suprapubic pressure, an assistant presses down *behind the woman's symphysis pubis* to help deliver the anterior shoulder of the fetus. In providing suprapubic pressure, the attendant is essentially dislodging the trapped shoulder from above the pubic bone. The birth attendant guides the assistant's use of suprapubic pressure.

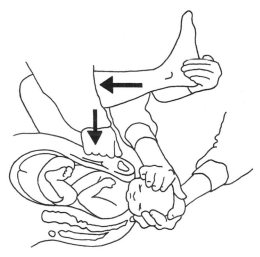

Fig. 8.8. Suprapubic pressure.

Fundal pressure is *not the same as suprapubic pressure* and is not appropriate in cases of shoulder dystocia. Fundal pressure is defined as mechanical pressure on the fundus (top) of the uterus and has been used to hasten the birth process. It is *not recommended for use during management of shoulder dystocia*, nor routinely at any time in the care of women in labor. In fact, the practice is considered obsolete and potentially hazardous in most developed countries.[47] There is some suggestion in the literature that, in low-resource settings where there is no other option, fundal pressure may be of use in emergency circumstances.[47] But, while fundal pressure does increase the force of expulsion by as much as 28%,[46] there is no evidence that it hastens birth.[47] Maternal risks of fundal pressure include uterine rupture and an increased incidence of severe perineal damage. Newborn risks include bone fracture and brain damage.[47]

The Gaskin maneuver

Moving a woman to the hands-and-knees position when delivery of the shoulder appears to be obstructed, now referred to as the "Gaskin maneuver," has been found useful in cases of shoulder dystocia.[39]

The hands-and-knees position appears to work by several mechanisms. First, the position allows the sacrum to move freely, which can increase the pelvic outlet sagittal diameter by 1 to 2 cm.[48] Further, the movement to this position appears to dislodge the impacted shoulders. Additionally, when there is bilateral impaction of the shoulders, the position may allow gravity to move the posterior shoulder forward over the sacral promontory. In this situation, it may be possible to attempt to deliver the posterior shoulder first, using gentle downward traction.

Somersault maneuver

Twenty-five percent of neonates are born with the umbilical cord wrapped around the neck, which is referred to as a "nuchal cord."[49] Common practice is for the birth attendant to slip the nuchal cord over the fetal head, prior to delivery of the shoulders if it is loose enough to allow for this simple maneuver. However, a small percentage of nuchal cords are too tight to allow for this action. A tight nuchal cord can delay progress during birth and may also limit circulation to the fetus during contractions, resulting in variable type fetal heart rate decelerations. One strategy to manage a tight nuchal cord at birth is to double clamp the cord and cut it, freeing the baby from this impediment. This strategy is effective but prevents the neonate from benefiting from both the oxygenated blood flow to the fetus prior to delivery and the placental blood transfusion following birth when cord clamping is delayed.

In order to avoid clamping and cutting a tight nuchal cord prior to the birth, the birth attendant can deliver the fetus using a somersault maneuver. This maneuver was first described by Schorn and Blanco.[50] The four steps in the process (Fig. 8.9) include unhurried shoulder delivery, flexion of the baby's head toward the mother's

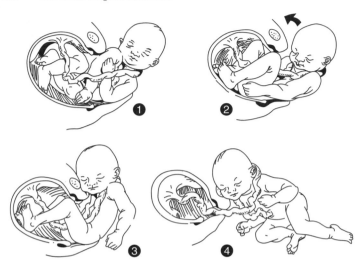

Fig. 8.9. Somersault maneuver. The somersault maneuver involves holding the infant's head flexed and guiding it upward or sideways toward the pubic bone or thigh, so the baby does a "somersault," ending with the infant's feet toward the mother's knees and the head still at the perineum. *1,* Once the nuchal cord is discovered, the anterior and posterior shoulders are slowly delivered under control without manipulating the chord. *2,* As the shoulders are delivered, the head is flexed so that the face of the baby is pushed toward the maternal thigh. *3,* The baby's head is kept next to the perineum while the body is delivered and "somersaults" out. *4,* The umbilical cord is then unwrapped, and the usual management ensues. [Mercer JS, Skovgaard RL, Peareara-Eaves J, Bowman TA. (2005). Nuchal cord management and nurse-midwifery practice. J Midwif Womens Health 50(5), 373–379. Reprinted with permission.]

8

thigh, maintaining the neonate's head near the perineum while allowing the body to deliver in a somersault manner, and finally unwrapping the baby from the cord. The use of the somersault maneuver allows birth attendants to safely manage tight nuchal cords while maintaining the benefits of the intact cord for the newborn.[49] Following the somersault maneuver, the birth attendant can delay cord clamping and watch for improvements in the color and tone of the fetus, who might be somewhat compromised due to the tight cord, thereby providing the benefits described in Chapter 7 (third and fourth stages, pages 228–229).

NONPHARMACOLOGIC AND MINIMALLY INVASIVE PHARMACOLOGIC TECHNIQUES FOR INTRAPARTUM PAIN RELIEF

Since the administration of medication can potentially alter a woman's ability to actively participate in the birth and since some women begin labor with a desire to avoid the use of pain medication and epidural anesthesia, it is important that birth care providers are well equipped with nonpharmacologic tools to relive pain.

Acupuncture

According to acupuncture theory, as taught in traditional Chinese medicine, acupuncture improves energy flow (*qi*) along the body's meridians (pathways for energy flow) and, when used during labor, reduces symptoms of pain, anxiety, and poor labor progress. Acupuncture involves the insertion of fine needles into the skin in order to stimulate specific points along the meridians (Fig. 8.10). The needles are then rotated, heated or electrically stimulated. The needles must be stimulated every 5 to 10 minutes to achieve *de qi*, essential to maximize the benefits.[51,p.294] *de qi* is perceived by the recipient as a tingling or numbness at the area of needle insertion and by the operator as tightness around the needle site.[52] Acupuncture appears to stimulate the release of beta-endorphins (endogenous analgesics). There also appears to be an additional relaxation effect when acupuncture is used during labor. Some midwives are trained to perform acupuncture in labor, and the use of acupuncture is popular in Sweden.[51] However, without trained professionals on staff, it can be difficult to arrange ready availability of a qualified acupuncturist during labor.

Ramnero and colleagues[53] conducted a controlled trial with a sample of 90 laboring women, with 51 randomized to receive acupuncture during labor and 49 who served as a control group. Women in the experimental group could use acupuncture alone or in conjunction with analgesia and anesthesia. When compared to women in the control group, women who received acupuncture experienced significantly fewer epidurals and significantly better relaxation (as measured by an 11-point numeric scale assessed at least once every hour and

8

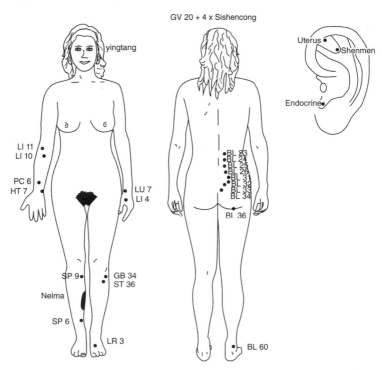

Fig. 8.10. All acupuncture points have Chinese names and those on the meridians also have names and numbers associated with the corresponding meridian. Two extra points located outside the specific pathways and named Yintang and Sishencong. Shenmen is an ear point, which corresponds to the lungs and is used for general analgesia and relaxation. [Redrawn based on Borup L, Wurlitzer W, Hedegaard M, Kosmodel US, Hvidman L. (2009) Acupuncture as pain relief during delivery: a randomized controlled trial. Birth 36(1), 5–12.]

15 minutes before and after the administration of analgesic agents).[53] Nesheim and associates[52] compared the use of intrapartum acupuncture in a sample of 106 parturients compared to a control group of 92 women who did not receive acupuncture. The trial was not blinded with the acupuncture administered by the same midwives who cared for the women during labor. Therefore, a second control group of 92 women who also did not receive acupuncture were chosen from the

general labor population in an attempt to control for this bias. The researchers found that women in the acupuncture group used significantly less analgesia, and reported high maternal satisfaction. In a more recent study, 607 healthy women in labor at term were randomized to acupuncture, TENS, or traditional analgesics groups.[54] In the acupuncture treatment group, 34 acupuncture points were used (see Fig. 8.10). Women in the acupuncture group used significantly fewer pharmacologic methods of pain relief than women in the other groups, and their infants had significantly higher 5-minute Apgar scores and umbilical cord pH values. The authors concluded that acupuncture is a favorable complementary option for intrapartum pain management.

Trials of the use of acupuncture to induce labor or augment labor contractions have produced mixed findings, and authors of systematic reviews have called for further well-designed randomized trials.[55]

Sterile water injections

When the baby is in an OP position, the laboring woman often experiences significant lower back pain, sometimes referred to as "back labor." Back labor, no matter what the cause, can be severely painful. Intradermal or intracutaneous sterile water injections injected into four specific points on the woman's back can be used as a nonpharmacologic approach for relief of back pain in labor. This is an underutilized intervention.[56] The mechanism of action is not fully understood but appears to be linked to the Gate Control Theory of pain relief.[57] More specifically, it appears that the sterile water acts as a mild irritant stimulating localized discomfort. The use of sterile water injections does not preclude the use of epidural anesthesia. Therefore, for women who would like to avoid epidural anesthesia, sterile water injections may be used in a stepwise attempt to address overwhelming back pain.

Formerly, the sterile water injections were administered intracutaneously (0.05 to 0.1 ml) and were considered to cause significant acute pain that lasted about 30 seconds, followed by 60 to 90 minutes of back pain relief.[57,58] More recently, *sub*cutaneous injections (0.5 ml) have been studied in comparison to *intra*cutaneous injections. A randomized controlled trial compared 0.5 ml of sterile water injected *subcutaneously* in each of the four sites to 0.1 ml injected *intracutaneously* in each site and 1 ml of placebo (saline solution) in each site. The subcutaneous injections were found to be as effective as intracutaneous injections in relieving back pain and significantly less painful during administration.[57] A more recent study confirmed this finding.[59] Therefore, experts now recommend giving subcutaneous sterile water injections rather than intradermal injections for back pain relief in labor.[57] Hutton and colleagues[60] conducted a meta-analysis of sterile water injections that included eight randomized controlled trials. They found that women who received the sterile water injections had a significant reduction in cesarean birth. This finding suggests broader benefits of sterile water injections and warrants further study.

Procedure for subcutaneous sterile water injections

Saline cannot be used for this procedure as it will have no effect.[57] Sterile water is drawn up into one or more tuberculin syringes (in an amount sufficient to allow for four injections of 0.5 ml each),[61] the skin is cleansed with isopropyl alcohol, and the water is injected subcutaneously into four points located in the sacral region of the back (Fig. 8.11). Even though subcutaneous injections are less painful than the intracutaneous injections, the discomfort of the procedure can be further reduced if two health professionals administer the injections simultaneously and administer them during, rather than between, contractions. Pain relief is often noticed within minutes.

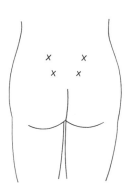

Fig. 8.11.   Sterile water injection points.

When sterile water injections are administered, the doula can help the woman into position and provide physical and emotional support during the uncomfortable procedure.

Nitrous oxide

Nitrous oxide mixed with oxygen is a noninvasive odorless gas used for labor analgesia. The woman administers it to herself via inhalation with each contraction or during painful procedures (such as manual rotation of the fetal head, manual removal of the placenta, and others). It is rarely used in the United States, but it is readily available to laboring women in many parts of the world for both home and hospital births.[62] Nitrous oxide has the advantage of a very short half-life, and when used as directed in the concentrations recommended for childbirth, nitrous oxide does not cause maternal or neonatal respiratory depression, prolonged labor, fetal malposition, or increased rates of operative vaginal or cesarean births.[62] Further, nitrous oxide can be used at the same time as other noninterventive approaches to labor care used by midwives.[62] In the future, midwives and consumers may promote the increased use of nitrous oxide in the United States.

Topical anesthetic applied to the perineum

Lidocaine gel, a topical anesthetic, has been studied and found to be safe and effective for perineal pain management during second stage labor.[63] When a woman experiences excessive burning that is disruptive to her spontaneous pushing efforts and warm compresses do not seem to help, the birth attendant or nurse can apply the gel to the internal and external tissues of the outer vagina and perineum. Studies of the use of lidocaine gel indicate that it is safe for both mother and fetus.[63] Similar topical anesthetics can be used to supplement injectable anesthetics administered after birth if perineal suturing is needed.

CONCLUSION

When labor progress slows, a variety of effective intermediate, pharmacologic, nonpharmacologic, and nonsurgical interventions may be used instead of turning immediately to more invasive procedures such as epidural anesthesia, instrumental vaginal birth, or cesarean delivery. These approaches may require the development of new skills by midwives and doctors. The application of new evidence-based skills may be rewarded by improved outcomes, including higher rates of vaginal births and maternal satisfaction. In addition, there are several skills that may be used by birth attendants to limit the duration of shoulder dystocia and minimize the adverse effects of this often unanticipated event that may occur during the final phase of labor. Ultimately, these outcomes may lead to lower maternity care costs, reduced recovery times for women and their babies, and, most important, women and babies who are ready to adjust together to this new phase in their lives.

REFERENCES

1. Greulich B, Tarrant B. (2007). The latent phase of labor: Diagnosis and management. J Midwif Womens Health 52(3), 190–198. doi:10.1016/jmwh.2006.12.007.

2. Kavanagh J, Kelly AJ, Thomas J. (2005). Breast stimulation for cervical ripening and induction of labour. Cochrane Database Syst Rev (3):CD003392. doi:10.1002/14651858.CD003392.pub2.

3. Razgaitis EJ, Lyvers AN. (2010). Management of protracted active labor with nipple stimulation: A viable tool for midwives? J Midwif Womens Health 55, 65–69. doi:10.1016/j.jmwh.2009.05.002.

4. Stein JL, Bardeguez AD, Verma UL, Tegani N. (1990). Nipple stimulation for labor augmentation. J Reprod Med 35, 710–714.

5. Curtis P, Resnick JC, Evens S, Thompson CJ. (1999). A comparison of breast stimulation and intravenous oxytocin for the augmentation of labor. Birth 26, 115–122.

6. Vincent M. (2005). Amniotomy: To do or not to do? Midwifery 8(5), 228–229.

7. Stewart P, Kennedy JH, Calder AA. (1982). Spontaneous labour: when should the membranes be ruptured? Br J Obstet Gynecol 89, 39–42.

8. Smyth RMD, Alldred SK, Markham C. (2007). Amniotomy for shortening spontaneous labour. Cochrane Database Syst Rev (4):CD006167. doi:10.1002/14651858.CD006167.pub2.

9. Varney H, Kriebs JM, Gegor CL, eds. (2004). The normal first stage of labor. In Varney's Midwifery, 4th edition (pp. 778–779). Sudbury, MA, Jones & Bartlett.

8

10. Fok WY, Leung TY, Tsui MH, Leung TN, Lau TK. (2005). Fetal hemodynamic changes after amniotomy. Acta Obstet Gynecol Scand 84, 166–169.

11. Senecal J, Xiong X, Fraser WD. (2005). Effect of fetal position on second-stage duration and labor outcome. Obstet Gynecol 105(4), 763–772. doi:10.1097/01.AOG.0000154889.47063.84.

12. Argani C, Ramin S, Satin A. (2009) Management of the fetus in occiput posterior position. UpToDate 17(3), 1–3.

13. LeRay C, Serres P, Schmitz T, Cabrol D, Goffinet F. (2007). Manual rotation in occiput posterior or transverse positions. Obstet Gynecol 110(4), 873–879.

14. Cargill YM, MacKinnon CJ. (2004). Guidelines for operative vaginal birth. J Obstet Gynaecol Can 26(8), 747–753.

15. Gibbs R, Danforth D, Karlin B, Haney A, eds. (2008). Danforth's Obstetrics and Gynecology, 10th edition. Philadelphia, Lippincott Williams and Wilkins.

16. Shaffer BL, Cheng YW, Vargas JE, Laros RK, Caughey AB. (2006). Manual rotation of the fetal occiput: predictors of success and delivery. Obstet Gynecol 194, e7–e9. doi:10.1016/j/ajog.2006.01.029

17. Reichman O, Gdansky E, Latinsky B, Labi B, Samueloff A. (2008). Digital rotation from occipito-posterior to Occipito-anterior decreases the need for cesarean section. Eur J Obstet Gynecol Reprod Biol 136(1), 25–28.

18. Frye A. (1995). Healing Passage: A Midwife's Guide to the Care and Repair of the Tissues Involved in Birth. Portland, OR, Labrys Press.

19. Beckmann MM, Garrett AJ. (2006). Antenatal perineal massage for reducing perineal trauma. Cochrane Database Syst Rev (1):005123. doi:10.1002/14651858.CD005123.pub2.

20. American College of Nurse-Midwives. (2005). Share with women: Perineal massage in pregnancy. J Midwif Womens Health 50(1), 63–64.

21. Davidson K, Jacoby S, Brown MS. (2000). Preventing lacerations during delivery. J Obstet Gynecol Neonat Nursing 29(5), 474–479.

22. Carroli G, Mignini L. (2009). Episiotomy for vaginal birth. Cochrane Database Syst Rev (1):CD000081. doi: 10.1002/14651858.CD000081. pub2.

23. Bloom SL, Casey BM, Schaffer JI, McIntire SS, Leveno KJ. (2006). A randomized trial of coached versus uncoached maternal pushing during the second stage of labor. Am J Obstet Gynecol 194, 10–13.

24. Schaffer J, Bloom S, Casey B, et al. (2006). A randomized trial of coached versus uncoached maternal pushing during the second stage of labor. Am J Obstet Gynecol 194(1), 10–13.

25. Roberts J, Hanson L. (2007). Best practices in second stage labor care: Maternal bearing down and positioning. J Midwif Womens Health 52, 238–245. doi:101016/j.jmwh.2006.12.011.

26. Sampselle CM, Miller JM, Luecha Y, Fischer K, Rosten L. (2005). Provider support of spontaneous pushing during the second-stage of labor. J Obstet Gynecol Neonat Nursing 34, 695–702.

27. DeJonge A, Lagro-Janssen ALM. (2004). Birthing positions: A qualitative study into the views of women about various birthing positions. J Psychosomat Obstet Gynecol 25, 47–55.

28. McKay S. (1981). Second stage labor: Has tradition replaced safety? Am J Nursing 81, 1016–1019.

29. Soong B, Barnes M. (2005). Maternal positions at midwife-attended birth and perineal trauma: Is there an association? Birth 32(3), 164–169.

30. Osborne K. (2010). Pushing techniques used by midwives when providing second stage labor care. (Unpublished doctoral dissertation.) Marquette University, Milwaukee, WI.

31. Myrfield K, Brook C, Creedy D. (1997). Reducing perineal trauma: Implications of flexion and extension of the fetal head during birth. Midwifery 13, 197–201.

32. McCandlish R, Bowler U, vanAsten H, Berridge G, Winter C, Sames L, et al. (1998). A randomized controlled trial of care of the perineum during second stage of normal labour. Br J Obstet Gynecol 105, 1262–1272.

33. Albers LL, Sedler KD, Bedrick EJ, Teaf D, Peralta P. (2005). Midwifery care measures in the second stage of labor and reduction of genital trauma at birth: A randomized controlled trial. J Midwif Women's Health 50, 365–372. doi:10.1016/j.jmwh.2005.05.012.

34. Roberts J. (2003). A new understanding of the second stage of labor: Implications for nursing care. J Obstet Gynecol Neonat Nursing 32, 794–801.

35. Roberts J, Goldstein S, Gruener J, Maggio M, Mendez-Bauer CA. (1987). A descriptive analysis of involuntary bearing-down efforts during the expulsive phase of labor. J Obstet Gynecol Neonat Nursing 16, 48–55. doi:10.1016/j.ejogrb.2006.12.025.

36. Hanson L. (2009). Challenges in spontaneous bearing down. J Perinat Neonat Nursing 23, 31–39.

37. Roberts J, Woolley D. (1996). A second look at the second stage of labor. J Obstet Gynecol Neonat Nursing 25(5), 415–423.

38. Simpson KR, James DC. (2005). Effects of immediate versus delayed pushing during second-stage labor on fetal wellbeing. Nursing Res 54, 149–157.

8

39. Mahlmeister LR. (2008). Best practices in perinatal nursing: Risk identification and management of shoulder dystocia. J Perinat Neonat Nursing 22(2), 91–94.

40. McFarland M, Trylovich C, Langer O. (1998). Anthropometric difference in macrosomic infants of diabetic and nondiabetic mothers. J Matern Fetal Med 7, 292–295.

41. Mehta S, Bujold E, Blackwell S, Sorokin Y, Sokol RJ. (2004). Is abnormal labor associated with shoulder dystocia in nulliparous women? Am J Obstet Gynecol 190, 1604–1607.

42. Baskett TF, Allen AC. (2007). Perinatal implications of shoulder dystocia. Obstet Gynecol 86(1), 14–7.

43. Camune B, Brucker M. (2007). An overview of shoulder dystocia: The nurse's role. Nursing Womens Health 11(5), 489–497.

44. Baxley EG, Gobbo RW. (2004). Shoulder dystocia. Am Fam Phys 69(7), 1707–1714.

45. Lathrop A, Winningham B, VandeVusse L. (2007). Simulation-based learning for midwives: Background and pilot implementation. J Midwif Womens Health 52(5), 492–498.

46. Buhimschi CS, Buhimschi IA, Malinow A, Weiner CP. (2001). Use of McRoberts' position during delivery and increase in pushing efficiency. Lancet 358, 470–471.

47. Verheijen EC, Raven JH, Hofmeyr GJ. (2009). Fundal pressure during the second stage of labor. Cochrane Database Syst Rev (4):CD006067. doi:10.1002/14651858.CD006067.pub2.

48. Meenan AL, Gaskin IM, Ball CA. (1991). A new (old) maneuver for the management of shoulder dystocia. J Fam Pract 32(6), 625–629.

49. Mercer JS, Skovgaard RL, Peareara-Eaves J, Bowman TA. (2005). Nuchal cord management and nurse-midwifery practice. J Midwif Womens Health 50(5), 373–379.

50. Schorn MN, Blanco JD. (1991). Management of the nuchal cord. J Nurse-Midwif 36, 131–132.

51. Martensson L, Wallin G. (2006). Use of acupuncture and sterile water injections for labor pain: A survey in Sweden. Birth 233(4), 289–296.

52. Nesheim BI, Kinge R, Berg B, et al. (2003). Acupuncture during labor can reduce the use of merperidine: A controlled clinical study. Clin J Pain 19, 187–191.

53. Ramnero A, Hansson U, Heiberg E. (2002). Acupuncture treatment during labour: a randomized controlled trial. Br J Obstet Gynecol 109, 637–644.

8

54. Borup L, Wurlitzer W, Hedegaard M, Kesmodel US, Hvidman L. (2009) Acupuncture as pain relief during delivery: a randomized controlled trial. Birth 36(1), 5–12.

55. Smith CA, Crowther CA. (2004) Acupuncture for induction of labour. Cochrane Database Syst Rev (1):CD002962. doi: 10.1002/14651858. CD002962.pub2.

56. Simkin P, Klein MC. (2009). Nonpharmacological approaches to management of labor pain. UpToDate 17(3), 1–14.

57. Martensson L, Nyberg K, Wallin G. (2000). Subcutaneous versus intracutaneous injections of sterile water for labour analgesia: A comparison of perceived pain during administration. Br J Obstet Gynecol 107, 1248–1251.

58. Simkin P, O'Hara MA. (2002). Nonpharmacologic relief of pain during labor: Systematic reviews of five methods. Am J Obstet Gynecol 186(5), S131–S151.

59. Bahasadri S, Ahmadi-Abhari S, Dehghani-Nik M, Habibi GR. (2006). Subcutaneous sterile water injections for labour pain: A randomized controlled trial. Austral N Z J Obstet Gynecol 46, 102–106. doi: 10.1111/j.1479-828X.2006.00536x.

60. Hutton EK, Kasperink M, Rutten M, Reitzma A, Wainman B. (2009). Sterile water injection for labour pain: A systematic review and meta-analysis of randomised controlled trials. Br J Obstet Gynaecol 116, 1158–1166. doi: 10.1111/j.1471-0528.2009.0221.x.

61. Martensson L, Wallin G. (1999). Labour pain treated with cutaneous injections of sterile water: A randomised controlled trial. Br J Obstet Gynecol 106, 633–637.

62. Rooks J. (2007). Use of nitrous oxide in midwifery practice: Complementary, synergistic, and needed in the United States. J Midwif Womens Health 52(3), 186–189.

63. Collins MK, Proter KB, Brook E, Johnson L, Williams M, Jevitt CA. (1994). Vulvar application of lidocaine for pain relief in spontaneous vaginal delivery. Obstet Gynecol 84(3), 335–337.

8

Chapter 9

The Labor Progress Toolkit: Part 1. Maternal Positions and Movements

Penny Simkin, BA, PT, CCE, CD(DONA),
and Ruth Ancheta, BA, ICCE, CD(DONA)

Maternal positions, 278
Side-lying positions, 279
Standing, leaning forward, 289
Kneeling positions, 290
Squatting positions, 297
Supine positions, 306
Maternal movements in first and second stages, 311
Other rhythmic movements, 323
References, 324

This Toolkit, which consists of two parts (Chapter 9 [Maternal Positions and Movements] and Chapter 10 [Comfort Measures]), contains descriptions of numerous techniques for enhancing labor progress and maintaining comfort in both the first and second stages.

Many of these techniques are designed to improve the biomechanical forces of labor: the powers, passage, and passenger. They include such techniques as the woman's use of her own body; the use of props

9

The Labor Progress Handbook: Early Interventions to Prevent and Treat Dystocia.
Edited by Penny Simkin, Ruth Ancheta

to support the woman in particular positions or movements; and the use of pressure or physical support by another person.

Many techniques are designed to reduce pain and enhance relaxation without the use of pain medications. When pain is reduced, the woman's tolerance of a prolonged labor is improved, which allows more time for the use of primary interventions. Without drugs, there are fewer, if any, side effects that might interfere with labor progress or adversely affect the woman or the baby.

Other techniques that reduce anxiety, fear, and distress may improve labor progress by decreasing maternal catecholamine production. Increased catecholamine production sometimes results in slowing of uterine contractions as well as fetal stress. Women who experience less anxiety and fear have lower catecholamine levels.

MATERNAL POSITIONS

This section contains descriptions of positions and specific features of each. We have arranged the positions in categories. The positions in each category cause similar physical changes. For example:

- Semisitting and side-lying positions are restful and gravity neutral. They may help an exhausted woman save her energy, especially if she has been up and walking for a long period. Also, if progress is rapid, neutralizing gravity may slow the labor to a more manageable pace.
- Upright positions take advantage of gravity to apply the presenting part to the cervix, improve the quality of the contractions, and enhance the descent of the fetus[1,2]
- Positions in which the woman leans forward tend to enhance fetal rotation or help maintain the favorable occiput anterior (OA) position and reduce back pain.[3–6]
- Asymmetric positions in which the woman flexes one hip and knee change the shape of the pelvis, enhance rotation, and reduce back pain.
- The exaggerated lithotomy position, used for several contractions in the second stage, may facilitate the passage of a "stuck baby" beneath the pubic symphysis.
- Dorsal positions tend to cause supine hypotension and increase back pain. Contractions are more frequent and painful, yet less likely to improve labor progress![1]

Side-lying positions

Pure side-lying semiprone (exaggerated Sims)

When: During first and second stages

How to do pure side-lying: The woman lies on her side with both hips and knees flexed and a pillow between her legs, or with her upper leg raised and supported (Figs. 9.1 through 9.3).

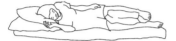

Fig. 9.1. Side-lying.

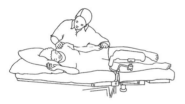

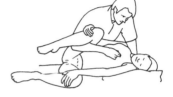

Fig. 9.3. Side-lying to push.

Fig. 9.2. Side-lying with leg in leg rest.

How to do semiprone (exaggerated Sims): The woman lies on her side with lower arm behind (or in front of) her trunk, her lower leg extended, and her upper leg flexed more than 90 degrees and supported by one or two pillows. She rolls partly toward her front (Figs. 9.4 and 9.5).

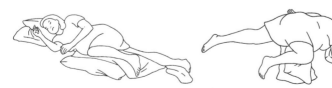

Fig. 9.4. Semiprone, lower arm forward.

Fig. 9.5. Semiprone, lower arm behind.

9

See the following for information on which side the woman should lie.

What these positions do

- Allow tired women to rest
- Are safe if pain medications have been used
- Are gravity neutral (can be used with a very rapid first or second stage)
- May relieve hemorrhoids
- May resolve fetal heart rate problems, if due to cord compression or supine hypotension
- Help to lower high blood pressure (especially left lateral positions)
- May promote progress when alternated with walking
- Avoid pressure on sacrum (unlike sitting and supine positions)
- In second stage, because there is no pressure on the sacrum (as there is with sitting), these positions allow posterior movement of the sacrum as the fetus descends.
- May enhance rotation of an occiput posterior (OP) baby

Note: Gravity effects are different when a woman is in pure side-lying or semiprone.

If side-lying, the woman with known OP fetus should lie on the same side as the fetal occiput and back ("baby's back toward bed"; (Fig. 9.6), This helps shift the fetus from OP to occiput transverse (OT). Ask the woman with an OP fetus to lie on the same side as the occiput for 15 to 30 minutes to encourage rotation from OP to OT; then ask her to change to kneeling and leaning forward for 15 to 30

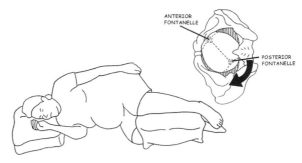

Fig. 9.6. Woman in pure side-lying on the "correct" side, with fetal back "toward the bed." If fetus is suspected or known right OP, woman lies on her right side. Gravity pulls fetal occiput and trunk toward right OT.

minutes (to encourage rotation from OT to OA). As can be seen in Figure 9.7, lying on the side opposite the fetal occiput actually uses gravity to take the fetus into direct OP.

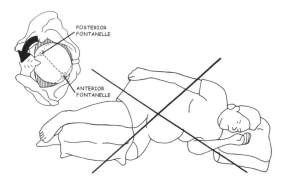

Fig. 9.7. Woman in pure side-lying on the "wrong" (left) side for suspected or known ROP fetus. Fetal back is toward the ceiling. Gravity pulls fetal occiput and trunk toward OP.

If the woman is semiprone (exaggerated Sims), she should lie on the side opposite the fetal occiput ("baby's back toward ceiling"; Fig. 9.8) for at least 15 to 30 minutes. In this position, her pelvis is rotated so that the pubis is pointing more toward the bed than with straight side-lying. This alters the effects of gravity so that the fetal trunk is encouraged to rotate to transverse and then to anterior.

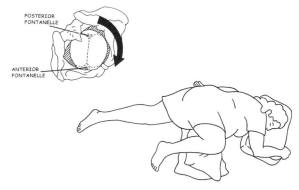

Fig. 9.8. Woman with OP fetus in semiprone on the "correct" side, with fetal back "toward the ceiling." If fetus is suspected or known right OP, the semiprone woman lies on left side. Gravity pulls the fetal occiput and trunk toward right OT, then right OA.

9

If the position of the occiput is uncertain (see discussion on pages 133–134) use trial and error, rotating through the six positions of the "roll-over," using progress or comfort in each position as an indicator of progress (Fig. 9.9).

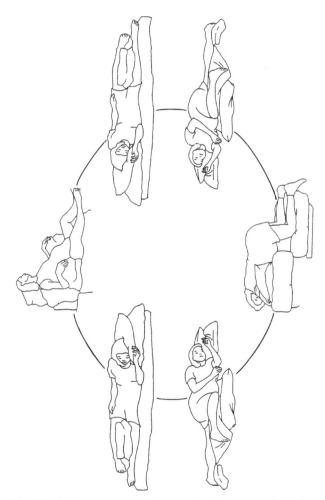

Fig. 9.9.   The "rollover sequence" for use when there are *no indicators of malposition*, or when it is *difficult to determine which side the fetal back is on.*

When to use side-lying positions

- As long as labor continues to progress well and the woman wants to use them
- When supine hypotension occurs
- When the woman has been given narcotics or an epidural
- When the woman has pregnancy-induced hypertension
- When the woman finds it comfortable in first or second stage
- When the woman is tired
- In second stage, if hemorrhoids are painful in dorsal positions
- In a rapid second stage, to neutralize gravity effect

When not to use side-lying positions

- When the woman refuses, due to increased pain or preference for another position. However, if it is explained that this position may improve labor progress, the woman may be willing to try it.
- When a gravity advantage is needed to aid descent, especially if second stage progress has slowed
- When she has been in side-lying for more than an hour without progress

The "side-lying lunge"

When: During first and second stages
How: With the woman in a semiprone position, the partner or doula stands facing the bed and places the woman's upper foot against the partner's hip. During contractions, the partner leans slightly against the woman's foot to flex her hip and knee more and hold the leg in a more flexed position (Fig. 9.10). It is important that the partner does not lean with all his weight, as it could overstretch the ligaments in the sacroiliac or hip joint and cause later pain and poor function. This is especially problematic if the woman has an epidural and is unable to feel discomfort from stretching.

9

What this position does

- Changes the shape of the pelvis, slightly opening the upper sacroiliac joint, and giving more room on the upper side of the pelvis
- Increases chances of rotation of an OP or asynclitic fetus
- Is comfortable and effortless for the mother

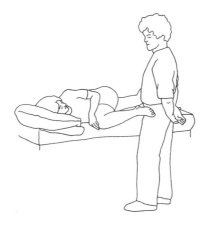

Fig. 9.10.   Side-lying lunge.

When to use the side-lying lunge

- When dilation or descent has slowed
- If a fetal malposition is suspected
- When the woman has an epidural, which does not allow her to maintain her upper leg in the flexed position without help and is limited in the positions she can use
- If the woman is too tired to do the kneeling or standing lunge, and it is desirable to alter pelvic shape

When not the use the side-lying lunge

- When a gravity advantage is needed to aid descent, especially if second stage progress has slowed
- When she has been in the position for more than an hour without progress

Sitting positions

Semisitting

When: During first and second stages

How: The woman sits with trunk at >45-degree angle with bed (Fig. 9.11).

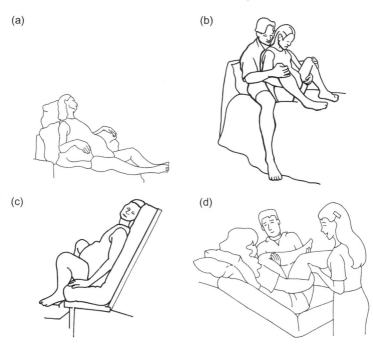

Fig. 9.11. (a) Semisitting. (b) Semisitting to push. (c) Semisitting with bed, back raised. (d) Semisitting with people supporting the woman's legs.

What this position does

- Provides some gravity advantage, compared with supine
- May be better than supine for:
  - increasing pelvic inlet dimensions
  - improving oxygenation of fetus
- Is an easy and restful position to assume
- Pressure on sacrum and coccyx may impair enlargement of the pelvic outlet.

When to use semisitting positions

- If progress is good, and the woman prefers it
- When the woman needs rest
- When an epidural is in place, as alternative to supine or side-lying

- For caregiver's convenience during second stage in viewing perineum

When not to use semisitting positions

- With known or suspected OP fetus
- If fetal heart rate reacts adversely
- If woman has hypertension and this position exacerbates it
- When the woman refuses, due to increased pain or preference for another position. However, once it is explained that this position might improve labor progress, the woman may be willing to try it.

Sitting upright

When: During first and second stages

    How: The woman sits straight up on bed, chair, or stool (Fig. 9.12).

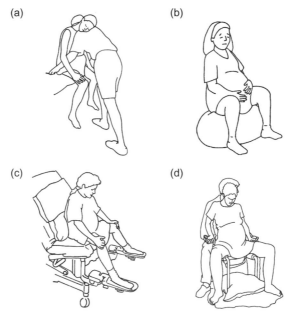

Fig. 9.12. (a) Sitting upright with partner support, in first stage. (b) Sitting upright on a birth ball. (c) Sitting upright to push. (d) Sitting upright on a birthing stool (adapted from photograph of the DeBy Birth Support).

What this position does

- Provides gravity advantage
- Allows a tired woman to rest, if she is well supported
- Allows for placement of hot pack on shoulders, low back, or lower abdomen or cold pack on low back
- Enables the woman to rock or sway in rocking chair or on birth ball

When to use upright sitting positions

- When the woman needs to rest
- When the woman has a backache
- When the woman finds it comfortable in first or second stage
- When active labor progress has slowed; sitting up is thought to be especially beneficial if her knees are lower than her hips[5]

When not to use upright sitting positions

- When the woman refuses, due to increased pain or a preference for another position. However, if it is explained that there is a chance that this position will improve labor progress, the woman may be willing to try it.
- When fetal heart rate is compromised in that position
- When she has an epidural and insufficient trunk strength to maintain position

Sitting leaning forward with support

When: During first and second stages

How: The woman sits with feet firmly placed, knees apart, and leans forward, arms resting on thighs or on a prop in front of her (Fig. 9.13, a and b), or she straddles a chair or toilet and rests her upper body on the back (Fig. 9.13, c and d).

What this position does

- Provides gravity advantage
- Is restful if the woman is well supported
- Relieves backache
- May enhance rotation from OP (better than supine and semisitting positions)

9

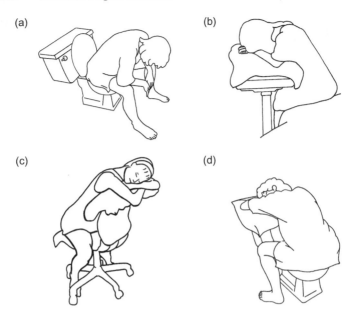

Fig. 9.13. (a) Sitting forward on a toilet. (b) Sitting, leaning on a tray table. (c) Straddling a chair. (d) Straddling a toilet.

- Aligns fetus with pelvis (see Fig. 2.2)[7]
- Enlarges pelvic inlet (compared with supine)
- Allows easy access for backrub

When to use sitting and leaning forward

- If woman is semireclining and labor is not progressing, to shift the weight of the fetal torso off the woman's spine
- When the woman has a backache
- When the woman finds it comfortable in first or second stage
- When active labor progress has slowed.

When not to use sitting and leaning forward

- When the woman objects, due to increased pain or a preference for another position. However, if it is explained that this position may improve labor progress, the woman may be willing to try it

9

- If labor progress does not improve after 6 to 8 contractions in this position.
- If epidural or narcotics interfere with her ability to maintain this position

Standing, leaning forward

When: During first and second stages
How: The woman stands and leans on the partner, on a raised bed, over a birth ball placed on the bed, or on a wall rail or countertop (Fig. 9.14). She may sway from side to side.

(a) (b)

(c) (d)

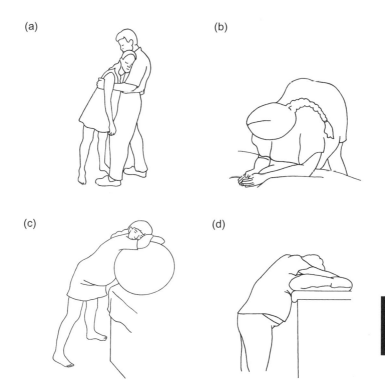

9

Fig. 9.14. (**a**) Standing, leaning on a partner. (**b**) Standing, leaning forward on bed. (**c**) Standing, leaning on birth ball. (**d**) Standing, leaning on counter.

What this position does

- Provides gravity advantage
- Enlarges pelvic inlet (compared with supine or sitting)
- Aligns fetus with pelvic inlet[5,7] (see Fig. 2.2)
- May promote flexion of fetal head
- May enhance rotation from OP or OT, especially if combined with swaying movements[5]
- Causes contractions to be less painful but more productive than in supine or sitting[1]
- Relieves backache by reducing pressure of the fetal presenting part on the woman's sacrum
- May be easier to maintain than hands-and-knees position
- If the woman is embraced and supported in the upright position by her partner, the embrace increases her sense of well-being and may reduce catecholamine production.
- May increase her urge to push in second stage

When to use standing and leaning forward

- When labor progress is slow or arrested
- When contractions space out or lose intensity
- When the woman has a backache
- When the woman finds it comfortable in first or second stage

When not to use standing and leaning forward

- When the woman objects, due to increased pain or a preference for another position. However, if it is explained that this position may improve labor progress, the woman may be willing to try it.
- When birth is imminent and the attendant does not want to deliver the baby in this position
- When epidural or narcotics interfere with the woman's motor control

Kneeling positions

Kneeling, leaning forward with support

When: During first and second stages

How: The woman kneels on bed or floor, leaning forward onto back of bed, on a chair seat, birth ball, or other support (Fig. 9.15).

(a) (b)

(c) (d)

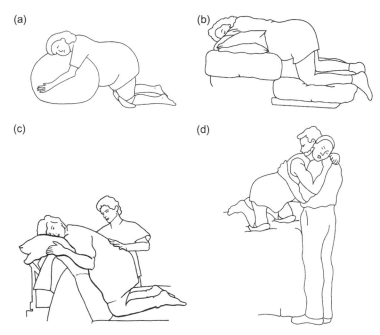

Fig. 9.15. (**a**) Kneeling, leaning on a ball, with knee pads. (**b**) Kneeling on foot of bed. (**c**) Kneeling over back of bed. (**d**) Kneeling with partner support to push, and knee pads.

What this position does

- Provides some gravity advantage
- Aligns fetus with pelvic inlet
- Enlarges pelvic inlet more than side-lying, supine, or sitting
- Allows easy access for back pressure
- Relieves strain on hands and wrists compared with hands and knees
- Allows easy movement (swaying, rocking)
- May relieve cord compression
- May cause soreness in knees (to prevent this, the woman can wear kneepads made for sports or gardening)

9

When to use kneeling and leaning forward

- When fetus is thought or known to be OP or otherwise malpositioned
- When the woman has a backache
- When labor progress has slowed in first or second stage
- When the woman is in a bath or pool if space allows
- When fetal distress is noted with supine or side-lying position
- When fetus is at a high station
- If the woman finds it comfortable
- To alternate with other positions for backache

When not to use kneeling and leaning forward

- When the woman has pain in her knees or legs
- If the woman is very tired
- When first or second stage is not progressing in the position
- If epidural or narcotics impair her motor control

Hands and knees

When: During first and second stages

How: The woman kneels (preferably on a padded surface), leans forward, and supports herself on either the palms of her hands or her fists (the latter being more tolerable if she has swollen hands or carpal tunnel syndrome) (Fig. 9.16). Knee pads may make her more comfortable.

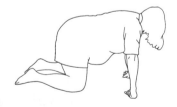

Fig. 9.16. Hands and knees.

What this position does

- Aids fetal rotation from OP or OT[7]
- May aid in reducing an anterior lip in late first stage

- Reduces back pain[7]
- Allows swaying, crawling, or rocking motion to promote rotation and increase comfort
- Relieves hemorrhoids
- May resolve fetal heart rate problems, especially if due to cord compression
- Allows easy access for counterpressure or double hip squeeze (pages 197, 354–357)
- Allows access for vaginal exams
- May cause the woman's arms to tire; to relieve, she rests upper body and head on a pile of pillows, chair seat, or birth ball

When to use hands and knees

- When labor progress has slowed in first or second stage
- When the woman has a backache
- When the fetus is thought or known to be OP
- When the woman finds it comfortable in first or second stage
- When an anterior lip slows progress

When not to use hands and knees

- When the woman objects, due to increased pain or a preference for another position. However, if it is explained that this position may improve labor progress, the woman may be willing to try it.
- When epidural or narcotics impair her motor control

Open knee–chest position

When: During prelabor, first and second stages

How: The woman goes to hands and knees, then lowers her chest to the floor, so that her buttocks are higher than her chest. In the open knee–chest position (Fig. 9.17) her hips are less flexed (>90-degree angle) than in the usual closed knee–chest position (Fig. 9.18). This more open position puts the pelvis at a very different angle from that when the knees are drawn up under her trunk.

9

What this position does

- Protects against fetal hypoxia/anoxia with prolapsed cord
- If used during the latent phase or any time before engagement, it allows repositioning of the fetal head. May need to hold this position for 8 to 10 contractions in a row or 30 to 45 minutes for this purpose. Gravity encourages the fetal head to "back out" of the pelvis and rotate or flex before reentering.
- May resolve some fetal heart rate problems
- May reduce an anterior lip
- Reduces back pain
- Relieves hemorrhoids

It is tiring. Pillows, shin padding, and support from the partner make the position easier.

When to use the open knee–chest position

- If there is a prolapsed cord
- When one suspects OP during prelabor or early labor; contractions "couple" (come in pairs close together), followed by a longer interval; or when they are short, frequent, irregular, and painful, especially in the low back and are not accompanied by dilation.[8] This position may be alternated with semiprone (exaggerated Sims) position. See pages 279–281 for further description.
- When the woman has a backache
- When it is necessary for the woman to avoid a premature urge to push
- When the woman has a swollen cervix or anterior lip
- If the caregiver is about to perform a digital or manual rotation of an OP head during first or second stage (see pages 246–250)

When not to use the open knee–chest position

- During a normally progressing second stage (works against gravity)
- If the woman becomes short of breath or has gastric upset or other discomfort
- If epidural or narcotics interfere with motor control

(a) (b)

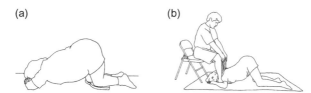

Fig. 9.17. (a) Open knee–chest position with knee pads. (b) Open knee–chest position, shoulders resting on partner's padded shins.

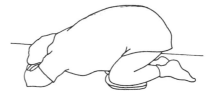

Fig. 9.18. Closed knee–chest position.

Closed knee–chest position

When: During first and second stages

   How: The woman kneels and leans forward, supporting herself on her hands, then lowers her chest to the bed, with her knees and hips flexed and abducted beneath her abdomen (see Fig. 9.18).

What this position does

- Reduces back pain
- Is less strenuous than hands-and-knees or "open" knee–chest position
- Spreads ischia, enlarging pelvic outlet (bispinous and intertuberous diameters)
- Relieves hemorrhoids
- May resolve some fetal heart rate problems
- Is an antigravity position, which may help reduce an anterior lip

When to use the closed knee–chest position

- When the woman has a backache
- When the woman has a swollen cervix or anterior lip

When not to use the closed knee–chest position

- In prelabor or early labor when fetal rotation is desired (instead, try open knee–chest with hips at >90-degree angle; see pages 293–295).

9

- When the woman objects, due to increased pain or a preference for another position. However, if it is explained that this position may improve labor progress, the woman may be willing to try it.
- If the woman becomes short of breath or has gastric upset or other discomfort
- During a normally progressing second stage (works against gravity)

Asymmetric upright (standing, kneeling, sitting) positions

When: During first and second stages.

How: The woman sits, stands, or kneels, with one knee and hip flexed, and foot elevated above the other (Fig. 9.19). Comfort guides the woman in which leg to raise. She should try both sides; one side may be much more comfortable than the other; the more comfortable side is probably the one to use.

(a)   (b)

(c)   (d)

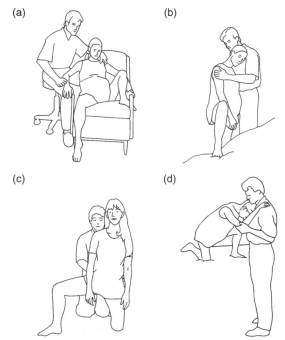

Fig. 9.19. (**a**) Asymmetric sitting. (**b**) Asymmetric standing. (**c**) Asymmetric kneeling. (**d**) Asymmetric kneeling with partner support.

What these positions do

- Exert a mild stretch on adductor muscles of the raised thigh, causing some lateral movement of one ischium, thus increasing pelvic outlet diameter
- May aid rotation from OP
- Reduce back pain
- Provide gravity advantage
- Allow the woman to "lunge" in this position, thereby causing the pelvic outlet to widen even more on that side (see pages 313–314)

When to use asymmetric upright positions

- When the woman has a backache
- When active labor progress has slowed
- When rotation is desired in first or second stage
- When the fetus is suspected to be asynclitic or otherwise malpositioned

When not to use asymmetric upright positions

- When the woman finds that these positions increase pain in her knees, hips, or pubic joint
- When she has an epidural or narcotics that may weaken her legs or impair her balance

9

Squatting positions

Squatting

When: Primarily during second stage, but any time the mother finds it comfortable

How: The woman lowers herself from standing into a squatting position with her feet flat on the floor or bed, using her partner, a squatting bar, other support for balance, if necessary (Fig. 9.20).

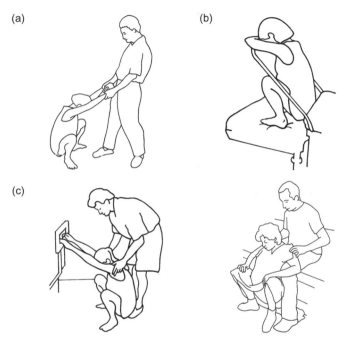

Fig. 9.20. (a) Partner aided squat. (b) Squatting with a bar. (c) Squatting holding a bed rail. (d) Squatting, supported by seated partner's legs.

What this position does

- Provides gravity advantage
- Enlarges pelvic outlet by increasing the intertuberous diameter
- May require less bearing-down effort than horizontal positions
- May enhance urge to push
- May enhance fetal descent
- May relieve backache
- Allows freedom to shift weight for comfort

- Provides mechanical advantage: upper trunk presses on fundus more than in many other positions
- May impede correction of the angle of the head, if the fetus is at a relatively high station and asynclitic. The pressure of the woman's upper torso on the fundus may reduce the space available for the fetus to "wriggle" into synclitism. (Positions that lengthen the trunk and relax the pelvic joints may be preferable. See *supported squat* and *dangle*.) However, if the fetal head is engaged and well-aligned in OA, squatting may hasten descent.
- If continued for a prolonged period, squatting compresses the blood vessels and nerves located behind the knee joint, impairing circulation and possibly causing entrapment neuropathy. As long as the woman sits back or rises to standing after every contraction or two, such problems are avoided. *Please note:* Women for whom squatting is a customary resting position do not have these potential nerve and circulation problems.

When to use squatting

- When more space within the pelvis is desired during second stage, especially when fetus is OA
- When descent is inadequate

When not to use squatting

- When there is lower extremity joint injury, arthritis, or weakness
- When an epidural has caused motor or sensory block in legs
- When using maximal prolonged breath-holding and straining (may increase likelihood of tears)

Supported squatting positions

When: During second stage

How to do the supported squat: During contractions, the woman leans with back against her partner, who places his or her forearms under her arms and holds her hands, taking all her weight (Fig. 9.21) She stands between contractions.

How to do the "dangle": The partner sits on a high bed or counter, feet supported on chairs or footrests, with thighs spread. The woman stands between the partner's legs with her back to her partner, and places her flexed arms over the partner's thighs. During the

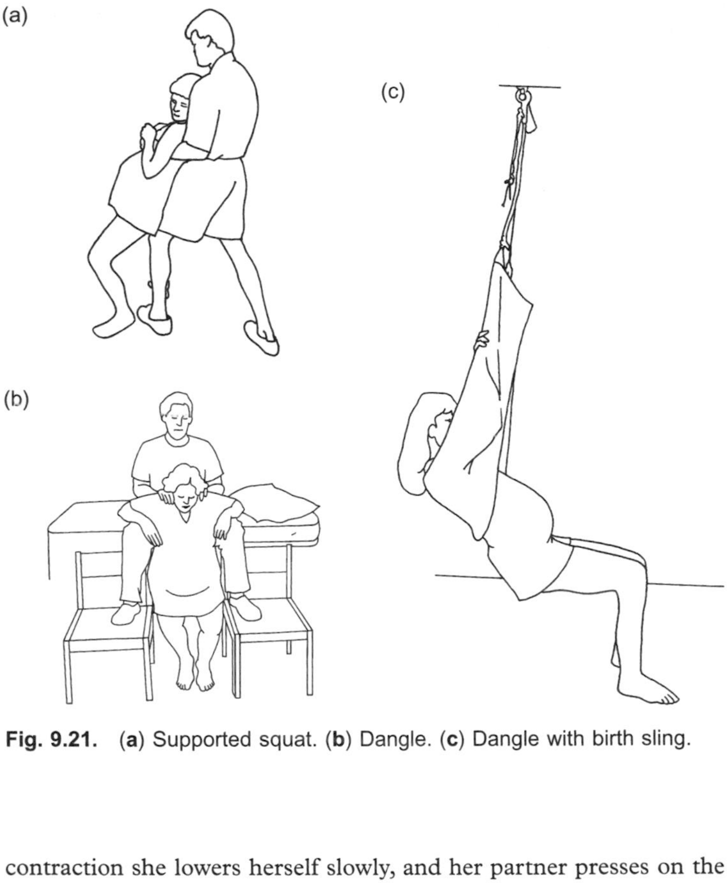

(a)

(c)

(b)

Fig. 9.21. (a) Supported squat. (b) Dangle. (c) Dangle with birth sling.

contraction she lowers herself slowly, and her partner presses on the sides of her chest with his thighs; her full weight is supported by her arms on his thighs and the grip of his thighs on her upper trunk (Fig. 9.21b). If the partner places his feet directly beneath his knees, the woman's weight is borne by his bones, rather than having him rely totally on his muscle strength. She bears down with her urge to push, and then stands between contractions.

A "birth sling," suspended from the ceiling, may also be used to support the woman (Fig. 9.21c). The dangle or use of a birth sling is much easier for the partner than the supported squat.

9

How to make a birth sling

A birth sling may be constructed of a length of sturdy cloth (folded to about 2 feet wide). It is looped so that each end is attached to an eye bolt in the ceiling or another strong support. It should be long enough that the woman can place it around her shoulders like a shawl and lower herself so that her knees are flexed and the sling bears all her weight. The woman grasps each side of the sling as she lowers herself. She can avoid direct pressure on her armpits by wearing the sling like a shawl and flexing her elbows (see Fig. 9.21c). Ensure safety by checking that the sling will not give way when there is weight in it, and be sure there is someone standing by the woman whenever she is using the sling.

A note for hospitals and birth centers if considering installing slings and birth ropes:

Some of the exercise equipment currently used in fitness centers may adapt well to use in the hospital or birth center as supportive devices for the dangle or other positions and movements. They utilize ceiling mounts and supportive straps that are designed to support many times the user's weight. We recommend exploring such options when considering installing birth slings or ropes.

What this position does

- Provides gravity advantage
- Elongates the woman's trunk: may help resolve asynclitism by giving fetus more room to reposition angle of head in pelvis
- Allows more mobility in pelvic joints than in other positions
- Allows fetal head to "mold" the woman's pelvis as needed
- Enables woman to feel secure and supported by the partner or sling, which may reduce catecholamines

The supported squat requires great strength in the support person, and it is tiring. To make it easier for the partner, he or she may lean back on a wall for support, making sure to maintain a straight back (not leaning forward at all), and alternating this with other positions.

If prolonged, may cause paresthesia (numbness, tingling) in woman's hands, from pressure of the partner's arms or thighs in her armpits (causing nerve compression in the brachial plexus). To

9

prevent this, suggest that the woman stand up and lean on her partner between contractions or try the dangle instead. The dangle allows the partner's legs or the birth sling to support all of the woman's weight, making it less tiring for the partner than the supported squat.

The dangle leaves the partner's hands free to stroke or hold the woman.

When to use supported squatting positions

- When more mobility of pelvic joints is needed
- When lengthening of the woman's trunk seems desirable, as with an asynclitic fetus
- In second stage, when fetal head is thought to be large, asynclitic, OP, or OT
- When descent is not taking place

When not to use supported squatting positions

- When the woman objects, due to increased pain or a preference for another position. However, if it is explained that this position may improve labor progress, the woman may be willing to try it.
- If the woman has weakness or pain in her shoulder joints
- When birth is imminent, unless the caregiver has agreed that delivery can take place in this position
- When the woman has an epidural or narcotics that interfere with her balance or the use of her legs
- When no one is available who is strong enough to support the woman or there is no birth sling available.

Half squatting, lunging, and swaying

When: During first or second stage

How: The woman stands and, holding onto a supporting device suspended from above (see the birthing rope, Fig 9.22a), lowers her body and leans back so that she is in a half squat (Fig 9.22b). She may raise one leg, as in the lunge, described on pages 313–314 (Fig. 9.22c), or sway from side to side with a feeling of security.

Note: The birthing rope shown here, originally designed to aid upper body stretching, attaches over a sturdy door, which remains

(a)

(b)

(c)

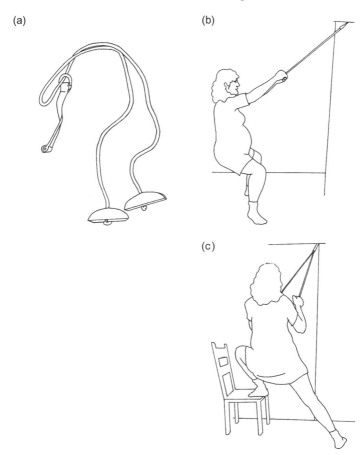

Fig. 9.22. (**a**) Birthing rope. (**b**) Half squatting with birthing rope. (**c**) Lunging with birthing rope. (Drawing of The Rope based on PrePak Products, Inc.)

9

closed during use. The apparatus hangs on the side of the door *oppo-site* the direction in which the door opens. The supportive rope enables the woman to maintain positions that would not be possible without it. *Caution:* A support person should remain close by to aid the woman with balance.

What this position and swaying movements do

- Provide gravity advantage
- Alter pelvic dimensions when the woman goes from standing to half-squatting, and when she sways from side to side in a half-squatting position, or with one leg raised.
- May facilitate fetal rotation and descent
- May be difficult for the woman to use if she is exhausted or has upper body weakness

When to use the half-squat with lunging or swaying

- When more mobility of pelvic joints is needed
- When the woman is unable to do a full squat
- When the fetal head is thought to be large, asynclitic, OP, or OT
- In second stage, when descent is not taking place

When not to use the half-squat with lunging or swaying

- If the woman refuses
- When birth is imminent, unless caregiver agrees that delivery can take place in this position
- When the woman has an epidural or narcotics that interfere with her balance or the use of her legs

Lap squatting

When: During second stage for four to six contractions followed by another position

How: The partner sits on armless straight chair; the woman sits on her partner's lap, facing and embracing her partner and straddling her partner's thighs. Her partner embraces her and, during contractions, spreads his or her thighs, allowing the woman's buttocks to sag between them. The woman keeps from sagging too far by bending her knees over her partner's thighs. The partner sits up straight and does not lean forward (Fig. 9.23). Between contractions, the partner brings his or her legs together so the woman is sitting up on them. A doula or another person holds the woman's wrists or hands to help support her. If the doula leans back, her weight can easily counterbalance the woman's weight to ease the work for the partner.

9

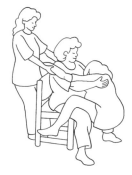

Fig. 9.23. Lap squat, with three people.

What this position does

- Provides gravity advantage
- Allows the woman to rest between contractions, while she is held by both her partner and the person holding her wrists or hands
- Passively enlarges the pelvic outlet
- Requires less bearing-down effort than many other positions
- Relaxes the pelvic floor
- May enhance descent if fetus is OA or repositioning of fetus is malpositioned
- Mechanical advantage: upper trunk presses on fundus more than in other positions
- May enhance the woman's sense of security, as she is held closely
- May be awkward for the caregiver (who must get on floor to view progress)
- May be tiring for the support person who bears woman's weight. The second support person's help in supporting the woman is an important safety precaution.
- May be less effective if fetus is asynclitic

When to use lap squatting

- When second stage progress has arrested
- When the woman has joint problems that make other squatting positions impossible
- When the woman is too tired to squat or dangle
- When all other positions have been tried

9

- Can be used with a light epidural. To do this, the woman sits on the side of the bed with her legs dangling and spread apart. The woman's partner sits on a rolling stool and rolls to the edge of the bed, which should be lowered to just above the level of the partner's lap. The partner faces the woman, with his or her arms encircling her hips, and the partner slides the woman off the bed onto his or her lap. The woman holds her partner around the neck and her partner holds her around her waist and rolls away from the bed. The doula (or another person) assists with the transfer of the woman from bed to the partner's lap, and then, standing behind the partner, takes the woman's hands, and the woman and doula hold each other's wrists securely. See earlier instructions on how to use this position during and between contractions.

When not to use lap squatting

- When the woman finds it impossible or much more painful
- When there is no strong support person available or the woman is too heavy to be supported
- When there is no third person available to help
- When the woman has a dense epidural and has no use of her legs

Supine positions

Supine

When: During first and second stages

How: The woman lies flat on her back or with her trunk slightly raised (<45 degrees). Her legs may be out straight, bent with her feet flat on the bed, in leg rests, or drawn up and back toward her shoulders (Fig. 9.24).

What this position does

- Allows use of the sheet to aid pushing (see later for sheet pull instructions)
- Allows easy access for vaginal exams
- Allows access if instruments are needed for delivery
- May cause "supine hypotension" in the woman, with resulting reduction in oxygen to the fetus

9

(a)

(b)

(c)

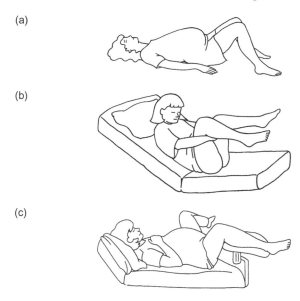

Fig. 9.24. (**a**) Supine with hips and knees bent. (**b**) Supine, head of bed somewhat elevated. (**c**) Supine with leg supports.

- May lead to illusion of cephalopelvic disproportion due to the reduced pelvic diameters characteristic of this position (often corrected by changing positions)
- Impedes rotation from OP or OT to OA
- Requires the woman to push against gravity
- Places the fetus in an unfavorable drive angle in relation to pelvis
- Causes contractions to become more frequent, more painful, but less effective than when the woman is vertical

When to use the supine position

- When necessary for medical interventions that cannot be done with the woman in another position
- When preparing for sheet pull (see later)

When not to use the supine position

- When medical interventions are not needed

Sheet pull

When: During second stage, during contractions (Fig. 9.25)

(a)   (b)

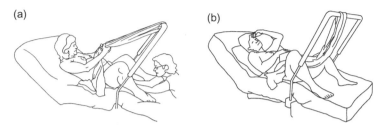

Fig. 9.25.   The sheet pull. (**a**) Pulling during contractions. (**b**) Resting between contractions.

How: The woman lies flat on her back or with her trunk slightly raised (about 30 degrees), with her knees flexed and feet either flat on bed or braced on the uprights of the squatting bar. A sheet or long shawl is looped either around the squatting bar, or around a bar at the foot of the bed, or it may be grasped at one end by a strong nurse, partner, or doula. The other end is held by the woman. When the contraction begins, the woman holds the sheet tightly and pulls on it while lifting her head and bearing down. It is important that she does not pull herself to sitting but remains quite flat. This maximizes use of her abdominal muscles and gives her leverage to bear down effectively. If the woman pulls herself to sitting, this reduces significantly her use of her abdominal muscles and defeats the purpose of the activity. If another person is holding the other end of the sheet, he or she should brace himself or herself so as not to get pulled over! At the end of the contraction, the woman lies back and rests.

What this position does

- Aids a woman who may be pushing ineffectively (due to an epidural or some other cause)
- May be advantageous over pushing in other supine positions but has most of the same disadvantages (supine hypotension and reduced fetal oxygenation, reduced pelvic dimensions that may restrict descent, reduced fetal rotation, gravity disadvantage).

When to use this position

- When the woman is unable to push effectively, especially with an epidural
- When, because of custom or hospital policy, the woman is restricted to a supine position for pushing
- When little progress has been made with other positions

When not to use this position

- When other nonsupine positions are possible
- When the fetal heart tones are nonreassuring
- When supine hypotension is present

Exaggerated lithotomy (McRoberts' position)

When: During second stage

How: The woman lies flat on her back, legs abducted and knees pulled toward her shoulders (by herself or by two other people, each one drawing one leg up toward one of her shoulders; Fig. 9.26).

What this position does

- May cause supine hypotension, with resulting reduction in oxygen supply to the fetus
- Removes any positive effects of gravity
- Is awkward and tiring for the woman
- Puts fetus in an unfavorable drive angle, with exceptions (see later)
- May be beneficial if the fetal head is "stuck" and cannot pass beneath the pubic arch when the woman is in other positions. Pulling the woman's knees toward her shoulders rotates her pelvis posteriorly, flattening her low back and moving her pubic arch toward her head.[9,10] This position may move the pubic arch over the fetus's head, allowing the fetus to slip under the arch and continue its descent (Fig. 9.26).

9

(a)   (b)

(c)

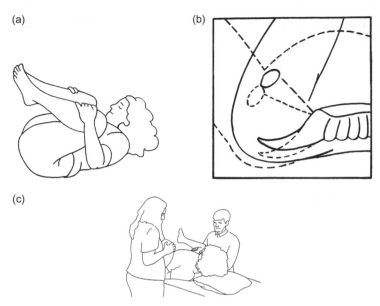

Fig. 9.26. (**a**) Exaggerated lithotomy (McRoberts' position).
(**b**) Exaggerated lithotomy (detail). (**c**) Exaggerated lithotomy (McRoberts')
with people supporting the woman's legs.

Precaution: If the woman has an epidural, there is danger of
injuring her pubic symphysis or sacroiliac joints by forcing her legs
back beyond safe limits. Without sensation, the woman cannot feel
the joint pain that would otherwise signal impending damage. Those
supporting her legs should resist the temptation to force her legs back,
as they could cause serious long-term damage.[11]

When to use exaggerated lithotomy

- When gravity positions and positions to enlarge pelvic diameters
  have been tried, but the fetus remains "stuck' at the pubis
- Before forceps or vacuum extraction are used

When not to use exaggerated lithotomy

- When other, less stressful positions have not been tried first

MATERNAL MOVEMENTS IN FIRST AND SECOND STAGES

This section contains descriptions of movements by the woman that may:

- Help resolve a fetal malposition such as OP, persistent OT, or asynclitism
- Enhance fetal descent by continually altering the shape and size of the woman's pelvic basin
- Reduce labor pain by allowing woman to find more comfortable positions and movements, to enable her to cope with the hours of contractions needed to dilate her cervix and press her fetus through her pelvis
- Increase the woman's active participation and decrease her emotional distress, contributing to fetal well-being (see page 29)

For information on how to monitor the fetal heart and contractions when women are moving around, see pages 37–44.

Pelvic rocking (also called pelvic tilt) and other movements of the pelvis

When: Primarily early first stage, but any time, if desired

How: On hands and knees, the woman "tucks her seat under" by contracting her abdominal muscles and arching her back, and then relaxes, returning her back to a neutral position (Fig. 9.27) (This is similar to the "Cat-Cow" exercise used in yoga.) It is done slowly and rhythmically throughout contractions when she has back pain and presumed OP or other malposition.

(a)   (b)

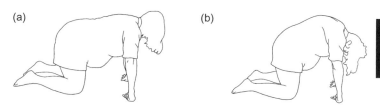

9

Fig. 9.27. (a) Pelvic rocking, first position: flat back. (b) Pelvic rocking, second position: flexed back with "seat tucked under".

(a)   (b)

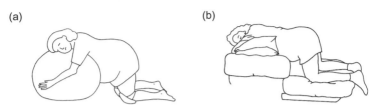

Fig. 9.28.   Pelvic rocking with support. (**a**) Resting upper body on ball. (**b**) Resting upper body on bed, with foot of bed lowered.

It will be easier on her arms and wrists if she does not bear her weight on her hands but rests her upper body on a support, such as a bean bag, chair, birth ball, or birth bed (Fig. 9.28).

Other pelvic movements, such as swaying hips from side to side, are also helpful. The birth ball allows the woman to roll her upper body on the ball—forward and back, side to side, and in circles—almost effortlessly.

Why pelvic rocking helps

If the woman adopts a hands-and-knees position, gravity encourages rotation of the fetus from OP to OA. The pelvic rocking movement around the fetal head may help to dislodge the head to enable rotation to OA[3,4,7] or correcting asynclitism. The position and movement reduce back pain, possibly by easing pressure of the fetal occiput on the woman's sacroiliac joint. For many women, this position is the only one they can tolerate when back pain is severe.

Advantages

- Gravity plus movement helps alter the position of the fetus's head within the pelvis, and encourages rotation from OP.
- Relieves back pain
- If the presumption of OP is in error, this exercise does not rotate the fetus to OP.

Disadvantages

- The woman's knees may become tired or sore. Knee pads help.

- The belts of the monitor may slip. A support person or caregiver may have to hold the transducer in place (see Fig. 2.6) or monitor intermittently. With some monitors, it is possible to insert a washcloth between the belt and the transducer (see Fig. 2.7), pushing the transducer more snugly against the abdomen to keep it from slipping.

The lunge

When: Primarily first stage, but also second stage if desired

Whenever labor progress is slow or has stopped, despite continuing contractions

How: Stabilize a chair so that it will not slide. The woman stands, facing forward with the chair at her side. She raises one foot, places it on the chair seat, and rotates her raised knee and foot to a right angle from the direction toward which she is facing (Fig. 9.29a). Keeping her body upright, she shifts her weight sideways (lunges),

(a) (b)

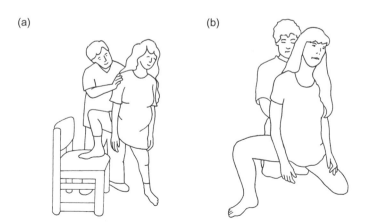

Fig. 9.29. (**a**) Standing lunge. (**b**) Kneeling lunge.

bending her raised knee, then returns to upright, continuing these rhythmic sideways lunges through each contraction. She repeats throughout several contractions in a row. She should feel a stretch in one or both inner thighs; if not, she should widen the distance between the foot on the floor and the foot on the chair. Her partner helps her with balance.

The lunge can also be done on a bed in the kneeling position (Fig. 9.29b).

Deciding which direction to lunge

If the fetus is known to be OP, the woman should lunge in the direction of the occiput (e.g, if the fetus is LOP, she lunges to the left). Lunging to this side will probably feel better.

Even if the baby is not believed to be OP and if the woman has no back pain, the lunge may be useful at any time when active labor progress has slowed. The changes in pelvic shape caused by the lunge may correct subtle fetal positional problems. The woman will probably find that lunging to one side feels better than the other. The side that feels better is probably the one that gives more room for the occiput to adjust.

Why the lunge helps

The elevated femur acts as a lever at the hip joint, "prying" one ischium outward. This creates more space in that side of the pelvis for the posterior occiput to rotate or the asynclitic occiput to resolve its position. Lunging also uses gravity to advantage.

Advantages

- Facilitates rotation
- Reduces back pain
- Allows the partner to provide physical and emotional support

9

Disadvantages

- The woman should have someone (partner, doula, or caregiver) close by to help her maintain her balance.
- The woman with joint pain or problems in her legs or hips should not do the lunge.

(a)   (b)

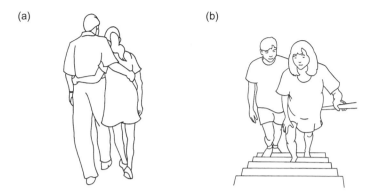

Fig. 9.30. (a) Walking. (b) Stair climbing.

Walking or stair climbing

When: Primarily first stage, but also second stage if desired

How: The woman walks or climbs stairs (Fig. 9.30), continuing during contractions if possible. If not, she leans on her partner or the railing. If she spreads her feet wide apart on each stair, in effect she is "lunging" and climbing stairs at the same time.

Alternatively, she may face the railing and climb the stairs sideways, one or two steps at a time.

Why walking and stair climbing help

Slight but repeated changes in the alignment of pelvic joints occur with each step (more so with stair climbing), encouraging fetal rotation and descent. Walking and stair climbing also use gravity to advantage.

Advantages

- Facilitates fetal rotation
- Often improves morale, especially if it provides a change of scene

Disadvantages

- May be tiring
- Stairs may be inconveniently located.

9

Slow dancing

When: Primarily first stage, but also second stage if desired

How: The woman stands facing her partner and leans on him or her, and they sway slowly from side to side. The partner embraces her and presses on her low back. She lets her arms hang relaxed at her sides or hooks her thumbs into her partner's back pockets or waistband. She rests her head on her partner's shoulder or chest. The partner remains upright; leaning forward for long periods may cause back pain. They can sway to their favorite music and she can breathe in the rhythm of the "dance." This is the most relaxing and least tiring way to maintain a standing position, since the woman is partially supported (Fig. 9.31).

Between contractions, they may continue slow dancing, or walk together, or she might sit until the next contraction.

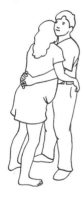

Fig. 9.31. Slow dancing.

Why slow dancing helps

Slight but repeated changes in the pelvic joints occur as she sways, encouraging fetal rotation and descent. The vertical position uses gravity to advantage.

Advantages

- The partner's embrace and support may reduce her emotional stress and her catecholamine production, enabling her uterus to work more efficiently.
- The partner, who knows and loves her more than anyone else, provides a kind of support that no one else can give, as well. For

partners who want to help but feel at a loss to know how, it is most gratifying.

- Rhythmic swaying movements are comforting and may enable her to relax her trunk and pelvic muscles.
- The partner can press on woman's lower back, providing counterpressure to relieve back pain.
- Can be done beside the bed, with monitors and intravenous lines attached to her body
- Good substitute for walking

Disadvantages

- The woman needs a partner with whom she feels comfortable "slow dancing."
- A large height discrepancy between the woman and her partner may make slow dancing challenging or impossible.
- Similar physical benefits can be gained if the woman leans and sways over a birth ball placed on a table or birth bed. She can also lean and sway on the bed, counter, or wall.

Abdominal stroking

When: Primarily first stage, but also second stage if desired

How: The woman gets into a hands-and-knees position. Her caregiver or partner stands beside her on the side opposite the fetal occiput. If this is unknown, abdominal stroking should not be used. The helper reaches beneath the woman's abdomen and, placing one hand on the woman's side, firmly and smoothly strokes across the woman's abdomen, toward the helper (in the direction toward which the occiput should rotate). For example, if the fetus is right OP, the helper stands on the woman's left side, reaches beneath her abdomen to her right side and strokes her abdomen toward the left. The stroking stops at about the middle of the woman's abdomen (Fig. 9.32). The stroking movement is done between contractions and is rhythmic in character. The stroke should be firm enough to lift the abdomen slightly; this usually feels very good to the woman.

9

Why abdominal stroking helps

Use abdominal stroking to help turn an OP baby if the position (left or right OP) is known. With gravity and external stroking of the

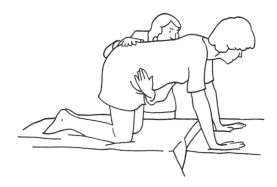

Fig. 9.32. Abdominal stroking for an right OP fetus.

abdomen in the direction the baby needs to rotate, the likelihood is increased that the baby will rotate.[3]

When to use abdominal stroking

- Whenever the fetus is clearly in an OP position and the direction of the occiput is known
- Can be used before labor or between contractions during early labor. Success is more likely if the head is unengaged.

When not to use abdominal stroking

- When fetal position is not known
- When the woman is unable to get into or remain in the hands-and-knees position

Abdominal lifting

When: Primarily first stage, but also second stage if desired

How: The woman stands upright. During the contraction, she interlocks the fingers of both hands beneath her abdomen and lifts her abdomen upward and inward, while bending her knees to tilt her pelvis[12] (Fig. 9.33). She maintains the lift throughout the contraction. Her partner may be able to assist with abdominal lifting by placing a woven rebozo, or shawl (5 to 6 feet long, 18 or more inches wide),

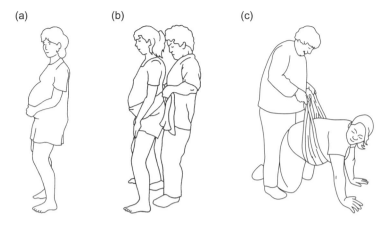

Fig. 9.33. (**a**) Abdominal lifting. (**b**) Abdominal lifting with a rebozo (shawl). (**c**) "Jiggle and jerk" with a rebozo.

around the woman, beneath her abdomen, crossing it in the back and lifting her abdomen for her.

Caution: In the rare instance that the umbilical cord is located low and anterior in the uterus, the abdominal lift might compress the cord. If so, the fetus may "protest" by increasing activity and the abdominal lift should be discontinued. The woman should be told that if she tries the abdominal lift in early labor before there is a nurse or caregiver present, she should discontinue it if her fetus becomes notably more active. It is also wise to periodically check the fetal heart tones during a contraction while the abdominal lift is being done. If the heart rate declines, discontinue the abdominal lift.

Why abdominal lifting helps

Abdominal lifting can help align the long axis of the fetus with the axis of the pelvic inlet. This improves fetal positioning and the efficiency of contractions. Abdominal lifting is particularly helpful for those women with:

- back pain in labor associated with a fetal OP position or such maternal conditions as:
- a pronounced curve in the low back ("swayback")

9

- pendulous abdomen (weak abdominal muscles)
- a short waist (from iliac crests to lowest ribs)
- some previous low back injuries

Advantages

- Reduces back pain
- Provides gravity advantage
- May be done at any stage of labor, from prelabor into the second stage
- Sometimes leads to rapid labor (especially in multiparas with pendulous abdomens)

Disadvantages

- Is tiring for the woman if she does it herself over a long period
- Since rapid progress sometimes occurs suddenly, this should not be done with strong active labor contractions until woman is where she intends to give birth

Abdominal "jiggling" with a rebozo (shawl)

The "jiggle and jerk" maneuver involves the use of a 5- to 6-foot-long rebozo, or woven shawl. The use of the rebozo for many purposes during pregnancy and birth began with traditional midwives in Latin America.[13] Correcting a malposition of the fetus during labor is one of its many uses. (Also see the Abdominal Lift, as discussed earlier.) Here is the technique:

- The woman leans forward from the hips (on hands and knees, kneeling over a birth ball, or standing and leaning forward on a raised bed or counter).
- The rebozo is folded to 12 to 18 inches wide and is placed the woman's mid-abdomen (with the center of the shawl over the center of her abdomen and the ends held behind her).
- The midwife or other caregiver stands straddling the kneeling woman (Fig. 9.33c) or just behind the standing woman, holding the ends of the rebozo, so that they are perpendicular to the woman's trunk.
- The caregiver then pulls on both ends of the rebozo to lift the woman's abdomen slightly toward her back. This will probably feel very good to the woman.

9

- Between or during contractions (whichever the woman prefers), the caregiver gently jiggles the woman's abdomen by alternately and rhythmically pulling up on one end of the rebozo and then the other. She can try doing this slowly or rapidly, so that she is "jiggling" the woman's belly.

- She occasionally (about every 10 jiggles or so) "jerks" one end of the rebozo, that is, she pulls up more forcefully (but never enough to cause pain), then resumes jiggling.

- If she knows that the baby is right OP, she should jerk the left end of the rebozo; if she knows the baby is left OP, she jerks the right end. If she is not sure, she takes turns.

- Over a period of a time (perhaps 30 to 45 minutes, or as tolerated by the woman), the fetus may resettle in a more favorable position.

Caution: We do not recommend this as a routine comfort measure for a doula or partner to use, unless done so with the knowledge and support of the midwife or doctor. Fetal heart tones should be checked periodically to ensure that the fetus is tolerating the procedure.

Over time, this technique becomes tiring for both the woman and the caregiver, who may wish to have another person take over. When the woman tires of it, it is time to try something else.

There are no known research studies of this technique, only anecdotal reports of success, and no known harmful effects.

The pelvic press

When: Second stage

How: With the woman standing, the partner, doula, caregiver, or preferably two people stand behind or beside her, and during a contraction, the person or persons press her iliac crests very firmly toward each other (Fig. 9.34). This should cause some movement in the pelvis, which slightly narrows the upper pelvis. The ilia pivot at the sacroiliac joints, causing the mid-pelvis and the pelvic outlet to widen. Combining the pelvic press with the squatting position will may give the greatest chance of increasing space within the pelvis. Within three or four contractions, there should be some evidence of rotation or descent.[4,5]

9
.

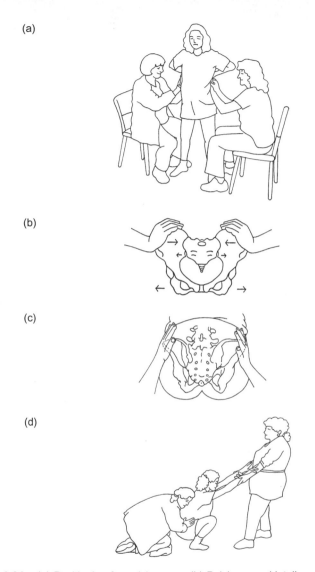

Fig. 9.34. (a) Positioning for pelvic press. (b) Pelvic press (detail, seen from front). (c) Pelvic press (detail, seen from rear). (d) Pelvic press, woman squatting.

How the pelvic press helps

The pelvic press is a technique for enlarging the mid-pelvic and inter-tuberous diameters in second stage. The added room may allow rotation and descent in cases of a malposition or "tight fit" at the pelvic outlet.

When to use the pelvic press

- In second stage, when there is a delay in descent or a caput forming (due to malposition or cephalopelvic disproportion)
- In second stage, when a woman reports severe back pain
- In second stage, if the woman is unable to squat

When not to use the pelvic press

- When the pelvic press causes severe bone or joint pain, as it might if the woman has arthritis or a previous injury to her pelvis
- When the woman has an epidural, because without sensation, joints could be damaged

Other rhythmic movements

When: First or second stage

How: Moving their bodies rhythmically often seems to occur instinctively in women who are coping well in labor. Rocking in a chair (Fig. 9.35a) or swaying while sitting on a birth ball (Fig. 9.35b) or while standing and leaning over a tray table (Fig. 9.35c) or birth ball that is placed on a bed (Fig. 9.35d) are examples of such rhythmic bodily movements. Furthermore, some women find rhythmic stroking or rocking by someone else or by themselves—stroking their own leg or hair, or their partner's arm, or an object—to be soothing. Moaning or self-talk in rhythm is similarly helpful. These behaviors are not planned. They occur spontaneously and instinctively when the woman feels safe. If a woman with slow labor progress is not spontaneously moving as described here, the caregiver might suggest that she try it, and guide her in such movements.

Why rhythmic movements help

- Rhythmic movements tend to be calming.
- Rhythmic movements may alter the relationships among fetus, pelvis, and gravity to promote progress.

9

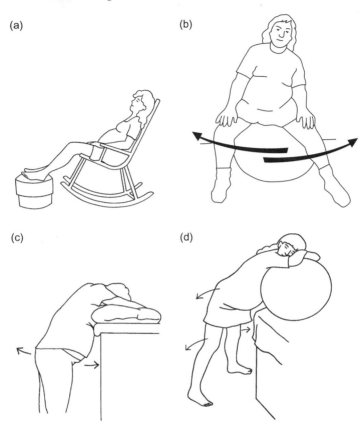

Fig. 9.35. (**a**) Sitting in a rocking chair. (**b**) Swaying on a birth ball. (**c**) Rocking, leaning on a counter. (**d**) Standing, swaying with a ball.

- When spontaneous, rocking is often an indication that the woman is coping well.

REFERENCES

1. Simkin P, O'Hara M. (2002). Nonpharmacologic relief of pain during labor: Systematic reviews of five methods. Am J Obstet Gynecol 186:S131–S159.

2. Lawrence A, Lewis L, Hofmeyr G, Dowswell T, Styles C. (2009). Maternal positions and mobility during first stage labour. Cochrane Database Syst Rev (2):CD003934.

3. Andrews C, Andrews E. (1983). Nursing, maternal postures, and fetal position. Nurs Res 32(6):336–341.

4. Hunter S, Hofmeyr G, Kulier R. (2007). Hands and knees posture in late pregnancy or labour for fetal malposition (lateral or posterior). Cochrane Database Syst Rev (4):CD001063.

5. Sutton J. (2001). Let Birth Be Born Again: Rediscovering and Reclaiming Our Midwifery Heritage. Bedfont, Middlesex, UK, Birth Concepts.

6. Fenwick L, Simkin P. (1987). Maternal positioning to prevent or alleviate dystocia in labor. Clin Obstet Gynecol 30(1):83–89.

7. Stremler R, Hodnett E, Petryshen P, Stevens B, Weston J, Willan A. (2005). Randomized controlled trial of hands and knees positioning for occipitoposterior position in labor. Birth 32:243–251.

8. El Halta V. (1995). Posterior labor: A pain in the back. Midwif Today 36:19–21.

9. Gherman R, Tramont J, Muffley P, Goodwin T. (2000). Analysis of McRoberts' maneuver by xray pelvimetry. Obstet Gynecol 95:43–47.

10. Henderson C, MacDonald S. (2004). Mayes' Midwifery, 13th edition. Oxford, Balliere Tindall.

11. Health T, Gherman R. (1999). Symphyseal separation, sacroiliac joint dislocation transient lateral femoral cutaneous neuropathy associated with McRoberts' maneuver. A case report. J Reprod Med 44(10):902–903.

12. King JM. (1993). Back Labor No More!!! Dallas, Plenary System.

13. Trueba G. (2001) Comfort Measures for Childbirth: The Rebozo Way (DVD). Guadelupe Trueba (gtrueba@prodigy.net.mx).

14. Davis E. (2004). Heart and Hands: A Caregiver's Guide to Pregnancy and Birth, 4th edition. Berkeley, Celestial Arts.

15. Gaskin I. (2003). Ina May's Guide to Childbirth. New York, Bantam Books.

9

Chapter 10

The Labor Progress Toolkit: Part 2. Comfort Measures

Penny Simkin, BA, PT, CCE, CD(DONA),
and Ruth Ancheta, BA, ICCE, CD(DONA)

General guidelines for comfort during a slow labor, 327
Nonpharmacologic physical comfort measures, 328
Heat, 328
Cold, 330
Hydrotherapy, 332
Touch and massage, 337
Acupressure, 345
Acupuncture, 347
Continuous labor support from a doula, nurse, or midwife, 347
Psychosocial comfort measures, 350
Assessing the woman's emotional state, 351
Techniques and devices to reduce back pain, 354
Counterpressure, 354
The double hip squeeze, 355
The knee press, 357
Cook's counterpressure technique No. 1: ischial tuberosities (IT), 359
Cook's counterpressure technique No. 2: perilabial (P-L), 361
Cold and heat, 363
Hydrotherapy, 365
Movement, 366
Birth ball, 367
Transcutaneous electrical nerve stimulation (TENS), 368
Sterile water injections for back pain, 371
Breathing or moaning for relaxation and a sense of mastery, 371
Bearing-down techniques for the second stage, 374
Conclusion, 376
References, 376

10

The Labor Progress Handbook: Early Interventions to Prevent and Treat Dystocia.
Edited by Penny Simkin, Ruth Ancheta
© 2011 by Penny Simkin and Ruth Ancheta; illustrations copyright Ruth Ancheta

Nonpharmacologic methods to relieve labor pain. *Note:* Please see Chapters 2 and 8 for general measures to aid labor progress.

In cases of dystocia, there is another important goal besides improving labor progress. That is to help the woman keep her pain within manageable limits, if possible, without interfering with her ability to move freely. This can sometimes be accomplished by using the nonpharmacologic pain relief measures described in this section.

We want to acknowledge the benefits of a well-timed epidural in serious cases of dystocia: as a precursor to painful interventions; as an aid for an exhausted mother to get some sleep; and possibly to create, in effect, a "mind–body split" in cases where deep-seated fear or anxiety is an underlying cause of dystocia. We hope this book will help prevent dystocia from becoming arrested labor, which often necessitates profound pain relief and obstetric interventions for a good outcome.

GENERAL GUIDELINES FOR COMFORT DURING A SLOW LABOR

The following are general comfort guidelines for slow labors:

- Frequent position changes (about every 20 to 30 minutes when progress is slow) shorten labor and may reduce the woman's pain significantly. See Chapter 9 for information on specific positions. When progress is adequate and the fetus tolerates the contractions well, there is no need to change anything.
- Rhythmic movement reduces both pain and anxiety. See Chapter 9, pages 323–324, for more information on why movement helps and specific movements to try. For information on monitoring the mobile woman's fetus, see Chapter 2, pages 37–44.
- Pressure techniques as shown on pages 354–361 reduce back pain.
- Heat and cold, as shown later in this chapter (pages 328–332, 363–365), reduce various types of pain.
- Hydrotherapy, as shown on pages 332–337, reduces muscle tension, pain, and anxiety dramatically for many women. Immersion in water also provides buoyancy (reducing the effect of gravity on the woman, not on the fetus), even distribution of hydrostatic pressure over the immersed parts of the woman's body, and warmth, often resulting in pain relief and more rapid progress in active labor.

10

- Techniques such as relaxation, naturalistic rhythmic breathing and moaning patterns, and bearing-down efforts give many women a sense of mastery over their pain and help them get through a long, potentially worrisome labor. See pages 371–375 for suggestions on the use of such techniques.
- An experienced doula or labor support provider brings to the woman or couple continuous emotional support, physical comfort, nonclinical advice, and assistance in getting information. The use of doulas is increasing, especially in North America, but also in many other countries, as scientific evidence of their benefit builds.[1] In settings where there is a commitment to maintaining normality and minimizing unnecessary interventions, doulas and caregiving staff have a more positive influence than in settings where usual care includes high rates of intervention use and cesarean birth.[1–2] See pages 347–350 for information on continuous support and doula care.

NONPHARMACOLOGIC PHYSICAL COMFORT MEASURES

Heat

How

- Apply a warm moist towel, heating pad, heated silica gel pack, heated rice pack or hot water bottle to lower abdomen, groin, thighs, lower back, shoulders, or perineum, or
- Direct a warm shower on her shoulders, abdomen, or lower back, or suggest she immerse herself in warm water (see Hydrotherapy) or
- Apply warmed blanket to her entire body.

How heat helps

Heat (Fig. 10.1) increases local skin temperature, circulation, and tissue metabolism. It reduces muscle spasm and raises the pain threshold.[3–4] Heat also reduces the "fight-or-flight" response (as evidenced by trembling and "goose bumps").[4–5] Local heat or a warm blanket calms the woman and also may increase her receptivity to a stroking type of massage that she cannot tolerate when her skin is sensitive or sore due to the fight-or-flight response.

10

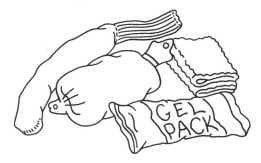

Fig. 10.1. Heat.

Please note: Rice-filled microwaveable packs can be purchased in many department stores, or they can easily be made by the woman by filling a large tube sock with 1.5 pounds (0.68 kg) of dry uncooked rice and stitching or tying closed the top of the sock. Placing the rice pack for 3 to 5 minutes in a microwave oven set on "high" or 10 minutes in a covered ceramic dish in a 180°F oven provides moist heat for up to 30 minutes. Adding lavender seeds or flowers to the rice makes for a lovely aroma. Rice packs can be reheated for the same woman but should not be reused by others.

Caution: If the rice pack is being reheated in a microwave oven that is also used to heat food, caution should be exercised to avoid contaminating the oven with the woman's body fluids. Place the rice pack in a glass or plastic container or consult your infection control department if this is a concern. Rice packs can also be frozen for use as cold packs.

A further caution: Compresses should not be uncomfortably hot to the person applying them. Women in labor may have an altered perception of temperature and may not react to excessive heat even if it is causing a burn. Wrap one or two (or more) layers of toweling or a plastic disposable bed pad around the source of heat as needed to ensure it is not too hot. The caregiver should test the temperature on his or her own inner arm to make sure it is tolerable.

Special cautions on the use of heat with a woman who has an epidural:

- One side effect of epidural analgesia is an alteration in thermoregulation (an imbalance between the generation of body heat

10

by the contracting uterus and the body's ability to dissipate it), that may lead to maternal temperature elevation and associated effects on the fetus.[6] If the woman's temperature is elevated, covering her with a warm blanket may further increase her temperature.

- Because a woman with an epidural lacks sensation, never place a hot or warm compress on the area of her body affected by the epidural (even if she reports pain in that area). It may cause a burn.

When to use heat

- When the woman reports or shows pain in a specific area
- When the woman reports or shows signs of anxiety or muscle tension
- When the woman reports feeling chilled
- In the second stage, warm compresses on the perineum enhance relaxation of the pelvic floor and reduce pain.

When not to use heat

- When the woman reports feeling uncomfortably warm or has a fever
- If staff are worried about potential harm from the heat

Cold

How

- Apply cold compresses to lower back, or perineum, using an ice bag, frozen gel pack or rice pack, latex glove filled with ice chips, frozen wet washcloth, cold can of soft drink, plastic bottle of frozen water, or another cold object (Fig. 10.2, a–c).
- Provide a large strap-on gel pack (available from sports medicine suppliers) for the low back (Fig. 10.2, d). This allows the woman to move or walk around.
- Use a cold moist wash cloth to cool a sweating woman's face, hands, or arms.
- Place a frozen gel pack or plastic bottle of frozen water against her anus to relieve painful hemorrhoids in second stage.

10

(a)   (b)

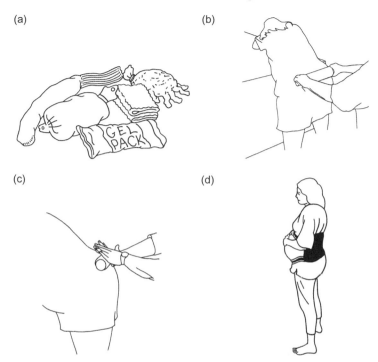

(c)   (d)

Fig. 10.2. (**a**) Cold. (**b**) Rolling cold with ice-filled pin. (**c**) Rolling cold with chilled soda can. (**d**) Strap-on cold pack.

Caution: Always put one or two layers of fabric or a disposable bed pad between the cold item and the woman's skin. This avoids the sudden discomfort that would occur with the direct application of cold to the skin and allows for a gradual and well-tolerated shift from feeling cool to feeling cold.

How cold helps

Cold is especially useful for musculoskeletal and joint pain. Cold decreases muscle spasm (works longer than heat). It reduces sensation in the area by lowering tissue temperature, which slows the

10

transmission of pain and other impulses over sensory neurons (explaining the often-noted numbing effects of cold). Cold also reduces swelling and is cooling to the skin.[4-5,7]

When to use cold

- When woman reports back pain in labor
- When woman feels overheated, is sweating, or has a fever during labor
- When hemorrhoids cause excessive pain
- After the birth, as a cold compress on the woman's perineum to relieve swelling or stitch pain

When not to use cold

- When the woman is already feeling chilled. Use heat first in this case.
- When the woman is from a culture in which the use of cold is a threat to the woman's well-being during labor or postpartum. Ask her if she prefers a hot pack, a cold pack, or neither.
- When the woman reports that the use of cold is not helping her or is irritating
- When the woman has an epidural, do not place a cold pack on the area of her body affected by the epidural. It may damage her skin.

Hydrotherapy

How

Shower: The woman stands or sits in the shower (Fig. 10.3), with water at a comfortable temperature, and directs the shower spray where she wants it (on her back or front). A hand-held shower head is more versatile in directing the spray than a fixed shower head.

Bath: She sits, kneels, or reclines in a tub of deep warm water with enough space for her to change position and perhaps for her partner to get in (Fig. 10.4, a–d).

Caution: Water temperature in the bath should not exceed 98–100°F or 37–37.5°C, because warmer water may raise the woman's temperature and cause fetal tachycardia.[8] The woman should leave

(a)   (b)

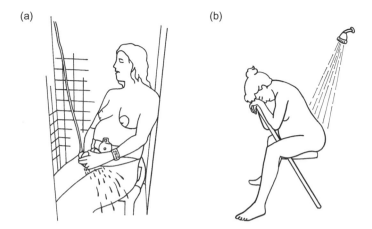

Fig. 10.3. (**a**) Shower on woman's abdomen (with telemetry). (**b**) Shower on woman's back.

the bath after 1.5 hours or so for 30 minutes. This ensures the greatest benefits of the bath. The woman can return to the bath after 30 minutes or so.[2,8–9]

How hydrotherapy helps

Hydrotherapy (shower or bath) reduces muscle tension, pain, and anxiety dramatically for many women.

The effects of immersion in water may be summarized as follows: Bathing provides buoyancy and warmth, both of which often bring immediate pain relief, relaxation, lowering of catecholamines, increase in oxytocin, and more rapid active labor progress. The extent of these effects depends on many variables, such as the water depth and temperature, the duration of the bath, cervical dilation on entry, the woman's cultural perceptions, and psychological factors. Benefits seem to be greatest if the water is at shoulder depth and at body temperature, if the woman waits until active labor before entering the bath, and if she remains in the water for a period up to about 1 to 1.5 hours.

10

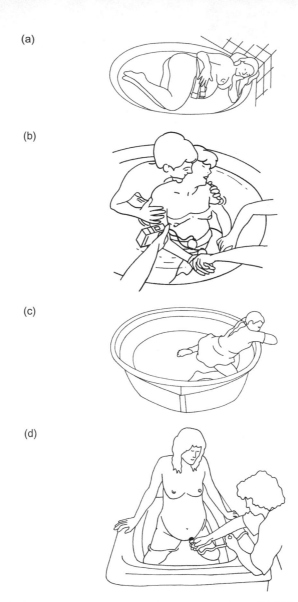

(a)

(b)

(c)

(d)

Fig. 10.4. Baths. (**a**) Side-lying with wireless monitors. (**b**) Sitting with hand held telemetry unit. (**c**) Kneeling in birth pool. (**d**) Monitoring out of water.

Why the woman should leave the water periodically

Fluid balance is altered by immersion in deep water. The hydrostatic pressure on the immersed parts of the woman's body (which increases with the depth of the water) presses tissue fluid into the intravascular space.[8] This increases her blood volume, especially in her chest, which triggers the gradual release of a fluid-regulating hormone, ANF (atrial natriuretic hormone). Over time, ANF inhibits functioning of the posterior pituitary gland, including production of vasopressin (another fluid-regulating hormone) and oxytocin.[8] Of course, the decrease in oxytocin production leads to slowing of labor. Leaving the water for 30 minutes after 1 to 1.5 hours reverses this effect.

How to monitor the fetus in or around water

With a *hand-held Doppler device*, use models designed for underwater use. If these are not available, the woman must lift her abdomen out of the water or step out of the shower as needed for intermittent monitoring (Fig. 10.4, d). The older *wired electronic fetal monitoring tocodynamometers and ultrasound transducers* ("belt monitors") are used underwater with telemetry units held out of the water in some hospitals with women who are monitored continuously (Fig. 10.4, b). These belt monitors are highly water resistant, and because the battery-powered telemetry units operate on very low voltage, many hospitals consider them safe for the woman and fetus.[10] The sensors are usually covered with waterproof gloves or long plastic bags. (These covers are used more to protect the equipment than the woman.)

Please note: Before trying this, please contact your hospital's biomedical services or engineering department regarding both safety and any potential equipment damage connected with underwater use of the specific equipment used in your hospital.

The newer *wireless remote waterproof tocodynamometers and ultrasound sensors* can be used for continuous monitoring in the shower or bath. They are attached by belts to the woman's abdomen but are self-contained and have no wires attached, as shown in Figures 10.3, a, and 10.4, a. These cause minimal interference with rest, bathing, or movement by the woman.

10

When to use hydrotherapy

- As a possible alternative to bedrest for women with pregnancy-induced hypertension[11]

Showers: Use in any phase of first stage labor or early second stage. *Immersion in bath:* Use after active labor is established (with one exception—see later). Because immersion in water often slows contractions when used before active labor,[8] a bath is sometimes recommended to stop preterm contractions or to slow exhausting prelabor contractions and give the woman some temporary rest. Entrance into the water before 5-cm dilation, however, has been associated with longer labor and greater need for oxytocin augmentation.[12] Barbara Harper, an American expert on water birth, suggests a less strict approach to timing of entry into the bath than awaiting 5-cm dilation—leaving the decision up to the woman. If the labor slows when she is in the water, then she gets out until her labor becomes established, which might occur before or after 5-cm dilation.[13]

- Immersion in deep water when one is in preterm labor, prelabor, or latent labor often stops contractions temporarily through the mechanism described earlier. This may be desirable if the woman is having preterm labor contractions or an exhaustingly long prelabor; otherwise, it is not desirable because it could suppress early labor progress. If the woman awaits active labor before entering the bath, dilation often speeds up and pain is reduced.[8]

When not to use hydrotherapy

Showers

- When the woman's balance or ability to stand is unreliable, due to medication or other reasons
- When there is a medical contraindication requiring restriction to bed

Immersion in a bath

- Before active labor is established (unless slowing of labor or temporary cessation of contractions is desired)

10

- When there is a medical contraindication such as bleeding or fetal distress
- When birth is imminent (unless the woman and practitioner are planning a water birth)
- When the woman has received narcotic medications or an epidural for pain

Effectiveness of hydrotherapy during active labor

A recent meta-analysis of randomized controlled trials compared outcomes of immersion in water with no immersion during the first stage of labor. It found significant reductions in both epidural use and reported pain in the women who used a bath during labor. There were no differences in operative deliveries, Apgar scores below 7 at 5 minutes, admissions to neonatal intensive care units, or neonatal infection rates.[9] A randomized controlled trial found that when dystocia has been diagnosed, bathing significantly decreases the need for labor augmentation with amniotomy and oxytocin.[14] Birth in the water is more controversial than laboring in water and has strong proponents and opponents. There are few randomized controlled trials of water birth,[9] but more scientific evaluation is needed to help resolve the controversy.

Showers have not been studied systematically, but clinical experience suggests many women experience enhanced maternal relaxation and significant reductions in pain.

Touch and massage

How

Various forms of touch, including patting or holding the woman's shoulder or hand, stroking her cheek or hair, even if brief, can convey to the woman a sense of caring, reassurance, understanding, or non-verbal support. Cultural views of this kind of touch vary, especially if it is not given by a family member, close friend, or a female. Women's personal comfort with this kind of touch also varies, so the caregiver must be tactful, ask permission, or observe for signs that the woman wants comforting touch (i.e., reaching for the caregiver's hand, responding positively to a fleeting pat after a clinical procedure). Caregivers also do not always feel comfortable giving this kind of touch and, if not, they should not do it.

10

Massage during labor is formalized touch with the intention of enhancing relaxation and relieving pain.[3] It may involve a specific part of the body, such as the hands, feet, scalp, shoulders, or back. It may involve light or firm stroking, kneading, or still pressure. It may include the use of the hands or any of a variety of massage devices. It may be done with or without oils, lotions, or powders.

Also see How to Give Simple Brief Massages for Shoulders and Back, Hands, and Feet on pages 339–345.

When to use touch or massage

- When the woman seems tense, frightened, or anxious
- When the woman describes pain in a specific area (i.e., the back, thigh, abdomen)
- When the woman's arms, legs, or feet ache or are tired from great effort
- When the caregiver wants to express empathy, or reassurance

When not to use touch or massage

- When the caregiver is uncomfortable or unskilled in its use
- When the woman does not want it, or it is not helping
- When there are cultural proscriptions against its use

Effectiveness of touch and massage

One trial of "reassuring touch" compared with "usual care" during transition found fewer expressions of anxiety and improved blood pressure in the group who received reassuring touch.[15] Two trials of massage by women's partners, who were taught to give 20- to 30-minute massages to the women several times during labor, found that the massage groups had less pain and anxiety and reported greater satisfaction with their childbirths than the control groups.[16–17] A fourth trial used a pain questionnaire to compare labor pain in one group of laboring women who received usual nursing care plus massages at three times in the first stage of labor, with a similar group who received usual care only. The massage group reported less pain up to 7 cm of dilation, at which time pain was assessed as the same in the two groups.[18]

10

How to give simple brief massages for shoulders and back, hands, and feet

A laboring woman may appreciate one or more brief (1- to 3-minute) massages of her shoulders, back, hands, or feet. They will soothe her and give her a little comfort break.

Follow these general guidelines.

- Always ask for permission and describe the massage you would like to do.
- Be sure your hands are clean and warm and that she is comfortable.
- Use unscented massage oil. Squirt a little on your hands and rub them together briskly to warm your hands.
- Once you begin, do not remove both hands until you are done. It is unsettling for her to relax into a massage, only to have the massager's hands disappear, and not know when or where they will go next.

Three-part shoulder mini-massage

When to use it

- Anytime during labor if she is tense—during or between contractions

When not to use it

- When she does not want to be touched or does not like the massage

How

The woman sits up, or leans forward and rests her head on her arms or a pillow. You stand behind her.

Part 1: Place your hands comfortably on her shoulders near her neck. Stroke firmly from her neck to her shoulders, then over her shoulders to her upper arms. Knead her upper arms a few times (let her tell you how firmly to stroke and knead), and stroke firmly back toward her neck. Do that three or four times.

10

Part 2: With your hands molded over the tops of her shoulders, "knead" or squeeze and release her shoulder muscles as firmly as she likes (ask her for feedback) for 1 to 2 minutes.

Part 3: Using the middle three fingertips of one hand, make some brief deep circle massages on spots on the tops of her shoulders and small areas along her spine. Circle in one area for 15 to 30 seconds, then move to another. She'll tell you her favorite places.

"Criss-cross" massage over the small of her back

When to use

- Anytime during or between contractions

How (Fig. 10.5)

(a)   (b)

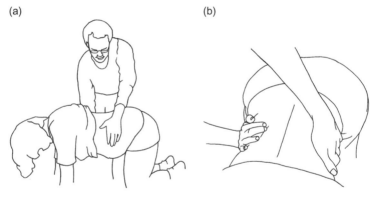

Fig. 10.5. (a) "Criss-cross" back massage. (b) Close-up view of "criss-cross" back massage. (Source: Simkin P. [2008]. The Birth Partner: A Complete Guide to Childbirth for Dads, Doulas, and All Other Labor Companions, 3rd edition. Boston, MA, Harvard Common Press. Reprinted with permission.)

The woman kneels on the bed or the floor leaning over the birth ball or other support. (If she is on the bed, you will be able to adjust the height of the bed so you can reach her back without strain.) Because her knees may get sore fairly quickly, it is a good idea for her to wear knee pads or to kneel on a soft pad. (The foam pads made for garden-

10

ers work very well.) You face her side. Look at her back and notice the place where her waist is narrowest. That is where you will place your hands—on each side at the narrowest part, below her ribs. Place your right hand on her side farthest from you, fingers pointing down. Place your left hand on her near side, fingers pointing up. Press her sides in quite firmly. She should like that feeling. Then, stroke your hands firmly up and across her back toward each other. Cross one hand over the other and move to the original starting spots on her sides. Maintaining the same pressure, press her sides in again, and repeat the crossover movement over and over as long as she wants. The inward pressure on her sides brings much relief. You may do this during or between contractions for as long as she likes.

Hand massage (Fig. 10.6)

This massage relaxes her hand all the way up her arm, while still giving her pain-relieving benefits of pressure on the palms of her hands.

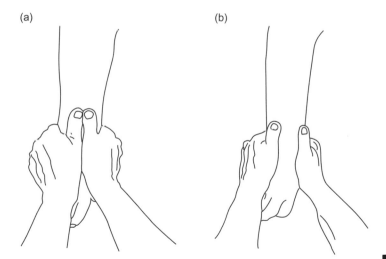

(a) (b)

Fig. 10.6. (a) Hand massage, thumbs together. (b) Hand massage, thumbs apart. (Source: Simkin P. [2008]. The Birth Partner: A Complete Guide to Childbirth for Dads, Doulas, and All Other Labor Companions, 3rd edition. Boston, MA, Harvard Common Press. Reprinted with permission.)

10

When to do it

- During or between contractions
- If she has been clenching her fists during contractions, or gripping the sheet or bedrail

How

Stand or sit facing her, a little above her. Ask her to relax her arm, and take her hand in both of yours. Grasp it so that your thumbs (from tips all the way to your wrist) are placed side by side on the back of her wrist. The pads of your fingers (*not* your fingernails) press into her palm.

Then, without moving your hands, increase your grip gradually and ask her to tell you when you are squeezing "hard enough." You may be surprised at how much pressure she likes. When she says it is enough, maintain that pressure, and slowly slide your thumbs apart and off her hand (Fig. 10.6). You are combining pressure on her palm with friction over the back of her hand. Replace your thumbs in the starting position and repeat 10 times or so.

Caution: If her hands are very swollen or if she has carpal tunnel syndrome (tingling or numbness in her hands that worsens with pressure), she will want very little pressure or she will not want you to do this massage at all.

Three-part foot massage

The purpose: to restore circulation and relieve foot aches and fatigue caused by prolonged standing and walking.

When to do it

- Between contractions and if she complains that her feet are hurting or getting tired

How

Part 1: "Breaking the popsicle" (Fig. 10.7)
    She sits on the bed with her feet extended, and you grasp one of her feet with both hands. Grasp it so that your thumbs, including the bases of your thumbs, are touching each other. The pads

(a)

(b)

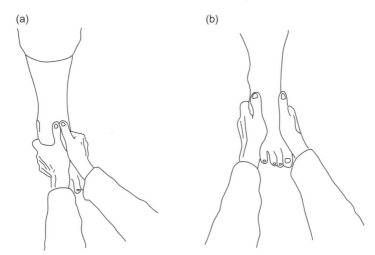

Fig. 10.7. (**a, b**) "Breaking the Popsicle" foot massage. (Source: Simkin P. [2008]. The Birth Partner: A Complete Guide to Childbirth for Dads, Doulas, and All Other Labor Companions, 3rd edition. Boston, MA, Harvard Common Press. Reprinted with permission.)

of your fingers (not your fingernails) press into the sole of her foot. Squeeze until she says that is firm enough. You may be surprised at how much pressure she wants. Maintain that pressure, and slowly slide your thumbs apart and off her foot (see the figure). You are combining pressure on the sole of her foot with friction over the back of her hand. Replace your thumbs in the starting position and repeat for 10 times or so.

Part 2: "Squeezing the apple" (Fig. 10.8)

If massaging her left foot, using your right hand, press the heel of your hand firmly into the arch of her foot and grasp her heel. Don't press your fingertips into her foot. Squeeze and release it several times, as if you were squeezing an apple or tennis ball.

Part 3: Deep circle massage with fingertips (Fig. 10.9)

(This description applies to massage of her left foot. You can adapt it to apply to her right.) Hold the sole of her left foot in your left hand. With the pads of the three middle fingers of your right hand, give her a deep circle massage in the "magic spot," on

10

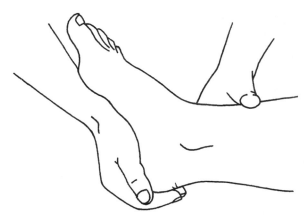

Fig. 10.8. "Squeezing the apple" foot massage.

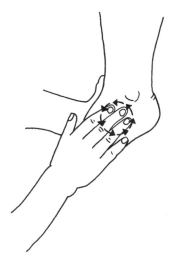

Fig. 10.9. Deep massage with fingertips.

10

the top of her foot just below her ankle. The spot is slightly off center toward the outside of her foot. Ask if you are rubbing a spot that feels good. Move around as necessary. Your fingers do not move on her skin; rather, you are moving her skin over her underlying muscles and bones. Do this for 30 to 60 seconds.

Once you have completed all three steps on one foot, repeat with her other foot. Then she will be ready to walk some more.

With a bit of practice, these massages are easily mastered and equip you to give comfort and kindness in a short time.

Acupressure

How

Pressure on the points illustrated in Figure 10.10 during labor is thought to enhance contractions, and possibly reducing labor pain.

1. Press firmly with a finger on the point for 10 to 60 seconds. Then rest for an equal length of time.
2. Repeat this cycle for up to six cycles. Contractions may speed up during that time.

Another technique is to apply an ice-filled washcloth to the *ho-ku* point (see Fig. 10.10) on the palm side of one hand and then the other for 20 minutes at a time.[19]

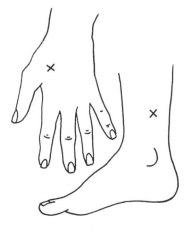

Fig. 10.10. Acupressure points: *ho-ku* point on hand (on the back of the hand, where the metacarpal bones of the thumb and the index finger come together); Spleen 6 point on ankle (on the tibia), four finger widths above the medial malleolus (inner ankle bone): apply pressure on the tibia and diagonally forward; this point will be very tender.

10

How acupressure helps

Acupressure is based on acupuncture theory, which states that specific health problems, including poor progress or excessive pain in labor, arise when there is a blockage of energy flow along particular meridians in the body. By releasing the blockage, harmony and smooth functioning return.

When to use acupressure

- When labor induction is considered necessary within a few days. The woman might try self-help measures to start labor, in hopes of avoiding induction, but only after discussing this with her doctor or midwife.
- In labor, when more frequent contractions are desired or needed
- When contractions are very painful but not accompanied by labor progress

When not to use acupressure

- During pregnancy before term (unless induction is being planned), because it may result in preterm labor contractions. We also suggest that the woman not even experiment with it on herself before labor.
- If she has not consulted her doctor or midwife

Effectiveness of acupressure

One controlled trial of acupressure compared pain ratings before and after ice massage on the *ho-ku* point. The women rated their labor pain lower after receiving the ice massage.[19]

Two randomized trials showed that acupressure decreased labor pain (measured by visual analog scale scores) compared to light skin stroking or no treatment/conversation only.[20–21] In one of the trials, analgesics were used by 5 of 36 women in the acupressure group versus 10 of 39 patients in the control group; the number of patients may have been too small to show a statistically significant change.

These small trials lend promise to the usefulness of acupressure, without findings of harm. Its effectiveness still is uncertain. However, the techniques are simple and, when used as described earlier, appear

10

to be free of harmful effects. They may therefore be worth trying when contractions are excessively painful and labor progress is inadequate.

Acupuncture

The ancient Eastern healing art of acupuncture is used on a limited basis in Western maternity care, primarily for the purposes of turning breech babies to vertex, relieving labor pain, and inducing labor. All these uses have been subjected to scientific evaluation. Other uses, such as augmentation of labor and control of blood pressure, have received little Western scientific scrutiny, although acupuncture is used for such purposes. See pages 267–269 for a discussion of acupuncture to relieve pain and induce labor and for a discussion of scientific findings regarding the use of acupuncture in labor.

Continuous labor support from a doula, nurse, or midwife

Until recently, nurses and midwives, along with women's partners, have been designated as the main people to provide support to laboring women. Professional staff were expected to add labor support to their long list of other tasks, and it was assumed that any knowledgeable professional could easily do this without instruction. Women's partners were assumed to be calm and capable enough to "coach" a woman through labor. More recently, doula research has shown that effective nonclinical labor support cannot be an "add-on" to other duties, nor can a loved one provide all the support a woman needs.[22–23] A doula is a person (usually a woman), trained and experienced in childbirth, who accompanies laboring women and their partners throughout labor and birth (Fig. 10.11). She provides continuous emotional support, physical comfort, and nonclinical advice and assists the laboring woman in getting the information needed to make informed choices regarding options. She is usually a lay person, although some nurses and childbirth educators have become doulas.

How the doula helps

The doula focuses on the woman through each contraction, offering reassurance, praise, encouragement, and comfort, as needed and

10

(a) 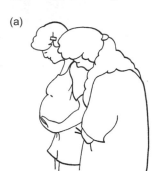   (b)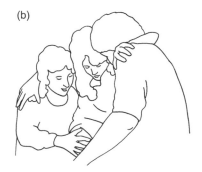

Fig. 10.11. (a) Doula supporting a woman. (b) Doula supporting a couple.

appropriate. She also guides, assists, and reassures the woman's partner. She rarely takes a break and remains with the woman until after the birth. Doulas usually do not work in shifts. The doula performs no clinical tasks. Her sole responsibility is the woman's and the partner's emotional well-being and the woman's physical comfort. Some hospitals and health agencies have doulas on staff to help women beginning when they are admitted, but most doulas contract privately with clients. Some work as volunteers; most charge a fee.

In North America, doulas are certified by DONA International (formerly Doulas of North America), the International Childbirth Education Association (ICEA), to Labor, formerly Association of Labor Assistants and Childbirth Educators, and the Childbirth and Postpartum Professional Association (CAPPA). The concept of the doula is growing rapidly in Europe, Australia, and New Zealand. Doulas UK represents and supports doulas in the United Kingdom.

When to use a doula

- A doula should be used whenever one is available and the woman wants her services. There are no known harmful effects when doulas, as described earlier, are in attendance.

When not to use a doula

- A doula should not be used when the woman prefers not to have one.

Effectiveness of doulas

A recent systematic review of 15 randomized controlled trials of continuous labor support included 12,791 women.[1] The researchers found that women who received continuous labor support benefited, but the greatest benefit was found in the trials in which the support provider was *not* a hospital staff member with clinical care responsibilities. Care by doulas and other nonclinical personnel resulted in 26% fewer cesareans, 41% fewer instrumental deliveries, 28% mothers who were less likely to use any pain medication, and 33% mothers who were less likely to be dissatisfied or to rate their birth negatively. Another systematic review of randomized controlled trials of continuous support by doulas or nurses in North America reported similar results.[2] Support begun in early labor provided greater benefit than support begun in active labor. The women who benefited most were those whose care was provided by doulas rather than by nurses, whose support was begun during early versus in active labor, and who were not accompanied by a loved one versus those who were accompanied by a loved one.

What about staff nurses and midwives as labor support providers?

"There are two common barriers to be overcome before nurses can provide skilled labor support to their patients: lack of time and lack of knowledge."[24]

While many maternity nurses and midwives enjoy and are skilled in the labor support role, others have little knowledge of these skills since labor support does not hold a high priority in most educational programs. Even the most knowledgeable and supportive nurses cannot always provide the kind of continuous care that contributes to improved obstetric outcomes, especially if they are responsible for more than one laboring woman or must assume other clinical or "indirect" patient care tasks that take her outside of the woman's room. The largest randomized controlled trial evaluating the effectiveness of nurses as labor support providers included 6,915 women who gave birth in 13 hospitals in the United States and Canada. All the participating hospitals had high rates of medical interventions. The supported group received continuous support from a specially trained nurse who had volunteered to provide the extra support. The control group received "usual care." There were very few differences in outcomes between the groups, except for slightly less use of continuous fetal monitoring, and more indicators of satisfaction with their births at 7 weeks post partum in the supported group. The authors propose that the lack of differences in outcomes between the supported and the usual care groups may be due to fact that the settings for the trial were highly interventive, relying heavily on continuous electronic monitoring, epidural analgesia, and induction and augmentation of labor.[25] The fact that the nurses were hospital employees who were accustomed to functioning within a high-intervention setting may also have influenced the lack of differences between the groups' outcomes.[1]

What about midwives? Continuous one-to-one care by midwives who focus on psychosocial aspects of childbirth has been shown to produce more favorable outcomes when compared with the usual care by obstetricians.[26] In North America, although the numbers of midwives and doulas are increasing, there are still relatively few of either group. About 8% of births in the United States are attended by midwives[27] (8% by family physicians and 79% by obstetricians[28]). Approximately 3% of births in the United States have doula support.[28] A recent Canadian survey of women's maternity experiences found that less than 4% of women received care from midwives, while 67% received care from obstetricians and 17% from family physicians (12% did not report or use other caregivers). This survey did not collect information on the use of doulas.[29] These figures illustrate that the favorable outcomes achieved by midwives are available to very few North American women, while in many other countries midwives are the primary care providers for the vast majority of childbearing women.

Nurses, many of whom are dedicated to supportive care, are often frustrated at the demands that take them from the woman's side. They tend to be very busy with multiple tasks and are often assigned more than one woman in labor. Also, they must give priority to their clinical responsibilities. These factors combine to leave many laboring women with little skilled emotional support or guidance for a low-intervention birth.

One can only speculate about how the lack of this kind of support contributes to the incidence of labor dystocia.

Psychosocial comfort measures

10

In Chapter 2, we discussed the importance of a peaceful environment for birth and showed how outside disturbances may interfere with the labor process. We also described the labor-inhibiting effects of disturbance, fear, and anxiety and how excessive production of stress hormones (catecholamines) can affect uterine and placental function. Chapter 2 also lists some basic and universal guidelines for helping women adapt to the labor environment and for adapting the labor environment to each woman.

In Chapter 9 and the previous section of this chapter, we provided many physical measures to improve comfort and progress.

This section presents specific psychosocial comfort measures that calm the laboring woman's distress and enhance her feelings of emotional safety.

Assessing the woman's emotional state[30]

It is not always possible to assess a woman's sense of well-being by observing her external façade. For example, a woman who is still and quiet during contractions may be as peaceful and confident as she appears, or she may actually feel as if she is "screaming inside" or "barely keeping the lid on"—moving a muscle or letting out a sound will open the dam of emotions and cause her to lose all sense of control. Another woman who is vocal and active may feel calm and safe as long as she can express and release her feelings or, as one woman said, "shout down the pain." Sometimes the best way to assess the woman's well-being is to ask her.

Occasionally ask her, between contractions, "What was going through your mind during that contraction?" Her answer may tell much about her emotional needs and whether she is coping well or is distressed. This knowledge will help those around her to provide appropriate emotional support. One unique and important study found that when women answered this question with indications of distressing thoughts (as opposed to answers that indicate that she is coping) during the latent phase (possibly indicating excessive catecholamine production), they were at increased risk for prolonged labor, nonreassuring fetal heart tones, intolerance of labor, and all the interventions that accompany such problems. This was *not* true when the women indicated distressing thoughts during active labor or transition. "We conclude that latent labor is a critical phase in the psychobiology of labor and that pain and cognitive activity (thoughts) during this phase are important contributions to labor efficiency and obstetric outcome."[31] Therefore, checking the woman's thoughts and

10

eliminating or reducing stressors are worthwhile goals, especially in early labor when a woman has little need for clinical care.

The following are specific ways to reduce stress and enhance the woman's emotional well-being.

Provide reassuring or comforting sensory stimuli

- music that the woman likes
- massage, backrub, touch
- lighting that suits the woman
- juice or frozen juice bars in a flavor she likes
- pleasant-smelling hand cream or massage oil
- making electronic fetal monitoring heart tones audible if the woman finds them reassuring; otherwise, turning them down

Provide reassurance and praise

- Ask what sensations the woman is having. Explain what causes them and reassure her that these sensations are normal. "Your body knows just what it's doing"; "I know this is difficult. It's because you're making good progress. It won't be much longer."
- Suggest comfort measures to her and her partner.
- Compliment her: "You're doing so well?"; "Don't change a thing"; "You're perfect."
- If she is interested, explain monitor tracings to the woman. Respect her wishes regarding information.
- Explain that the vocal woman next door says it helps her cope or push when she yells. And, if culturally appropriate, you might add, "You might also find that helpful at some point."
- Help her reframe distressing thoughts, especially in early labor: "Can you imagine your strong contractions doing exactly what they are supposed to do—open your cervix and bring your baby to you?"

Reduce fear-inducing stimuli and actions

- Close the woman's door and that of any vocal women.
- Minimize interventions if the woman does not want them (especially painful or invasive ones).

- Ask other staff to make sure they cannot possibly be overheard by any laboring women when discussing their patients. Information and vocabulary that are emotionally neutral to staff members may be frightening to the woman.
- If the woman is accompanied by someone who seems to make her anxious, ask her privately if she would like that person to leave the room. Send him or her on an errand, or suggest they get a snack. If necessary, ask that person to wait elsewhere.
- If older children are present, they should be accompanied by their own support people, so the woman and her support person(s) can focus on coping with the labor.
- Avoid bringing unnecessary staff members into the woman's room.
- Provide a more private, less-inhibiting environment:
  - Remember that nudity or being scantily clad is threatening or embarrassing for some people. Offer an extra gown or robe to cover the woman's back. Some women feel more like themselves if they wear their own clothing in labor, while some want to remove all clothing.
  - Keep curtain and/or door closed.
  - Knock before entering and encourage other staff to do the same.
  - Sometimes women need privacy, a small space, and freedom from disturbances to adjust psychologically to the demands of labor. Encourage the woman to spend some time in the bathroom with the door closed. Labor progress sometimes improves after some private time. Many women who are "holding back" during second stage can relax their pelvic floors on the toilet.
- If you are concerned that the baby may be born suddenly, instruct the woman to push the call light in the bathroom if she feels a lot of pressure.
- Encourage and reinforce the woman's spontaneous coping behaviors, such as rhythmic movements, sounds, and position changes. ("You are good at finding the positions and sounds that work for you.")
- If you are not sure whether a specific behavior is helping the woman or is simply a sign of distress, ask nonjudgmentally. ("Does it help to shake your hands during the contraction?")
- Encourage the use of hydrotherapy. Many women "let go" in the shower or bath.

10

- If the woman is silent, in her own world, try not to disturb her with questions or procedures.
- If the woman loses rhythm in her movements, breathing, or vocalizing, help her get it back with eye contact, speaking in soothing rhythmic tones, nodding your head, or moving your hand rhythmically, so that she can follow the rhythm that you give her (which should mimic closely the rhythm she had).
- For ways to support women in pre-labor and latent first stage, see pages 109–111. For information on emotional dystocia in active first stage labor, see pages 160–169. See pages 215–219 for information on emotional dystocia and "holding back" in second stage labor.

TECHNIQUES AND DEVICES TO REDUCE BACK PAIN

Counterpressure

How

- The woman's partner applies steady pressure throughout the contraction on the woman's sacrum with the heel or fist of one hand (Fig. 10.12).
- The woman tells the partner where to push (wherever the pain is most intense) and how hard to push.
- If needed, the partner places his other hand on the front of the woman's hip (over the anterior superior iliac spine) to help her keep her balance.

(a)　　　　　　　　　　　　(b)

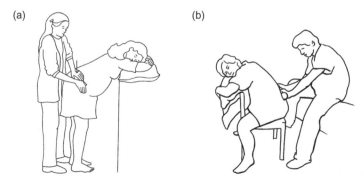

Fig. 10.12. (a) Counterpressure. (b) Counterpressure with tennis balls.

10

How counterpressure helps

- It is not clear exactly how or why counterpressure eases back pain in labor. It may change the shape of the pelvis enough to ease pain caused by the pressure of the occiput posterior or asynclitic baby's occiput on the sacroiliac joints. Judging from its popularity with women, every caregiver should know and be able to teach partners how to do counterpressure.

When to use counterpressure

- When the woman reports back pain.

When not to use counterpressure

- When the woman reports counterpressure is not helping, or when she finds it distracting.

The double hip squeeze

How

One or two people may perform the double hip squeeze. If there is one partner, he or she places his or her hands on the outsides of the woman's hips, over the woman's gluteal muscles (well below her iliac crests, over the "meatiest" part of her buttocks), and presses inward toward the center of her pelvis with the whole palms of his or her hands (not just the heels of the hands) steadily throughout the contraction (Fig. 10.13). As with counterpressure, the woman decides how much pressure she needs and exactly where he should place his hands. This is hard work for the partner. If this is too difficult to continue for as long as the woman needs it, it helps to have another person there to do the two-person double hip squeeze (see later). If there is no other person to help, then one-handed counterpressure may be used for a few contractions to allow the partner a break. Then he should resume the double hip squeeze if the woman finds it more helpful.

The two person double hip squeeze. The woman kneels over a birth ball, the seat of a chair, or on the lowered foot portion of a birthing bed over a pile of pillows placed on the mid-portion of the bed. Two

10

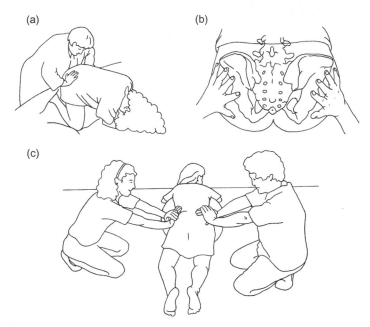

Fig. 10.13. (**a**) Double hip squeeze. (**b**) Double hip squeeze (detail, seen from rear). (**c**) Double hip squeeze with two support people.

people stand, one on either side of the woman. Each person places one open hand on the side of her hip above and medial to her hip joint. Their other hand covers the first hand. Then, at the same time, they lean in to put bilateral pressure on her hips. The pressure remains steady and equal through the contraction. Between contractions, they remove their hands and rest. The two-person double hip squeeze is much easier for those who must do it.

Note: This is different from the "pelvic press," which is used in cases of deep transverse arrest, persistent occiput posterior, or borderline cephalopelvic disproportion. See pages 321–323 for a description.

How the double hip squeeze helps

It is not clear how or why the double hip squeeze eases back pain in labor. The pressure may change the shape of the pelvis as does coun-

10

terpressure (see the preceding section). It may slightly reduce the stretch in the sacroiliac joints, easing the strain on those ligaments caused by internal pressure of the malpositioned fetal head.

Note: The authors consider it a poor prognosis if a woman needs maximum pressure in the double hip squeeze (i.e., requiring all the strength of her partner) to obtain relief. We believe that such extreme pressure may indicate that the fetal head is deeply engaged in its malposition or complicated by an accompanying problem, such as a nuchal hand, and less likely to self-correct spontaneously than when moderate or minor pressure is sufficient to relieve pain. In fact, one may wonder if the extreme hip pressure might decrease the volume in the pelvic basin and actually impair self-correction of the malposition. This possibility should be researched because the double hip squeeze seems very effective in relieving back pain, but it should not come at the cost of preventing rotation!

Other measures (e.g., the open knee–chest position [Chapter 10, pages 293–295], abdominal lifting [pages 318–320], the knee press [pages 357–359], or the use of cold [page 363] or heat [page 364] or the pelvic press in second stage [Chapter 9, pages 321–323] or an epidural) may be preferable to maximal pressure in the double hip squeeze.

When to use the double hip squeeze

- When the woman reports back pain.

When not to use the double hip squeeze

- When the woman reports that it is not helping.

The knee press

How

If the woman is seated: The woman sits upright on a straight chair with her low back against the back of the chair. She places her feet flat on the floor and her knees a few inches apart. (If her feet do not reach the floor, books or other supports can be placed beneath each foot [Fig. 10.14].)

Her partner or doula kneels on the floor in front of her and cups his hands over her knees. Locking his elbows in close to his trunk, and

10

(a)

(b)

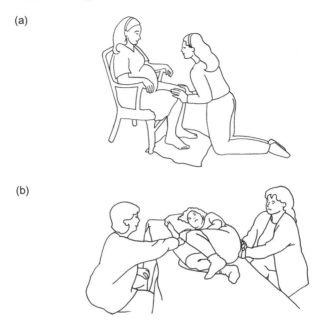

Fig. 10.14. (a) Knee press, seated. (b) Knee press, lateral.

rising off his haunches, he leans toward the woman throughout each contraction, allowing his upper body weight to apply pressure on her knees, directed from his hands straight back toward her hip joints. She feels a slight release in her low back and relief of back pain.

If the woman is side-lying, with one or two pillows supporting her upper knee: Two partners are needed. Only the upper knee is pressed. The woman flexes her upper knee and hip joints to 90-degree angles. One partner presses on the woman's sacrum during contractions to stabilize her. The other partner cups the woman's top knee in his or her hand and presses on that knee directly toward her hip joint.

How the knee press helps

10

Pressure directed via the femur straight into the flexed hip joint or joints alters the configuration of the pelvic basin, releasing the sacro-iliac joints and relieving low back pain.

When to use the knee press

- When the woman has back pain

When not to use the knee press

- When the woman reports the knee press is not reducing her pain

When the woman has joint pain, inflammation, or damage in her knee joints

Cook's counterpressure technique No. 1: ischial tuberosities (IT)

Authors' note: We are grateful to Lisa-Marie Sasaki Cook, RN, for teaching us the following two counterpressure techniques. The following descriptions are adapted from her unpublished manuscript.[32]

How

- The woman lies on her side or on hands and knees with hips flexed to 90 degrees, which allows partner or caregiver to palpate her IT ("sit-bones") and then apply pressure on both spots with thumbs, heels of the hands, fists, or tennis balls during or between contractions. The woman gives feedback on where and how hard to press, and when on her hands and knees, she can also "lean" into the pressure as feels comfortable (Fig. 10.15).

How Cook's IT counterpressure helps

The ITs are points of attachment for many muscles, including hamstring muscles, hip rotators, and adductors. Also, three major pelvic ligaments are connected to the ITs. As the fetal head descends through the pelvis, these muscles and ligaments undergo significant pressure, resulting in pelvic pain, especially during contractions. Direct manual counterpressure to the ITs provides an opposing force, decreasing the pain in the pelvis.

When done between contractions, women may be better able to relax within the pelvis.

10

(a)

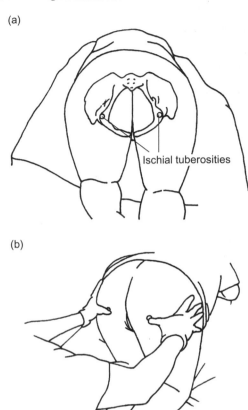

Ischial tuberosities

(b)

Fig. 10.15. (a) Bony landmarks for Cook's ischial tuberosity (IT) counterpressure. (b) Hand placement for Cook's IT counterpressure.

In Chinese medicine, the IT points are known as acupuncture points UB36 (Urinary Bladder 36) or by the Chinese name *Chengfu,* which translates into English as "receiving support." UB36 is described as being located at the midpoint of the inferior gluteal fold. This point, when activated, is said to alleviate pain in the lower back and gluteal region, sciatica, and other conditions.

When to use Cook's IT counterpressure No. 1

- During any phase of labor—early, active, transition, and second stage prior to crowning, especially when a woman complains of back pain or pelvic pressure, with or without an epidural
- When a woman has a premature urge to push before complete dilation with a cervical lip or swelling

When not to use Cook's IT counterpressure No. 1

- When the woman states that this counterpressure is not helping or is unpleasantly distracting
- When the woman complains that it causes discomfort
- When she has the following contraindications:
  - Preexisting symphysis pubis problems
  - Past pelvic trauma (accident, violence, obstetric trauma, etc.) that may have damaged the pelvic girdle area

Cook's perilabial counterpressure technique No. 2

Late in the second stage, the caregiver presses externally with thumbs or fingers just outside the woman's labia against both inferior pubic rami to counteract the forces of the fetal head against the pubic arch and pelvic musculature.

Note: It is not appropriate for the doula to use this technique unless she is asked to do so by the caregiver.

How

With the laboring woman in a semisitting position with knees drawn up and spread apart, or side-lying, or squatting, the caregiver uses thumbs or index fingers from both hands or, in a single-handed technique, one thumb and index or middle finger to provide counterpressure just outside the external labia toward the inferior rami of the pubic arch (Fig. 10.16). The points can be located by palpating the prominent adductor longus tendons and pressing just posterior to their insertion sites against the bony inferior pubic rami.

The woman tells the caregiver how hard to press and whether it is more effective when used during or between contractions. With the two-handed technique, the care provider is still able to support the

10

(a)

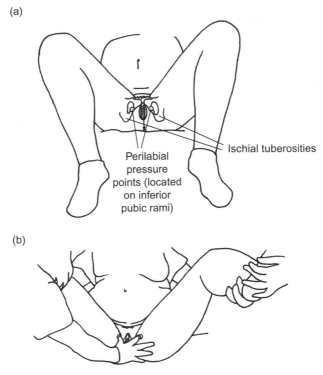

Perilabial
pressure
points (located
on inferior
pubic rami)

Ischial tuberosities

(b)

Fig. 10.16. (a) Location of Cook's perilabial counterpressure points with inferior pubic rami as reference points. (b) Placement of caregiver's fingers for the one-handed Cook's perilabial counterpressure technique.

perineum while providing pain relief using counterpressure with the upper hand to the descending rami.

How Cook's perilabial counter-pressure No. 2 helps

As the fetal head descends toward the pelvic outlet and approaches crowning, the perineal muscles and ligaments of the pelvic floor and the skin and mucosa of the vagina are stretched, causing burning and stinging in her vagina (the "rim of fire"). The counterpressure at the

10

inferior rami counteracts the force of the fetal head against the pubic arch and soft tissue to decrease the pain.

When to use Cook's perilabial counterpressure No. 2

- During or between contractions or continuously
- When the woman has an uncontrollable premature urge to push before compete dilation with a cervical lip or swelling
- During late second stage when the woman is pushing and the head is approaching crowning
- At crowning when the woman is trying not to push in order to protect her perineum from lacerations

When not to use Cook perilabial counterpressure No. 2

- When the woman states that this counterpressure is not helping or is unpleasantly distracting
- When the woman complains that it causes discomfort
- When she has the following contraindications:
  - Preexisting symphysis pubis problems
  - Past pelvic trauma (accident, violence, obstetric trauma, etc.) that may have damaged the pelvic girdle area

Cold and heat

Cold and rolling cold: See pages 330–332, for the rationale and complete instructions; see also Figure 10.17.

Note: Always place one or two layers of cloth between the woman's skin and the cold object to protect her skin from possible damage and to avoid the sudden shock of a freezing object directly placed on her skin.

Pressing and rolling a cold can of juice or soft drink over the woman's low back is sometimes appreciated more than steady pressure in one area.

When to use cold for back pain

- When the woman has musculoskeletal pain (especially low back pain)

10

(a)   (b)

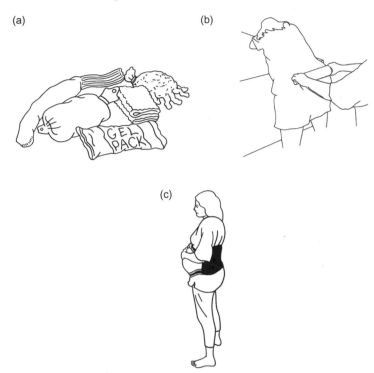

(c)

Fig. 10.17.   (**a**) Cold. (**b**) Rolling cold. (**c**) Strap-on cold pack.

When not to use cold for back pain

- If the woman is already chilled
- If she does not want cold used (for personal or cultural reasons)
- If she prefers heat
- If the woman has an epidural, *do not* place a cold object on any area with altered sensation (cool cloths would be safe)

10   *Warm compresses*

See pages 328–330 for more information.

When to use warm compresses

- If she has low back pain and prefers a warm pack to a cold pack

When not to use warm compresses

- If the woman has a fever

Caution: The woman's temperature sense may be distorted when she is in labor. The cold or warm compress should be wrapped in a towel or pad, and before placing it on the woman's skin, the caregiver should test the temperature of the compress on his or her own inner forearm to be sure the cold or heat is tolerable.

- If the woman has received an epidural, do not place a cold or warm compress on any part of her body where sensation is altered.

Hydrotherapy

Note: Hydrotherapy (Fig. 10.18) often results in dramatic pain reduction and may enhance labor progress. See pages 332–337 for instructions on hydrotherapy.

(a)   (b)

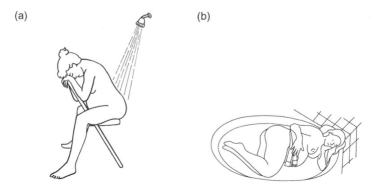

Fig. 10.18. (**a**) Shower on woman's back. (**b**) Bath.

10

Movement

The use of positions and movement were explained in Chapter 9. The lunge (Chapter 9, page 313), slow dancing (Chapter 9, page 316), walking (Chapter 9, page 315), pelvic rocking, pelvic tilt (page 311), swaying, rocking (Chapter 9, page 323), open knee–chest position (Chapter 9, page 293), the abdominal lift (Chapter 9, page 318), and abdominal stroking (Chapter 9, page 317) all encourage fetal rotation, and some also relieve back pain. See Figure 10.19.

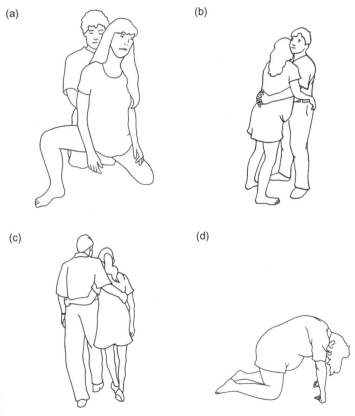

Fig. 10.19. (**a**) Kneeling lunge. (**b**) Slow dancing. (**c**) Walking. (**d**) Pelvic rocking, back rounded in flexion.

10

Birth ball

The birth ball (Fig. 10.20) is an excellent aid to movement and relaxation during labor. It is a physical therapy ball. Unlike large balls made for children's use, physical therapy balls are made to support adult weights. Such balls usually have a 300-lb (136-kg) weight limit, but you should check with the seller or manufacturer if this information is not included with the ball. The most widely used sizes are 65 cm and 75 cm in diameter. For women below 5 feet 3 inches tall, a 55-cm ball is a good size; for women between 5 feet 3 inches and 5 feet 9 inches, the 65-cm ball is a good size; for women taller than 5 feet 10 inches (178 cm), a 75-cm-diameter ball is a better choice. Birth balls can be inflated to varying degrees of firmness and differing diameters, according to the woman's comfort. (Unfortunately, there

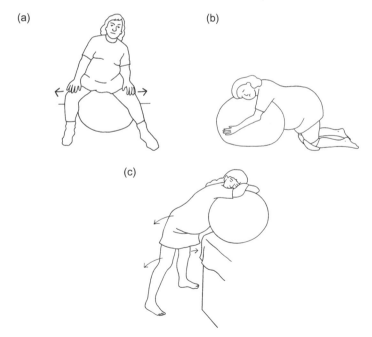

Fig. 10.20. (**a**) Sitting, swaying on a birth ball. (**b**) Kneeling on a birth ball, with knee pads. (**c**) Standing, swaying with ball.

10

is wide variation in the actual inflated size of the balls from one manufacturer to another. One manufacturer's "65-cm ball" may be much smaller than another manufacturer's. To some extent, this can be corrected by the amount of inflation. Furthermore, the balls do stretch over time and with use.)

The round shape of the ball makes swaying (while sitting on it or leaning over it) almost effortless. It is a comfortable alternative to the hands-and-knees position. Cover the ball with a waterproof bed pad, towel, or blanket. The ball can be cleaned with the same disinfectant used on the birthing bed mattress.

Other inflated devices—peanut or egg shaped—are available, but they are limited in versatility compared with the ball.

Caution: The first few times a woman sits on the ball, she may feel a bit unsteady. She should hold on to the bed or her partner until she is totally secure. Also, as she lowers herself to sit on the ball, she should hold it to be sure it does not roll away! Once she is seated, her feet should be in front of her, about 2 to 2.5 feet apart. If she is insecure while sitting on the ball, she can still use it while kneeling or standing, as shown in Figure 10.20, b and c. Some childbirth classes provide balls to try before labor. Some hospitals also have them to use during labor.

(Many parents buy a ball for their own use in labor and afterward. The ball is very useful for soothing a fussy baby, when the parent sits on the ball with the baby nestled into his or her shoulder and bounces gently. This is much easier on the parent's back than walking with the baby.) It is also a useful aid for postpartum exercise.

Transcutaneous electrical nerve stimulation (TENS)

A TENS unit is a hand-held battery-operated device that causes transmission of mild electrical impulses through the skin where they stimulate nerve fibers. TENS units (Fig. 10.21) are available for sale or rent from physical therapy clinics and from medical equipment rental companies and, in many countries, from chemists or drugstores.

How

The four reusable stimulating pads, or electrodes, are placed on the low back on the paraspinal muscles on either side of the spine, two with their top edges at the level of the lowest ribs and two with their

(a) (b)

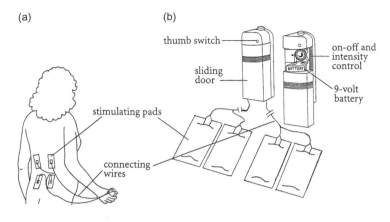

thumb switch

on-off and intensity control

sliding door

9-volt battery

stimulating pads

connecting wires

Fig. 10.21. (a) TENS in use. (b) British TENS unit designed for childbirth.

bottom edges slightly above the level of the gluteal cleft (Fig. 10.21, a), and held in place by adhesive on the pads. TENS units have adjustable parameters that vary with the model used: the most common British units, designed for childbirth, are simple and can be adjusted for intensity and for mode (continuous or burst, off and on). Alternating the mode after a contraction helps keep the woman from habituating to one kind of stimulation, which diminishes its effectiveness over time. The unit comes with instructions. Other more versatile and complex units, with more adjustable parameters, are also available. The woman or her partner increases the intensity of the nerve stimulation during contractions, and then decreases it and changes the sensation between contractions. In the U.K. model, this is all done with a thumb switch. (American models do not come with the thumb switch, which is awkward because the partner has to turn two dials to change the stimulation between and during contractions.) The woman feels a "buzzing," prickly or tingling sensation, that is always kept below painful levels.

Fetal monitoring: Rarely, the TENS unit interferes with transmission of ultrasound fetal monitor signals. If this is a problem, it can be dealt with by discontinuing the stimulation temporarily so that

10

clear signals are obtained, or discontinuing the monitoring if there is no medical reason to have continuous fetal monitoring.

How TENS helps

TENS stimulates tactile nerve endings and inhibits awareness of pain, as described in the Gate Control Theory of Pain.[33] TENS may also increase local endorphin production. It appears to have greater benefit if started early in labor, especially if the woman has back pain.

TENS allows the woman complete mobility, and a sense of control, in that she or her partner controls the use of TENS.

When to use TENS

- TENS is more effective when started in early labor, so it makes sense for the woman to obtain her TENS unit and be instructed in its use before labor begins. Then she can begin using it early in labor before going to the hospital.
- Throughout labor as long as the woman finds it helpful
- TENS appears to be most beneficial with women who have back pain.

When not to use TENS

- When using hydrotherapy (although she may remove the electrodes while in the water and replace them when she gets out)
- When woman reports that the TENS is not helping. (She may want to turn it off for a while without removing it. She may discover that the contractions are more painful without it.)
- If there is any irritation of the woman's skin at the sites of the electrodes

Effectiveness of TENS

A systematic review of trials of TENS for management of labor pain (19 randomized trials, 1671 women) included 15 trials where TENS was applied to the back, 2 trials with application to acupuncture points, and 2 trials with application to the cranium.[34] Overall, there was no significant difference between TENS and control groups in pain ratings, although the 2 trials of TENS applied to acupuncture

10

points indicated reduction in severe pain. Some studies reported lower use of added pain medications in the TENS groups than in the control groups. No adverse events were reported. Despite the lack of objective evidence of pain reduction with the most common applications of TENS, the majority of women using it were satisfied and stated they would use it again in a future labor.

TENS may be more effective for relief of back pain than labor pain in general, but only a few observational studies have investigated this possibility.[3]

The satisfaction expressed by women with TENS appears to relate to benefits other than pain relief. TENS allows the woman to be in control of the intervention, allows ambulation, has no effects on her mental state, and provides an inexpensive option for those who wish to avoid medications. There are no known side effects from TENS when used as directed for normal healthy individuals.[3]

TENS provides modest benefits in reduction of pain relief medications and is a satisfying option for many women who use it. Its efficacy when applied in early labor and in relieving back pain deserves further study. Women's individual preferences regarding its use should be respected.

Sterile water injections for back pain

Intracutaneous or subcutaneous injections of sterile water (sometimes called sterile water blocks) are an effective method of reducing back pain.[35–36] and are easily performed by clinical personnel. The use of saline injections does not have the same benefit.

See Chapter 8 for a complete discussion of sterile water injections for back pain.

BREATHING FOR RELAXATION AND A SENSE OF MASTERY

Breathing rhythmically during contractions, sometimes combined with moaning, is a widespread labor coping ritual.[30] Many women have already learned some breathing techniques from books or childbirth preparation classes.[37] The caregiver should ask them what they learned and encourage them to use what is already familiar. Many women discover their own unique rhythms of breathing and numerous other coping rituals, especially in active labor (see The Essence

10

of Coping, Chapter 5, pages 159–160). Women who have their own rituals do not need correction or instruction. They need support and freedom from disturbance (within the realistic context of clinical care). However, women who do not know what to do may feel overwhelmed and out of control, anxious, or tense. They can be taught simple effective breathing rhythms and assisted in using them during contractions.

Simple breathing rhythms to teach on the spot in labor

How

We recommend that the caregiver be able to teach both slow and light breathing. These can be taught quickly between contractions.

Slow breathing should be initiated at the point in labor when the woman cannot walk or talk through the peaks of her contractions. Teach her to "sigh" her way through the contractions with full, easy, audible breaths that may or may not be accompanied by moaning. Combine breathing with imagery. Here are some examples:

"Every out breath is a relaxing breath."

"Send each in-breath to a tense area and on the out-breath, send that tension away …"

"Imagine that each breath is another step up the mountain that is your contraction. When you get to the peak, you can breathe your way down."

"Let's count your breaths as you go through the contractions. Then (assuming the contractions follow a fairly consistent pattern) we'll be able to tell when you are about halfway through. It will make your contractions seem shorter."

Light breathing is reserved for a time in active labor when the woman becomes discouraged or finds that the slow breathing is no longer helping very much, even with your encouragement and help. Teach her to breathe more shallowly and more quickly but still at a speed at which she is comfortable through the contractions (for example, one quick light in-breath followed by an audible out-breath every 1 to 3 seconds. She pauses briefly after each out-breath to keep from breathing too fast). It may be easier for the woman if you pace her

10

with rhythmic hand or head movements, and talk to her soothingly and in the rhythm of her breathing: "Good ... that's the way ... just like that ... that's right ... yes. ..." Hyperventilation is unlikely if you pace her and encourage her to keep her inhalations silent and shorter than her exhalations, which should be audible or accompanied by moaning. (If hyperventilation occurs, the woman may need to breathe in and out of her cupped hands, a paper bag, or a surgical mask until the symptoms—light-headedness, gulping for air— disappear. Help her slow her breathing and move less air, while maintaining a steady rhythm.) You can continue the use of guided imagery if she responds well to it. Most women, after being helped with rhythmic breathing through several contractions, can then continue without guidance.

Of course, you will want her to adapt these rhythmic patterns in whatever way suits her best.

Note: If the woman is in advanced labor when she arrives, it may be impossible to teach her very much. If she lacks rhythm in her breathing or moaning, help her find a rhythm. Get her to look at your hand, move your hand up and down in rhythm, and say (in the same rhythm), "Breathe with my hand ... that's right ... stay with it ... good ... ," etc.).

How breathing techniques help

Breathing in a consistent rhythmic pattern is self-calming; it encourages tension release and a sense of well-being. This rhythmic self-calming behavior helps to quiet the cortical activity of the brain, putting the woman in a more instinctual state of mind.

When to use breathing techniques

- Whenever the woman seems distressed by her contractions
- If she has not mastered any other techniques for coping with labor pain

When not to use breathing techniques

- If the woman is successfully using other coping or breathing techniques
- If she resists trying them, or cannot respond to your teaching

BEARING-DOWN TECHNIQUES FOR THE SECOND STAGE

See Chapter 6 for phases of second stage, when to ask a woman to begin pushing, a description of the scientific evidence for making spontaneous pushing (rather than Valsalva maneuver pushing), the default mode, maternal positions to facilitate rotation and descent, and suggestions to help women push more effectively when they have received epidural anesthesia.

See Chapter 8, pages 246–250 and 252–267 for evidence-based lower-technology clinical interventions to promote second-stage labor progress when second stage is slow.

Spontaneous bearing down (pushing)

Spontaneous bearing down is unplanned and unrehearsed by the woman before birth, and undirected during the birth. The woman's strong involuntary urge to push usually compels her to bear down effectively in synchrony with strong contractions.

How

When the contraction begins, the woman begins breathing in any way that is satisfying to her, and bears down when she has the reflexive urge, for as long and as forcefully as her urge demands. Each bearing-down effort usually lasts no more than 5 to 7 seconds.[38-40] The woman may hold her breath, moan, release air, or bellow during contractions, and breathe quickly and lightly for several seconds between bearing down efforts. This breathing helps ensure adequate fetal oxygenation.

Note: Although some experts prescribe "open glottis pushing" (releasing air during bearing-down efforts), we are reluctant to prescribe any specific pushing techniques during contractions; rather, we support spontaneous behavior, and only if that is nonproductive do we suggest corrective actions, described later.

Self-directed pushing

Sometimes, due to fear, pain, or "holding back," women's spontaneous bearing-down efforts are ineffective, and self-directed pushing is more productive.

10

How

Self-directed pushing is used when the woman has a spontaneous urge to push but her bearing-down efforts are unfocused, ineffective, and "diffuse," without apparent progress for 30 minutes. Often her eyes are clenched shut, and she seems afraid or unwilling to bear down into her pelvis.

First, the caregiver encourages the woman to try a new position. Gravity-enhancing positions seem to help the woman focus her attention. If that does not help, the caregiver may instruct the woman to open her eyes and direct her gaze and her efforts downward toward her vaginal outlet. Without any further direction, the woman frequently responds impressively, becoming much more effective in her bearing-down efforts.

Lastly, the caregiver may have to tell the woman to "Push to the pain and right through it. It hurts less on the other side."

Directed pushing

How

With "directed pushing," the woman is instructed precisely as to when, how, and how long to push. She is usually expected to hold her breath and strain for 10 or more seconds at a time with only one short breath between bearing-down efforts. This technique is sometimes referred to as the "purple pushing," which describes the color of her face after a few contractions of this type of pushing.

There are potential risks to this type of pushing. See Chapter 6, pages 178–179 and Chapter 8, pages 257–258, for a discussion of these risks. To reduce these risks, the woman should be directed to hold her breath for no more than 5 to 7 seconds at a time, to take several breaths between bearing-down efforts, and to use a position other than lying on her back.

When to use directed pushing

Directed pushing is used if the woman is anxious and asks for help ("I can't do it! What am I supposed to do?"). It is also used when a woman has an epidural but should be delayed until the fetal head is visible at the vaginal outlet, or the woman feels an urge to push. (See Chapter 6, pages 182–186, second stage.) Directed pushing is also

10

used if there is a medical problem requiring that the baby be born right away or if instrumental delivery is probable.

CONCLUSION

The comfort measures described in this chapter exemplify the non-pharmacologic approach to labor pain relief. They reduce pain while maintaining a sense of mastery and participation by the woman. They make it possible for the woman to use the positions and movements (described in Chapter 9) to maintain labor progress and, one hopes, to reduce the likelihood of a cesarean for dystocia.

REFERENCES

1. Hodnett ED, Gates S, Hofmeyr GJ, Sakala C. (2007). Continuous support for women during childbirth. Cochrane Database Syst Rev (3), CD003766. doi:10.1002/14651858.CD003766.
2. Simkin P, O'Hara, M. (2002) Nonpharmacologic relief of pain during labor: Systematic reviews of five methods. Am J Obstet Gynecol 186, S131–S159.
3. Simkin P, Klein M. (2009). Nonpharmacological approaches to management of labor pain, parts 1 and 2. UpToDate, 17(3), 1–11.
4. Lehmann JF. (1990). Therapeutic Heat and Cold, 4th edition. Baltimore, Williams and Wilkins.
5. Nanneman D. (1991). Thermal modalities: heat and cold. A review of physiologic effects with clinical applications. Am Assoc Occup Health Nurses J 39, 70–75.
6. Lieberman E, O'Donoghue C. (2002). Unintended effects of epidural analgesia during labor: A systematic review. Am J Obstet Gynecol 186, S31–S68.
7. Enwemeka C, Allen C, Avila P, Bina J, Munns S. (2002). Soft tissue thermodynamics before, during, and after cold therapy. Med Sci Sports Exerc 34, 45–50.
8. Odent M. (1997). Can water immersion stop labor? J Nurse Midwif 42, 414–416.
9. Cluett E, Burns E. (2009). Immersion in water in labour and birth. Cochrane Database Syst Rev (2), CD000111. doi:000110.001002/14651858.CD14000111.pub14651853.
10. The Royal Australian and New Zealand College of Obstetricians and Gynaecologists. (2008). College Statement 24: Warm Water Immersion during Labour and Birth. East Melbourne, Australia.

11. Katz VL, Ryder RM, Cefalo RC, Carmichael SC, Goolsby R. (1990). A comparison of bed rest and immersion for treating the edema of pregnancy. Obstet Gynecol 75(2), 147–151.

12. Eriksson M, Mattsson LA. Ladfors L. (1997). Early or late bath during the first stage of labour: A randomised study of 200 women. Midwifery 13, 146–148.

13. Harper B. (2005). Gentle Birth Choices. Rochester, VT, Healing Arts Press.

14. Cluett E, Pickering R, Getliffe K, Saunders N. (2004). Randomized controlled trial of labouring in water compared with standard of augmentation of dystocia in first stage of labour. BMJ 328, 314–320.

15. Sommer P. (1979). Obstetrical patients' anxiety during transition of labor and the nursing intervention of touch. (Doctoral dissertation.) Dallas, Texas Women's University.

16. Field T, Hernandez-Reif M, Taylor S, et al. (1997). Labor pain is reduced by massage therapy. J Psychosom Obstet Gynaecol 18, 286.

17. Chang MY, Wang SY, Chen CH. (2002). Effects of massage on pain and anxiety during labour: A randomized controlled trial in Taiwan. J Adv Nurs 38, 68.

18. Chang MY, Chen CH, Huang KF. (2006). A comparison of massage effects on labor pain using the McGill Pain Questionnaire. J Nurs Res 14, 190.

19. Waters B, Raisler J. (2003). Ice massage for the reduction of labor pain. J Midwif Womens Health 48, 317–321.

20. Chung UL, Hung LC, Kuo SC, Huang CL. (2003). Effects of LI4 and BL 67 acupressure on labor pain and uterine contractions in the first stage of labor. J Nurs Res 11, 251.

21. Lee MK, Chang SB, Kang DH. (2004). Effects of SP6 acupressure on labor pain and length of delivery time in women during labor. J Altern Complement Med 10, 959.

22. Klaus MH, Kennell JH. (1997). The doula: An essential ingredient of childbirth rediscovered. Acta Paediatr 86, 1034–1036.

23. Bertsch TD, Nagashima-Whalen L, Dykeman S, Kennell JH, McGrath S. (1990). Labor supported by first-time fathers: Direct observation with a comparison to experienced doulas. J Psychosom Obstet Gynecol 11, 251–260.

24. Hodnett E. (1996). Nursing support of the laboring woman. JOGNN 25(3), 257–264.

25. Hodnett E, Lowe N, Hannah M, et al. (2002). Effectiveness of nurses as providers of birth support in North American hospitals: A randomized controlled trial. JAMA 288, 1373–1381.

26. Butler J, Abrams B, Parker J, Roberts JM, Laros RK. (1993). Supportive nurse–midwife care is associated with a reduced incidence of cesarean section. Am J Obstet Gynecol 168, 1407–1413.

27. Martin, JA, Hamilton, BE, Sutton, PD, Ventura, M, Mathews, T & Osterman, MJK. (2010). Births: Final Data for 2008. National vital statistics reports; vol 59 no 1. Hyattsville, MD. Retrieved from http://www.cdc.gov/nchs/VitalStats.htm.

28. Declercq E, Sakala C, Corry MP, Applebaum S. (2006). Listening to Mothers, II: Report of the Second National U.S. Survey of Women's Childbearing Experiences. New York, Childbirth Connection.

29. Chalmers B, Dzakpasu S, Heaman M, Kaczorowski J. (2008). The Canadian Maternity Experiences Survey: An overview of findings. J Obstet Gynaecol Can 30(3), 217–228.

30. Simkin P. (2002). Supportive care during labor: A guide for busy nurses. JOGNN 31, 721–732.

31. Wuitchik M, Bakal D, Lipshitz J. (1989). The clinical significance of pain and cognitive activity in latent labor. Obstet Gynecol 73(1), 35–42.

32. Cook L. (2010). Cook's counterpressure as a comfort method in labor. Unpublished manuscript and personal communication. Birthing Basics, www.birthingbasics.net.

33. Melzack RD. (1973). The Puzzle of Pain. New York, Basic Books.

34. Dowswell T, Bedwell C, Lavender T, Neilson JP. (2009). Transcutaneous electrical nerve stimulation (TENS) for pain relief in labour. Cochrane Database Syst Rev (2), CD007214. doi:10.1002/14651858.CD007214.

35. Hutton EK, Kasperink M, Rutten M. (2009). Sterile water injection for labour pain: A systematic review and meta-analysis of randomised controlled trials. BJOG 116, 1158.

36. Mårtensson L, Wallin G. (2008). Sterile water injections as treatment for low-back pain during labour: A review. Austral N Z J Obstet Gynaecol 48, 369–374.

37. Simkin P, Whalley J, Keppler A, Durham J, Bolding A. (2010). Pregnancy, Childbirth, and the Newborn: The Complete Guide, 5th edition. Deephaven, MN, Meadowbrook.

38. Beynon C. (1957). The normal second stage of labour: A plea for reform in its conduct. J Obstet Gynaecol Br Commonw 64(6), 815–820.

39. Roberts J, Hanson L. (2007). Best practices in second stage labor care: Maternal bearing down and positioning. J Midwif Womens Health 52, 238–245. doi:101016/j.jmwh.2006.12.011.

40. Hanson L. (2009). Challenges in spontaneous bearing down. J Perinat Neonat Nursing 23, 31–39.

Epidural Index

Epidurals in general, 128, 182–6
Advantages of, 128, 146, 165, 327
Effects on fetal position, 129, 149, 156, 182–5
Effects on progress, 129, 149, 182–5, 189
And operative delivery rates, 149
Variation in degrees of maternal mobility, 184

In first stage labor
And emotional dystocia, 327
If fetus is malpositioned, 149, 182–5

In second stage labor
Bearing down with, 183–4
  Care plan, 183
Delayed urge to push—Options:
  Delayed pushing ("Laboring down"), 183–4
  Adjusting dose, 185
  Removing time limit for second stage, 185–8
  Sheet pull, 306

Using EFM for biofeedback, 186
Maternal positions that may be usable with epidurals, 138–9, 147–9, 182–5, 187, 191, 198, 305–6, 308–10
When the fetus is malpositioned, 138–9, 145
  Drawbacks of supine, semi-sitting vs. lateral positions with OP fetus,
  Recommending which side the woman should lie on, 138–9
Manual or digital repositioning of fetus by doctor or midwife, 145, 246–50, 319

Precautions with epidurals
Avoiding hydrotherapy, 336–7
Avoiding pelvic press, 242
Preventing joint, nerve injuries when using lithotomy or semisitting positions, 214, 310

The Labor Progress Handbook: Early Interventions to Prevent and Treat Dystocia.
Edited by Penny Simkin, Ruth Ancheta
© 2011 by Penny Simkin and Ruth Ancheta; illustrations copyright Ruth Ancheta

When using and heat or cold,
329–32

**The option of trying other
measures first**
Trying non-pharmacological
measures to deal with
pain, 153–4, 56, 337

Trying non-pharmacological
ways to augment
contractions (to avoid
increased pain
associated with synthetic
oxytocin regimens),
45–6, 135–6, 154, 156,
337

Index

3 Rs, (essence of coping in active labor), 26, 160, 216

abdomen, pendulous, 24, 118–9,143, 320

abdominal lifting, 119, 140, 144, 203, 318–20, 357
  precautions for, 119, 144, 319

abdominal shape, as a sign of OP, 52, 54

abdominal "jiggling", 319–20,
  precautions for, 320

abdominal stroking, 104, 140, 317–8, 366

abuse, survivors of,
  needs of, during labor, 112–3, 161, 164–5, 216
  vaginal exam with, 69

active labor, prolonged,
  definitions of, 22, 125–6
  management of, 126–8
  possible causes, 127–33

active management of labor, 122, 126, 229–32

acupressure, 46, 154, 345–7
  avoiding before term, 346

acupuncture, 154, 267–9, 347

ambulation, *see* walking

American College of Nurse-Midwives, 88

American College of Obstetricians and Gynecologists, 3, 37

artificial rupture of membranes (AROM), 17, 18, 107, 127–8, 140, 156, 165, 246
  as a possible factor in dystocia, 134–5, 246
  need for more study, 135
  risks, 135, 246

Association of Women's Health, Obstetric and Neonatal Nurses, 88

assessments,
  caput, 80, 82
  cervix, prenatally, 64–6
  cervix in labor, 66–8, 70–2, 177
    see also cervix
  contractions, 81–4
    see also contractions
  descent,
    abdominal assessment of, 73–5

The Labor Progress Handbook: Early Interventions to Prevent and Treat Dystocia.
Edited by Penny Simkin, Ruth Ancheta
© 2011 by Penny Simkin and Ruth Ancheta; illustrations copyright Ruth Ancheta

ssessments (*cont'd*)
  vaginal assessment of,
      72–3, 75, 80
  dilation, 70, 126–7, 177
  effacement, 65, 70
  fetal well-being, 16, 28, 86–94,
      153, 247, 311
  fetal position, prenatally, 52–64
  fetal position, in labor, 66,
      69, 76–9, 133–4
    accuracy of clinical
        assessments vs.
        ultrasound during
        labor, 79
  fetal weight, 57, 64,
    as an estimation, 64
    prediction equation, 64
  flexion, 79
  maternal well–being, 84–6
  membranes, 71
  molding, 80
  pelvis, 80,
  presenting part, 72
  progress in first stage, 94–6, 125
  progress in second stage, 96,
      174, 185, 186–8
  synclitism/asynclitism, 76–9
  woman's emotional state, 85–6,
      160–6, 112–3, 215
  urge to push, 146
  see also emotional dystocia
      and maternal coping,
      signs of
asymmetrical dilation, *see*
      cervical lip
asymmetrical positions and
      movements, 141–2,
      192, 196, 203,
      283–4, 296, 313–4
    see also lunge

asynclitism, 24, 35, 76–79,
      116–120
  in latent labor, 116–20
  in active labor, 127–8, 130–1
  and AROM, 134–5
  and cervical lip, 250
  maternal positions for, 117–8,
      136–42, 200, 203,
      284, 288–94,
      296–306
  maternal movement for, 144,
      311–316, 319–324
  in pre-labor and latent labor,
      115–8
  repositioning *see* manual or
      digital rotation of
      the fetal head
  signs of, 76–7, 79
  in second stage, 200–203
  see also malposition
augmentation, *see* contractions,
      inadequate

Baby-Friendly Initiative, 236–7
back pain,
  measures to alleviate, 103–6,
      114, 119–21, 136–45,
      188, 191, 354–61
  in pre-labor and latent labor,
      103–6, 114, 119–21
  in active labor, 136–45
  in second stage, 188, 191
  as a clue to progress, 94
  as a clue to malposition,
      CPD, 129, 20
  nuchal hand and, 204
  TENS for, 114, 136, 368–71
  see also malposition; occiput
      posterior (OP) *and*
      occiput transverse

bearing down, 174, 176–7, 374–6
  delayed, 183–5
  diffuse, 180–1, 216–7, 375
  directed, 13, 178–9, 182, 203, 258, 375–6
    directed by clinician, 258
  epidural, effect on, 182–5
  epidural, helping women push with, 185–7
  fear as an impediment to, 216–9
  "holding back", 217
  "laboring down", *see* bearing down, delayed
  with a malpositioned fetus, 190–203
    see also malpolsition, maternal positions and movements for
  premature urge *see* urge to push
  relaxing the perineum and, 218–9
  self-directed, 181, 374–5
  spontaneous, 17, 19, 67, 96, 176–7, 179–81, 186, 188, 203, 250, 253, 257–8, 271, 374
    verbal support for, 253–4,
  "trial pushes",146
  see also Quick Epidural Index; second stage, urge to push *and* Valsalva Maneuver
bed rest in late pregnancy, 114, 336
"Belly Mapping", 60–3
birth ball, 32–3, 38, 137, 156–7, 286, 289, 291, 312, 320, 324, 367

precautions for, 368
birth plan or preference list, 31–2, 238
birth rope, 301–2
  precautions for, 302
birth sling, 194, 300–1
  precautions for, 302
bladder, emptying,
  before examinations and procedures, 57, 68, 248
  every hour or two, to reduce pain and facilitate progress, 34, 261
breast crawl, 236
breastfeeding, 12, 17, 19, 20, 27, 28, 226–8, 230, 234–8
Bishop score, various interpretations of, 65–6
breathing,
  in latent labor, 110, 114
  in first stage, 114, 159, 165–6
    when to begin, 110
  naturalistic, 328,
  in second stage, 177, 216, 218
    see also bearing down
  supporting and teaching, 371–3
  through contractions in second stage, 183–5

caput, 72–3, 80, 96, 135, 200, 323
cardinal movements, 35, 108–9
  effect of epidural on, 149, 183–5

care plans (flowcharts),
  little or no progress in labor, 7
  anxiety or distress in labor,
      165
  prolonged prelabor or latent
      phase, 107
  prolonged active phase, 128
  occiput posterior/asynclitism
      in active first stage,
      140
  premature urge to push, 146
  complete dilation, with no
      epidural, 180
  diffuse pushing with no
      epidural, 182
  complete dilation with
      epidural, 183
  occiput posterior/asynclitism
      in second stage, 203
carpal tunnel syndrome, 292,
      342
catecholamines, 27–30, 112,
      158, 162, 301, 333,
      351,
cephalopelvic disproportion
      (CPD), 22, 24, 94,
      127, 129,
  clues to, 76, 80, 132
  and AROM, 134, 246
  and dorsal positions, 211–4
  caused or made worse by
      malposition, 129,
      132–3
  suspected in active labor, 22,
      135–6
    maternal positions for,
        146–7
  suspected in second stage,
      177–8, 188, 190–1,
      205–14

    maternal positions and
        movements for, 188,
        190–1, 205–14
    see also assessments, fetal
        weight
cervical dystocia, 24, 65, 71,
      245
cervical lip, 71, 129, 146,
      156–8, 250–1, 363,
  and asynclitism, 250
  interventions for, 250–1
  manual reduction of, 250–1
  positions for, 293–5,
  possible other interventions,
      158
cervix,
  assessing prenatally, 64–6
  assessing during labor, 66–8,
      70–2, 177
  difficult to find, 71
  dilation, 32–3, 64–8, 70–2,
      95–6, 102, 177
  effacement, 65, 70–1, 95,
      102, 106, 108,
      112–3, 245, 248,
  as a factor in dystocia, 24, 65,
      71, 245
  position of, 108–9
  remodeling of, 65, 111
    see also cervix, ripening
  retraction of, 81, 175–6
  rigid os (stenosis), 24, 71, 129
    manual stretching of , 245
  ripening of, 65–6, 106, 108,
      113
  scarred, 24, 113
  swollen, 71, 146, 156–7, 292,
      294–5
  "zipper" cervix, 71
  manual stretching, 250

cesarean birth, 3, 11, 13, 17, 22–3, 37, 64, 73, 107, 110, 126, 128, 134–5, 140, 149, 151–2, 162, 165, 177, 203, 205, 217, 219, 246–8, 250, 257, 270, 328, 349
potential to reduce cesarean rate using:
longer time frame before diagnosing dystocia, 22–23
sterile water injections, 270
clinical interventions, low-technology, 242–72
intermediate-level interventions, 243
for use by clinical personnel only, 243
tertiary care, referral or consultation, 243
see also doulas, role during clinical interventions
prelabor and latent labor interventions, 244
nipple stimulation, 244
management of cervical stenosis or "zipper" cervix, 245–6
therapeutic rest, 244–5
active labor and second stage interventions, 245–51
artificial rupture of the membranes (AROM), 246
digital or manual rotation of the fetal head, 246–50

manual reduction of a persistent cervical lip, 250–1
fostering normality in second stage labor,
guiding women through crowning of fetal head, 254–5
hand skills to protect the perineum, 255–6
maternal birth positions 253–4
perineal management in second stage, 252–3
prenatal perineal massage, 251–2
differentiating perineal massage from other interventions, 256–7
when progress in second stage remains inadequate, 257–8
duration of second stage labor, 257–8
directing bearing down efforts, 258
hand maneuvers and anticipatory management for intrapartum problems
shoulder dystocia, 258–65
precautionary measures, 260–1
shoulder dystocia maneuvers, 261–5
warning signs, 261
nuchal cord, somersault maneuver, 265–7

clinical interventions, low-
technology (*cont'd*)
non-pharmacologic and
minimally invasive
pain relief, 267–271
acupuncture, 267–9
nitrous oxide, 271
subcutaneous sterile
water injections,
269–71
topical anesthetic on
perineum, 271
cold,
for hemorrhoids, in second
stage, 332
for pain relief, 33, 136, 140,
198, 283, 330–2,
363–5
precautions when using,
331–2
to reduce swollen cervix,
330
consultation and referral, 16,
93, 93, 243
continuous support, 328,
347–50
from doulas, 347–9
from nurses and midwives,
349–50
contractions,
assessing, 81–4, 125, 74–6,
146–153
inadequate, 24, 146–51, 215
and dehydration, 150–1,
and exhaustion, 151
and immobility, 147–8
and medication, 149
and uterine lactic acidosis,
151–3
also see emotional dystocia

irregular or coupling
contraction pattern,
as a sign of possible
malposition, 115,
116, 100, 120, 132,
in pre-labor or latent phase,
95
non-pharmacological ways to
stimulate, 24, 45–6
acupressure, 46,154
breast or nipple
stimulation, 45–6,
153,
heat on fundus, 46
hydration, 45,150
hydrotherapy, 45, 154–6
movement and positioning,
45,153
prevent/alleviate fear, 24,
29, 31–3
touch, 45
non-progressing, 102
patterns in latent and active
second stage, 174–5,
177
pre-labor, 102, 106–7
progressing, 102
tetanic, 153, 177,
cooperation between patients
and caregivers, 5–6,
30–3, 60–3, 66–9,
86, 112–3, 151–2,
230, 238
coping with labor pain, *see*
maternal coping
cord
compression, 91, 94, 179, 246
positions to help prevent
or reduce. 280, 291,
293

clamping and cutting,
        228–30, 232, 237,
nuchal, and somersault
        maneuver, 229
counterpressure,
    on the back, 197, 293, 317,
        354–5
    Cook's counterpressure on
        iscial tuberosities,
        359–61
    Cood's perilabial
        counterpressure
        361–3
cultural factors, 4, 7–8, 158–9,
        162–3, 166, 332,
        337, 353
    non-clinical factors influencing
        care, 9–11, 23

deflexed head and CPD, *see*
        flexion of fetal head
        on chest
dehydration
    see hydration and dehydration
"difficult" patients, 164
diffuse pushing *see* bearing
        down
dilation,
    as a feature of normal labor,
        21–2, 95
    assessing, 70, 126–7, 177
    asymmetrical, 250
    when cervix is scarred, 15, 92
    and definitions of dystocia,
        21–3
    and definitions of labor onset,
        102–3
    and hydrotherapy, 154, 336–7
    one of many ways to progress
        in labor, 108–9

in pre-labor and latent phase,
        106–7
    as a sign of active labor, 125
    as a sign of readiness to push,
        176–7
double hip squeeze, 195–7, 355–7
    distinguished from pelvic
        press, 195
doulas, 10, 12, 52, 243, 328,
        347–50
    role during clinical
        interventions, 234,
        238, 243, 246, 248,
        254, 263, 271,
drinking in labor, *see* hydration
        and dehydration
drive angle, 35–6, 213, 307, 309
drug–induced rest, 102, 107,
        115
dystocia,
    and cesarean rates, 3, 23,
        135, 152, 250,
    etiologies of,
        cervical, 24, 65, 71, 111–2,
            129, 245
        emotional, 4, 24, 112–3,
            129, 215–9
        extrinsic, 4,
        fetal, 4, 24, 112, 127, 204,
        iatrogenic, 4, 24, 111, 127,
            147–9, 182–5
        intrinsic, 4
        maternal, 4, 24, 129, 150–3
        pelvic, 4, 24,
        unknown, 129, 153–6
        uterine, 4, 24, 82, 129,
            see also contractions,
            inadequate
    various definitions of, 21–3,
        101–3, 125–7, 174–8

early interventions,
  and their place in the care of
        laboring women, 4,
        6–7, 8,14, 127, 129,
        188, 200, 278
  see also, interventions/actions,
        primary, secondary
        and tertiary
eating in labor, 34, 84, 85
  also see hydration and
        dehydration
effacement,
  assessing, 65, 70–1, 95,
  AROM done after 100%
        effaced, 246
  when cervix is scarred,
        112–3
  and definitions of labor onset,
        102
  one of many ways to progress
        in labor, 108,
  in pre-labor and latent phase,
        95
  also see Bishop Score
emotional dystocia, 4, 24,
        85–6,112–3, 129,
        160–8, 215–9
  assessment, 162, 216, 351–2
  common fears, 162, 216–7
  as distinguished from
        "holding back", 217
  effects on fetus, 29
  physiology of, 29, 112
  predisposing factors, 112,
        163, 216–7
  preventing, 31–2, 85–6,
        110–11, 349, 352–4
  ways to help, 132 , 163–8,
        217–9
  see also abuse, survivors of

environment, effect on labor
        progress, 4, 28, 31,
        34, 86, 158, 226,
        230, 253, 350–1,
        353
  see also emotional dystocia
epidural, 128, 182–6 *see also*
        Quick Epidural
        Index
  adjusting dose, 185
  advantages of, 128, 146, 165,
        327
  bearing down with, 183–4,
    care plan for, 183
  delayed bearing down, 183
    possible benefits of delayed
        bearing down plus
        lateral position, 184
  effect on fetal position, 129,
        149, 156, 182–5
  effect on progress, 129, 149,
        182–5, 189
  maternal mobility, variations
        in, 184
  maternal positions that may
        be usable with
        epidurals, 138–9,
        147–9, 182–5, 187,
        305–6, 308–10
  non-pharmacological ways to
        augment
        contractions (to
        avoid increased pain
        associated with
        synthetic oxytocin
        regimens), 23, 45–6,
        153–4, 156, 337
  precautions,
    avoiding hydrotherapy
        336–7

avoiding pelvic press, 242

protecting joint and nerve injuries when using lithotomy and semi-sitting positions, 214, 310

when using heat and cold, 329–32

removing time limit in second stage, 185–8

sheet pull, 306

trying other measures first, 153–4, 156, 337

upon request, 149

used more in recent years, 22

exhaustion, 24, 84, 109, 112, 114, 128–9, 151, 160, 162, 179, 215–6, 244,

"failure to progress", 3, 22, 125, 250

fear, 24–5, 28–32, 69, 112, 129, 160–3, 167, 216–8, 278, 327, 351–2, 354

fetal ejection reflex, 28–30,

fetal influence on labor, 23

fetal attitude *see* flexion of fetal head on chest

fetal monitoring, 37–44,

audible vs. silent, 352

auscultation, 24, 37, 87–91

comparison with EFM, 37

brief, when using abdominal lifting or abdominal "jiggling", 99, 119, 144, 319, 321

and cesarean and instrumental delivery rates, 37

continuous, 7, 17, 19, 37–40, 42–4, 86–7, 89–91,111, 248,

explaining, 163, 357

as feedback to aid bearing down in second stage, 186

and hydrotherapy, 41–4, 335,

intermittent, 41, 87, 313, 335,

risks, 24, 37

telemetry, 42–4, 335,

and TENS, 369–70

three-tiered system, 91–3

without immobilizing the woman, 35–44

fetus,

pre-term, 65, 66, 90, 93, 228, 235

post-term, 66, 93

cervical ripening, role in pre- and post-term births, need for study, 66

"fight or flight" response, 28–30

using heat to reduce, 328

se e *also* "tend and befriend" response

flexion of fetal head on chest, 35, 79, 96, 109, 142, 183, 200,

after epidural, 183,

effect of maternal dorsal and semi–sitting positions, 142–3

maternal positions to promote, 289–90,

fourth stage, *see* third and fourth stage

fundal pressure,
  distinguished from
          suprapubic pressure,
          264

gestational age, 93–4, 179
gravity, 8, 19, 35, 104, 114,
          117–20, 131, 136,
          138, 139, 142–3,
          145, 156, 178, 181,
          188, 191, 230, 254,
          265, 289–3
  as an aid to progress, 117–20,
          131, 138–9, 145, 156,
          158, 178, 206–7, 212,
          278, 280–3
    -negative ("anti–gravity")
          positions, 156, 178
    -neutral positions, 156,
          158, 214, 278, 280,
    -positive, 181, 191, 193
  and shoulder dystocia, 265
  and protecting the perineum,
          254
  and birth of the placenta, 230

head compression, 135, 179
heat,
  to augment contractions, 46
  for pain relief, 328–30, 363–5
  precautions when using, 329,
          365
  to reduce "fight or flight"
          response, 328
hemorrhoids, 280, 283, 293–5,
          330, 332
hopelessness, 112, 114, 216
hydration and dehydration, 24,
          34, 45, 84, 85, 128–9,
          146, 150–1, 215

hydrotherapy, 140, 155–6, 327,
          332–7, 365
  for anxiety and distress, 164
  depth of bath, 336
  and fetal monitoring, 41–4,
          335
  for labor augmentation, 154,
          337
  for pain relief, 154, 199, 337
  precautions, 336–7
    leaving water periodically,
          335
    timing of, 154, 336–7
    when not to use, 336–7
hypertension, 111, 114, 147,
          283, 286, 336
hypotension, supine, 44, 142,
          147, 179, 212, 214,
          278, 280, 283, 306,
          308, 309

iatrogenic dystocia, *see* dystocia,
          etiologies of,
          iatrogenic
  see also hydration and
          dehydration; fetal
          monitoring,
          continuous
  and positions, maternal,
          dorsal, problems
          with
ice massage, 346
induction of labor, 17–9, 24,
          65, 107, 113, 153,
          350
  breast stimulation for, 153
  acupressure for, 346
  see also contractions,
          inadequate *and*
          oxytocin, synthetic

informed consent, 10, 38, 134, 248,
instrumental deliveries *see* operative deliveries
interventions/actions, primary, secondary (intermediate) and tertiary, 6–7, 242
intradermal sterile water injections, *see* sterile water injections

knee press,136, 198, 199, 357–9

labor and birth, normal, definitions and descriptions of, 16–21
active, 95–6, 125–6
latent phase, 95, 102–3, 106
second stage, 96
fostering, 251–7
movement as a component, 20
psychosocial outcomes of, 20
work, strenuous, as a component, 20
see also dystocia, various definitions of
labor onset, various definitions of, 102–3
"Laboring down," *see* bearing down, delayed
latent phase of first stage, definitions of, 102–3
latent phase of second stage, 174–7
lactic acidosis, uterine, 24, 151–3
Leopold's maneuvers, 52, 57–9
lordosis, lumbar, 129

lunge, 128, 187, 195–6, 203, 210, 302–4
instructions, 141–2, 313–4
precautions for, 313–4
side-lying,139–40, 283–4
see also movements, maternal

macrosomia, 64, 94, 113, 129, 132, 135, 205,
and AROM, 134, 246
see also cephalopelvic disproportion (CPD) *and* assessing fetal weight
malposition, and AROM, 134
as a cause of dystocia, 4, 24, 35, 52, 112, 129–33, 188–9
clues to, 52–63, 134
and contraction patterns, 133
and maternal dorsal positions, 35–6, 188
see also positions, maternal, dorsal, problems with
and epidurals, 149, 182–5
maternal positions and movements for, 35
in pre-labor and latent phase, 115–20
in active labor, 136–48
in second stage, 188–95
and operative delivery rates,129, 149
preventing *see* Optimal Fetal Positioning
see also back pain; occiput posterior; occiput transverse *and* asynclitism

malpractice, 11
manual reduction of a persistent
    cervical lip, 158
manual or digital rotation of the
    fetal head (manual
    repositioning), 145,
    246–50, 319
massage, *see* touch and massage
    see also ice massage, perineal
        massage
maternal coping, 25–6, 67, 95,
    110–13, 126, 129,
    158–60, 166, 215–6,
    225–7, 236, 323–4,
    351, 353, 37–2,
    coping scale, 26
    signs of coping,
        in first stage, 95, 158–60,
            166, s*ee also*, 3Rs
        in second stage, 215–6,
        in third and fourth stages,
            225–7, 236
maternal distress, 24, 46, 85
    preventing, 30–5, 112–3,
        161–2, 350–4
    see also emotional dystocia;
        hormones of labor
maternal movements, *see*
        movements,
        maternal
maternal positions, *see* positions,
        maternal
maternity care practices,
    comparison of US/UK/
        Canada, 8–11, 32,
        149, 247,
meconium, 86, 93–4, 228, 244
medication, 27, 128, 146, 149,
        164–5, 337, 349,
        371,

benefits, 27, 128, 146, 164–5
and intensity of contractions,
        149
and malposition,
    see also epidural, effect on
        fetal position
    and maternal positions that
        may be usable with
        epidurals
as a possible contraindication
        to hydrotherapy, 337
narcotics, 128, 140, 149, 165
nitrous oxide, 271
used less by women with
        doulas, 349
used less by women using
        TENS, 371
topical anesthetic on
        perineum, 271
see also epidural; drug-induced
        rest, *and* the Quick
        Epidural Index
midwifery model of care, 20,
        23, 126–7, 158, 230
moaning, *see* vocalization
molding, 15, 73, 80, 96, 108–9,
        135, 200, 205
monitoring, fetal, *see* fetal
        monitoring
movements, maternal,
    as an aid to progress, 35, 42,
        45, 200, 202,
        311–24
    as a comfort measure,
        136–44, 311–24
    see also 3Rs of labor coping
    effect on oxygen supply to
        fetus, 35, 311,
    effect on maternal pelvis 4,
        24, 35

and fetal monitoring *see* monitoring, fetal

positions and movements for suspected malposition or CPD in active labor, 134–43

suspected malposition or CPD in second stage, 188–95

specific movements, abdominal "jiggling" with a rebozo 320–1

precautions when using, 321

abdominal lifting, 318–20

precautions when using, 319

abdominal stroking, 317–8

lunge, 313–4

other rhythmic movements, 323–4

pelvic press, 321–3

precautions for, 323

pelvic rocking, 311–2

slow dancing, 316

walking and stair climbing, 316–7

see also optimal fetal positioning

neocortex, role in labor progress, 29, 34, 158

newborn, *see* third and fourth stage labor

nipple stimulation *see* contractions, inadequate, non-pharmacological ways to stimulate

nuchal hand, 204

see also back pain

observation, 5–6, 25, 30, 60, 67, 92, 129, 160, 163–4, 176, 179, 203, 204, 228, 238, 351,

occiput posterior (OP), 24, 35, 53,127

in active labor, 129–32

in second stage, 188–9

and AROM, 134–5

and cervical lip, 250

determining direction of, 54–63, 133–4,

disadvantages of supine and semi–sitting positions for, 143, 188, 212–3

see also positions, maternal, dorsal, problems with

increased incidence with epidurals, 149

and long pre-labor or latent phase, 112

maternal positions for active labor, 136–41,

maternal positions for second stage, 190–5

and premature urge to push, 144

preventing, 103–6

re-positioning *see* abdominal lifting; abdominal stroking *and* manual repositioning

and side-lying positions, 138–9

signs of, 54–9, 132–3

see also back pain; malpositions *and* positions, maternal

cciput transverse (OT),
persistent, 78, 132–3
in active labor, 132–3
and AROM, 134–5
deep arrest and epidurals,
183–5
deep arrest and pelvic press,
321–3
identifying, 168–9, 201(if
both OT and
asynclitic)
see also assessments, fetal
position
maternal positions for,
in active labor, 136–9
in second stage, 190–5
see also positions, maternal
and rotation
Optimal Fetal Positioning, 62,
103, 136
oxytocin
endogenous, 27–9, 45, 153,
176, 184–5, 226,
228, 236, 246, 267,
333, 335
synthetic, 13, 17, 37, 22–4,
87, 107, 111, 126–9,
133–5, 140, 147,
152–4, 177, 165,
177, 180, 183, 205,
219, 231, 244, 337,
reduced need for among
women using water
immersion? 154
trying nipple stimulation,
cautiously, to
augment labor, in
low-risk women,
before giving oxytocin,
244–5

when there is uterine lactic
acidosis, 151–3
also see third and fourth
stages,placenta,
uterotonic
medications

pain, 16, 24–7, 84, 95, 346
as a factor in progress, 4, 278
excessive, reasons for, 4,
34–5, 111–3, 332
intensity scale and coping
scale, 26
pain vs. suffering, 24–5, 27
patience, 22–3, 85, 126–7, 164,
205
pelvic dystocia, 24, 127–8, 205
pelvic floor damage, 213
pelvic press, 195–6, 203, 321–3,
precautions when using, 323
distinguished from double
hip squeeze, 195,
356
pelvic rocking, 311–3
also see movements, maternal
pelvis,
effect of movement on, 4, 24,
35
see also maternal
movements
effect of position on, 24,
35–6, 139, 141, 192,
195, 200
late pregnancy changes in,
35–6
perineal lacerations, 204
perineal massage, 251–2
differentiated from other
interventions 256–7
perineum, supporting, 256,

policies, effect on labor
        progress, 4, 8, 9, 34,
        38, 111,151, 156,
placenta, *see* third and fourth
        stages/ third stage/
        placenta
positions, maternal,
  as an aid to progress, 35, 118,
        120, 203
  categories of, 278
    asymmetrical, 278
    dorsal positions, 278
      and drive angle, 35–6,
        213, 307, 309
      and instrumental
        deliveries, 211–3
      problems with, 35–36,
        142–3, 211–3, 278
      forward-leaning, to
        reposition fetus or
        reduce back pain,
        278
      in active labor, 137, 145
      in late pregnancy, 103–6
      in pre-labor and latent
        phase, 117, 120
      in second stage, 190
      gravity negative ("anti-
        gravity"), 156, 294
      gravity neutral, 278
      gravity positive, ("gravity-
        enhancing"), 278
      horizontal, 278
      for tired women, 152
  specific positions:
    asymmetrical, 278
      asymmetrical upright,
        296–7
      asymetrical horizontal
        (side-lying lunge), 284

dangle and birth sling,
        299–301
exaggerated lithotomy
        (McRoberts') use of,
        309–10
  precautions for, 310
hands and knees, 309–10
knee-chest positions,
  open, 293–5
    and hemorrhoids, 294
  closed, 295–6
kneeling leaning forward
        with support, 290–2
roll-over sequence, 148, 282
semi-sitting, 285
sheet pull, 229–31
side-lying, (lateral and
        semi–prone),
        279–81
  which side to lie on if
        fetus is
        malpositioned, 281
side-lying lunge, 284
sitting
  leaning forward, 287–8
  upright, 286–7
squatting positions,
        297–302
  precautions for half-
        squatting, 303–4
  precautions for lap
        squatting, 305–6
  precautions for
        supported squatting,
        301–2
standing leaning forward,
        289
supine, 306
  see also dorsal positions,
        problems with

positions, maternal (*cont'd*)
    Why focus on maternal
        position? 35–36
post-traumatic stress disorder
    (PTSD), 25, 30
pre-labor and latent phase,
    prolonged, 87
    definitions of, 102
    "false" labor, 106, 113
    general suggestions for,
        103–7, 108–11,
        115–21
        see also contractions,
            irregular or coupling
    management styles for,
        102–3, 106–7,
        113–121
    "over-reacting" to labor,
        110
    possible causes, 111–3
    therapeutic rest, 244
premature rupture of the
    membranes
    (PROM) 132,
previous back injury, 119
previous trauma, effect on labor
    progress *see*
    emotional dystocia
psychosocial comfort measures,
    30–5, 112–3, 161–2,
    350–4
    see also emotional dystocia
        and vaginal exams,
        instructions for
pushing *see* bearing down
"pushing postions" as
    distinguished from
    "delivery positions",
    185–7, 211–3

relaxation, 31, 33, 110, 114,
    154, 216, 218, 248,
    249, 252, 267, 278,
    328,
    as one of the 3 Rs, 75–6,
        118–9, 143, 320,
        371–3
respect, 4, 27, 30, 32–3, 165–6,
    263, 352, 371
resting the uterus, 151–2
restriction to bed, 13, 111,114,
    184,
    minimizing, 38–44, 111, 114,
        336
rhythm, 25–6, 159–60, 216,
    327–8, 354, 371–3
    as one of 3Rs, 75–6, 118–9,
        143, 320
ritual, as one of 3rs, 25–6,
    159–60, 216, 371–2
rollover sequence, 148, 282
rotation,
    encouraging in pre- and early
        labor, 103–4,
        119–20
    after an epidural, 149, 183–4
    after AROM with a
        malpositioned fetus,
        134–5
    in latent phase of second
        stage, 176
    lack of, as a factor in
        dystocia, 127, 129,
        132
    manual and digital rotation,
        246–50
    positions to encourage,
        103–6, 136–42,
        190–5

six ways to progress in labor, 87–9
Royal College of Obstetricians and Gynaecologists, 18, 37
Royal College of Midwives, 18

second stage,
  definition of, 146
  epidural during, 156–61
  fear as an impediment to progress, 188–92
  management styles for, 146–7, 150–62
  phases of, 147–51
  positions for, *see* positions, maternal
  prolonged latent phase of, 150
  prolonged, possible causes, 162, 188,
  pushing during latent phase, 149–50
  time limits on, 159, 161–2
  Valsalva maneuver during, 178–81, 256, 374
  verbal support during, 253
  see also bearing down
sheet pull, 308–9
short waist, 119, 129
  see also abdominal lifting
shoulder dystocia, 94, 214–5, 258–65
  precautionary measures, 260
  warning signs, 261
  maneuvers, 261–5
  see also supra-pubic pressure, distinguished from fundal pressure

six ways to progress in labor, 32, 108–9
  see also movements, maternal, *and* positions, maternal
slow dancing, 32, 38, 195–6, 211, 316–7, 366,
Society of Obstetricians and Gynecologists of Canada (SOGC), 17, 37, 88, 247,
station, assessing,
  see assessments, descent
sterile water injections for back pain, 136, 140, 199, 269–71, 371
supine positions *see* dorsal positions
suprapubic pressure, 261–2
  distinguished from fundal pressure, 264
survivors of abuse, *see* abuse, survivors of

"tend and befriend" response, 30
third and fourth stages, 225–238
  overview, 225–6
  mutual regulation by mother and newborn, 225–7, 236
  skin-to-skin contact, 230, 234–8
  third stage:
    definition, 225
    family integration, 225–7, 235
    hemorrhage, 231–4
    hormones of, 225–7

ird and fourth stages (*cont'd*)
  newborn,
    assessments, 237–8
    behavior at birth, 225
    blood volume, 228
    delayed cord clamping,
      228–9
    early behavior, 225
    meconium, 228
    sensory experience, 225
    suctioning, 227–8
    transition, 225–8
  placenta,
    active management,
      229–34
    expectant management,
      229–34
    guarding the uterus, 231
    hemorrhage, 229, 231–4
    uterine massage, 231
    uterotonic medications,
      230–4
  fourth stage:
    Baby-friendly breastfeeding
      practices, 236
    Ten steps to successful
      breastfeeding, 237
    definition, 234
    keeping mother and baby
      together, 234–8
    procedures done with baby
      in mother's arms,
      238
    routine newborn
      assessments, 237–8
time as an ally, 5, 205
touch and massage, 33, 45, 165,
    337–45
  and endogenous oxytocin
    production, 45

mini-massages of shoulders,
    back, hands, feet,
    339–45
to reduce anxiety and pain,
    338
transcutaneous electrical nerve
    stimulation (TENS)
    for back pain, 114,
    136, 368–71
  not for use during
    hydrotherapy, 370
trial and error, 5, 23, 76, 129,
    130, 134, 141, 188,
    194, 282
trust, ways to enhance, 5–6,
    30–3, 60–3, 66–9,
    86, 112–3, 151–2,
    230, 238

UK/US/Canada, differences in
    maternity care,
    8–11
ultrasound predictions of fetal
    size, 205
ultrasound to identify fetal
    position,
  before manual or digital
    rotation, 247
  during pregnancy, 59, 60, 64,
    72, 76
  during labor, 79, 104, 129,
    133, 134, 138, 140,
urge to push,
  absence of, during latent
    phase of second
    stage, 174–77
  bearing down with, 180, 216,
    374–5
  delayed, reasons for, 174,
    183–6

and epidural anesthesia,
183–6
see also Quick Epidural
Index
premature
as a sign of possible
malposition or CPD,
133, 144–5
ways to deal with, 144–6,
294, 361–3
ways to enhance, 177,290,
298
see also second stage, latent
phase of
uterine dystocia, 24, 82, *see also*
contractions,
inadequate
uterine massage, 230–3

vaginal birth after cesarean
(VBAC), 3, 217
vaginal exams,
and abuse survivors, 69
fear of, 69
indications for, 66–7
instructions for, 66–72
positions for, 68
reactions to, in early labor, 69
timing of, 66, 67
see also assessments
Valsalva maneuver, 178–81,
253, 256, 374
history of prescribing, 178
problems caused by, 178–80
alternatives, when women
have epidurals,
182–6
visualization, 31, 33, 114, 163,
165,
vocalization, 33, 114, 159–60,

walking and stair climbing, 35,
42, 114, 147, 177,
280, 315–7
compared to AROM plus
oxytocin, 147
see also movements, maternal
woman as key to solution, 5
woman-centered care, 10
World Health Organization
(WHO), 4, 16–7,
73–4